# Statistical aspects of community health and nutrition

# Statistical aspects of community health and nutrition

Dr. AK Nigam

**WOODHEAD PUBLISHING INDIA PVT LTD**

New Delhi

Published by Woodhead Publishing India Pvt. Ltd.
Woodhead Publishing India Pvt. Ltd.,
303, Vardaan House, 7/28, Ansari Road,
Daryaganj, New Delhi - 110002, India
www.woodheadpublishingindia.com

First published 2016, Woodhead Publishing India Pvt. Ltd.


Woodhead Publishing India Pvt. Ltd. ISBN: 978-93-85059-10-0
Woodhead Publishing India Pvt. Ltd. e-ISBN: 978-93-85059-58-2

Typeset by Mind Box Solutions, New Delhi
Printed and bound by Replika Press Pvt. Ltd.

# Contents

# Foreword

The book is in response to meet the immense gap being felt by students and programme managers of public health, public health nutrition, agriculture as well as development specialist in adequately and appropriately understanding the application of the principle of statistical tools or to critically examine a survey design or finding. The book is written in a simple and easy to understand form. It focuses on guiding students, research workers, programme persons and other interested groups to insight into the correct usage of statistical principles and tools, interpreting data, improving skills in designing surveys and evaluations, undertaking qualitative and quantitative surveys, enhancing the knowledge of positive dimensions and limitations of the techniques used for the assessment of maternal, infant and neonatal mortality as well as the nutritional status. In addition, the book offers extensive information on statistical issues pertaining to measurement of hunger and food security, hunger mapping, diseases in community clusters, randomized response technique for sensitive characteristics, small area estimation and gender disparity. Special attention has been paid to present a balanced view of value and limitations of various survey techniques commonly used in public health and nutrition.

Dr Arun K. Nigam has over 50 years of wide ranging experience and has contributed significantly in the subject of development statistics, especially in the field of public health, food and agriculture and nutrition. Dr. Nigam completed his masters in Mathematical Statistics from Lucknow University and PhD from Banaras Hindu University. Dr Nigam was the Professor and Head, Training & Basic Research at the Indian Agricultural Statistics Research Institute of Indian Council of Agricultural Research (ICAR) and in this capacity provided leadership in conducting research in the fields of design of experiments and sample surveys. Dr Nigam's interest in the subject of public health nutrition has been evident since mid-90s when he, as the Director of the Institute of Applied Statistics and Development Studies (IASDS), conducted the state-based women and child nutrition survey for the

Department of Women and Child, State Government of Uttar Pradesh (UP). Under Dr. Nigam's leadership, the findings of 1998 for the first time in India presented the regional malnutrition scenario in the state of UP and through the regression analysis of raw data highlighted the significance of early age of child, women's health-nutrition status and access to sanitation as the highest risk factors associated with undernutrition in children.

Academics in university settings, public health specialists, nutritionists, development specialists, students and research workers will find the book a unique reference for improving understanding of statistical tools and its appropriate application in public health and nutrition research, surveys, evaluation and in program designing. It is hoped that this comprehensive book will serve as a valuable resource for enhancing knowledge towards appropriate usage of statistical tools.

It provides me immense satisfaction and indeed a great pleasure to write the foreword for this book.

**Dr Sheila C. Vir**

*Senior Public Health Nutrition Consultant & Director, Public Health Nutrition and development Centre, New Delhi*

*22nd April 2015*

# Why this book

From a theoretical statistician specializing in design of experiments and sampling theory, I had to switch over in 1987 to applications of statistics through research projects at the Institute of Applied Statistics and Development Studies (IASDS). My encounter with nutrition and health started with a research project from UNICEF in which IASDS carried out the first-ever study to assess nutritional status of children and women in Uttar Pradesh. The nutrition related data collected in the project led to a follow up study on in-depth analysis. This allowed me to get in closer contact with the nutrition specialist Dr. Sheila Vir of UNICEF. The interaction culminated with a specialized publication on nutritional status and its correlates which was owned and published by Department of Women and Child Development, Government of Uttar Pradesh with UNICEF support in 1999.

The above publication was a milestone in the life of IASDS and health and nutrition projects from leading national and international agencies started pouring in. These studies enabled me to interact with health and nutrition experts not only within the country but even from other countries. Within no time, I was also recognized as an expert in statistical aspects of these subjects resulting into contracts from leading agencies as Consultant.

For the past many years I was being motivated by Dr. Sheila Vir to write a book based upon my long experience in the area of community health and nutrition. The present write up is a result of this motivation. The book is neither a conventional textbook nor a critical review on the topic. It is instead an attempt to discuss the topic based upon my experiences and interactions while handling projects of IASDS. Though the book primarily addresses the concerns of research managers, it is likely to be equally useful to students, faculty and research workers. The book, however, assumes the first level knowledge of statistical methodology.

The book describes common flaws in the methods employed thus far and the ways to overcome these. It also gives some statistical methods which are very promising but have hardly been used in India. These are Geo Hot Spot Technique for diseases in community clusters, Randomized Response Technique for sensitive characteristics, Principal Components for data reduction and Small Area Estimation for inadequate sample size. Each of these techniques is explained through live data examples though some minimal theory is also described. The purpose of discussing these techniques is to make the reader aware of their potentials. However, the help of a statistician is required for using the techniques. For all of these excepting the randomized response, the analyses are computer intensive requiring software like SAS, SPSS, R, etc.

Though many of the useful topics have been discussed, there have omissions as well. The intention is not to present an exhaustive coverage of topics on community health and nutrition which do not have serious statistical concerns. Some of the areas which have not found place are morbidity and disease burden, family planning and unmet needs, management of low birth weight and severely undernourished and obese children, bio-chemical aspects, surveillance and HIV transmission. A similar concern is the extent of female feticide and child labor engaged in hazardous activities in industries like carpet, glass, etc. There is no methodologically sound estimate of either of the two, female feticide or child labor engaged in hazardous activities.

I owe a lot to Dr. Padam Singh, former Additional Director General, ICMR and Director, National Institute of Medical Statistics in whose company I started appreciating the intricacies of statistical aspects of community health and nutrition. This happened during several years when we worked together on some important research projects. Dr. V. K. Srivastava formerly of King George Medical University, not only involved me in several joint studies, but was always available to me for help, support and advice.

I must also thank Prof. Aloke Dey, NASI Senior Scientist Platinum Jubilee Fellow, for his help and support right since the formative stage. He advised me on the content and style of some chapters which added lot of value to the write-up. Thanks are also due to Dr. Neeraj Tiwari of Kumaun University for his advice on the write-up, particularly on Geo Hot Spots. I would also like to thank Dr. Ravindra Srivastava, Director, IASDS, for his valuable advice from time to time and for going through the manuscript. I also benefitted from time to time discussions with IASDS staff, Dr. P. P. Tewari, Ms. Reeta Saxena and Dr. Shruti Shukla.

Finally, the write-up would not be complete, if I do not make special mention of my wife Dr. Sushma. Without her care and support, it would not have been possible to complete this book. I must appreciate my sons Manish, Sumit and Sachin for their constant motivation, help and encouragement.

**A K Nigam**
*Institute of Applied Statistics and Development Studies*
*30 April 2015*

# 1

# Quantitative research methods

## 1.1 Community health and nutrition

In any investigation on health and nutrition in a community, one looks for questions like purpose of the study, whether to generate new information or for proving a hypothesis. Some typical examples of the first category may be: What is the prevalence of anemia among adolescent girls? What should be the recommended dietary allowance (RDA) for Indians according to age, sex, occupation categories? What is the dietary intake of adolescents, or assessing the nutritional status of under-4 years of age children? For proving a hypothesis, the examples could be the testing whether nutritional status is different according to gender, age, tribes or socio-economic groups. Some of the research methodology discussed here and what follows in the next chapter are discussed in Nigam and Singh (2011).

The community level studies are observational type in which the researcher collects information on the attributes or measurements of interest, but does not influence events. An example would be a study of prevalence of anemia among children. Community level studies are usually survey based. By contrast, in an experimental study, the researcher deliberately influences events and investigates the effects of the intervention. Clinical trials are of this category. While stronger inferences can be made from experimental studies under controlled conditions than from observational studies, community level studies are also necessary to have insight into characteristics of large populations. Two contrasting examples explain the two approaches. While the effect of iron supplementation to pregnant women versus anemia level could be studied in an experimental framework, a community level study can attempt to substantiate the experimental findings among a large class of pregnant women.

## 1.2 Research methodology

An important component of development is the situational analysis like current status of exclusive breastfeeding or mid-day meal program. Another component is impact assessment – studying changes in prevalence levels of any indicator. It broadly involves formative analysis/baseline/monitoring/

concurrent evaluation/ semi-annual assessment/ endline. Monitoring and evaluation are very important tools of development research. While monitoring is like concurrent evaluation or mid-term assessment for identifying the weaknesses and taking remedial measures for improving the program, evaluation is like impact assessment after project is completed.

It may now be desirable to introduce the reader to some basics needed at this stage. Systematic research involves a sequence of steps. These have been highlighted in Figs. 1.1 and 1.2. While Fig. 1.1 gives stages of development study, Fig. 1.2 gives stages of impact studies. Details of different components of quantitative and qualitative research methodology are discussed in the present and the following chapters.

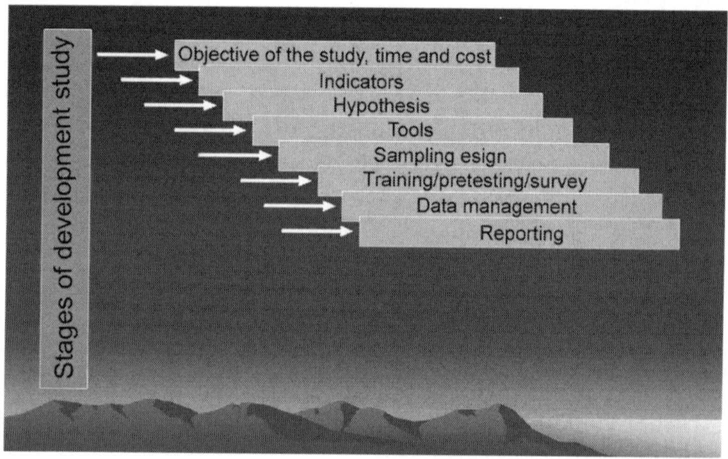


**Figure 1.1** Stages of development study

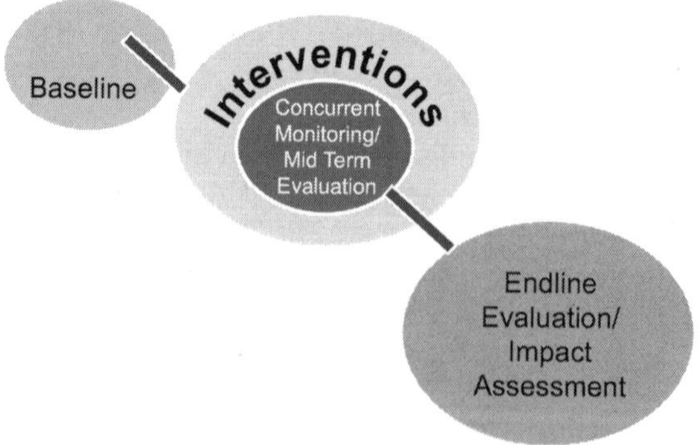


**Figure 1.2** Stages of impact assessment

## 1.3 Basic statistical tools

Every research study requires some basic statistical tools. An excellent source on these is the book by Snedecor and Cochran (1989). Before we proceed further it may be necessary to describe some of these tools.

### 1.3.1 Bar diagrams

It is easy to comprehend the important features of a data set if these are summarized in some form. Most common methods of summarization of data sets are percentages, trends, bar diagrams and averages. While each one of these summarization techniques is extremely useful, these can sometimes be misleading if not properly used. Figure 1.3 is a typical bar diagram depicting percent distribution of adult males and females by body mass index (BMI) grades.

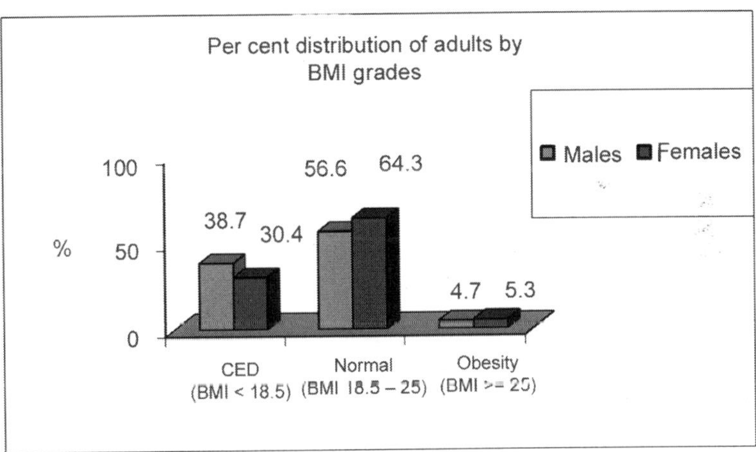


**Figure 1.3** % distribution of adults by BMI grades

### 1.3.2 Percentages

Summarizing the data in percentages, deciles, etc., are also very common. While percentage implies one-hundredth, decile is one tenth and median is fiftieth percentile. A one-time percentage reflects the overall current status; for instance, the prevalence of underweight among children below 5 years of age is 47 percent. But two or more time percentages reflect the changes over time. If the anemia prevalence in the pre-intervention stage is 78 percent and in the post-intervention stage is 71 percent, then there is a change (improvement) by 7 percentage points because of intervention.

Percentage computed in two different ways convey different meanings. This can best be explained through an example on antenatal checkups. Take the example of pregnant women from scheduled tribes and backward categories that had 3 or more antenatal checkups. Among the women who had 3 or more antenatal checkups if the percentage is worked out as scheduled tribes or backward categories women divided by the total number of women from both the categories, then it means that interest is to compare the feature between two categories. On the other hand, if the percentage is worked out as scheduled tribes women divided by total number of scheduled tribes women who had antenatal check up or backward categories women divided by total number of women of backward categories who had antenatal check up, then it conveys the feature among each of the two categories of women.

## 1.3.3 Trends and patterns

An analysis of trends is a way of comprehending longitudinal data. The graph below gives a typical trend analysis of sex ratios in the state of Uttar Pradesh in India. Sometimes the analysis of trends and patterns reflects some important features of data. We discuss these later in Section 1.16.

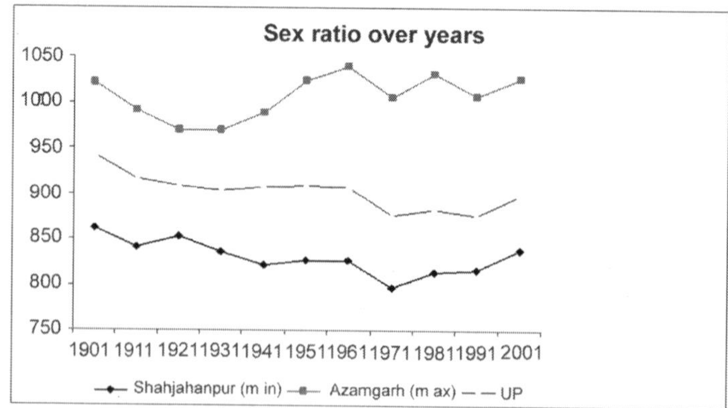


**Figure 1.4** Sex ratio over time

## 1.3.4 Averages

Amongst the most commonly used measures of central tendency are arithmetic mean, median and mode. Arithmetic mean in its simplest form is given by total of all observations divided by total number of observations. Median is the middle most value of the distribution. Mode is the most frequent value. Though arithmetic mean is very simple to compute and comprehend, it is a useful tool only when data are symmetric. In case of skewed (non-symmetrical) data, median is a better measure than arithmetic mean. As the median is the 50th percentile, half of the values are higher than the median, and the remaining half are lower. The median is less affected by outliers (extreme data points) than the mean, so with a skewed distribution it will give a better representation of the centre. Skewness means lack of symmetry in the distribution of the observations.

If $x_1, x_2, \ldots, x_n$ are n observations then arithmetic mean is given by

$$\bar{x} = \sum x_i /n = (x_1 + x_2 + \ldots + x_n)/n$$

For a frequency distribution type data with $x_i$ having frequency $f_i$ or for data with weights $w_i$, it is given by $\sum f_i x_i / \sum f_i$, or $\sum w_i x_i / \sum w_i$..

Another measure which is normally used for computation of index numbers is the geometric mean. It is the antilogarithm of the arithmetic mean of the logarithm of all values. It is a better measure of central tendency when data follow a lognormal distribution (long tail). Specifically, the geometric mean is useful in analyzing exponential trends and population growth. It also dampens the effects of extreme data points.

Arithmetic mean was being used by National Nutrition Monitoring Bureau (NNMB) for average weights/heights by single ages. As the distribution of weights/heights for a given age is skewed with some extreme values, median is more appropriate here. Some other examples of skewed data sets are income, consumption and expenditure, and dietary intakes. An insight into dietary intake data of NNMB and other agencies reveals that the data are asymmetrical and also have extreme values. Some of the mean intakes, both at household and individual level, also have large standard errors. This clearly suggests using median as the average intake instead of mean.

### 1.3.5 Variance

Variance measures how far a set of observations is spread out. A variance of zero indicates that all the values are all identical. Variance is therefore a measure of the amount of variability or scatter in numerical data when compared to the mean, or average. If $x_1, x_2, \ldots, x_n$ are n observations, then variance $\sigma_x^2$ is given by $\sum [x_i - \bar{x}]^2 /n$. Here is the arithmetic mean. Further, $\sigma_x$ which is square root of variance $\sigma_x^2$ is called standard deviation.

Covariance is the joint variation between two sets of observations: $x_1, x_2, \ldots, x_n$ and $y_1, y_2, \ldots, y_n$. It is denoted by $\sigma_{xy}$ and is given by

$$\sum [x_i - \bar{x})] [y_i - \bar{y})]/n$$

A closely related concept to variance is the coefficient of variation which represents the ratio of the standard deviation to the mean. Higher the coefficient of variation, greater is the dispersion in the variable. It is easily realized that coefficient of variation is free from unit of measurement. This makes it an extremely useful tool to compare two different series of observations.

## 1.4 Common probability distributions

This section is devoted to the common probability distributions which are important tools in the analysis of data. Before proceeding further it is important to understand the concept of a random variable.

### 1.4.1 Random variable

A random variable is a function that associates a unique numerical value with every outcome of an experiment. The value of the random variable will vary from trial to trial as the experiment is repeated. There are two types of random variables: discrete and continuous. A discrete random variable has distinct integer values. Numbers of persons in a family, number of students in a class or number of students with weight less than 50 kg are some examples of discrete variable. A continuous random variable is one which takes an infinite number of possible values. Continuous random variables are usually measurements like height, weight and the energy content of a drink. E*xpected value* of a random variable is intuitively the long-run average *value* of repetitions of the experiment it represents. The mean of a random variable is referred to as its expected value, and is denoted by E(x).

### 1.4.2 Probability distributions

We begin with the notion of a random experiment. An experiment with two or more possible outcomes and whose result cannot be predicted in advance is called a random experiment. For example, suppose a group of 20 individuals are classified according to their blood groups, viz. O, A, B and AB. The number of individuals in each group can be any integer between 0 and 20, subject to the fact that the frequencies over all the groups add up to 20. As another example of a random experiment, suppose a newly discovered vaccine against a disease is given to 30 persons. These 30 persons are then observed for a period of 6 months to see how many of these have developed the disease. Clearly, the number of affected persons may vary between 0 and 30.

Probability distributions are a fundamental concept in statistics. A study of outcomes of a random experiment leads to probability distributions. Some uses of probability distributions are to calculate confidence intervals for parameters and to calculate critical regions for hypothesis tests. Confidence interval is a type of *interval estimate* of a *population parameter*. It is an observed interval calculated from the observations, which when repeated includes the parameter of interest 99 percent of the times. Thus the confidence level is 99 percent that the true value of the parameter is in the confidence interval. These aspects are discussed further in Section 1.7.

A probability distribution assigns a *probability* to each *measurable subset* of the possible outcomes of a random *experiment*, *survey*, or procedure of *statistical inference*. A probability distribution can either be *univariate* or *multivariate*. A univariate distribution gives the probabilities of a single *random variable* taking on various alternative values; a multivariate distribution is a joint probability distribution and gives the joint probabilities of a set of two or more random variables.

Among important univariate distributions the normal distribution, also called Gaussian, is the most important continuous distribution. It is extremely useful and is often used in the *natural* and *social sciences* for real-valued *random variables* whose distributions are not known. Another useful distribution is the *Bernoulli distribution*, which takes value 1 with probability p and value 0 with probability q = 1 − p. While the *binomial distribution* describes the number of successes in a series of independent Yes/No experiments all with the same probability of success, the *Poisson distribution* describes the number of rare successes in a series of independent Yes/No experiments with different success probabilities.

The normal distribution is immensely useful because of the central limit theorem, which states that under mild conditions the mean of many random variables independently drawn from the same distribution is distributed approximately normally, irrespective of the form of the original distribution. Physical quantities that are expected to be the sum of many independent processes (such as measurement errors) often have a distribution very close to the normal. Moreover, many results and methods (such as propagation of uncertainty and least squares parameter fitting) can be derived analytically in explicit form when the relevant variables are normally distributed.

The Gaussian distribution also called the bell curve is symmetrical with mean, median and mode located in the centre. An extremely useful property of this distribution is that about 68 percent of values drawn from a normal population are within one standard deviation away from the mean; about 95 percent of the values lie within two standard deviations; and about 99.7

percent are within three standard deviations. A variable which follows the normal distribution is said to be normally distributed and such a variable is called a normal variate.

Other commonly used distributions are t, F and $\chi^2$. Student's t-distribution (or simply the t-distribution) is a continuous probability distribution that arises when estimating the mean of a normally distributed population in situations where the sample size is small and population standard deviation is unknown. Whereas a normal distribution describes a full population, t-distributions describe samples drawn from a full population; accordingly, the t-distribution for each sample size is different, and the larger the sample, the more the distribution resembles a normal distribution.

The t-distribution plays a role in a number of widely used statistical analyses, including the t-test for assessing the statistical significance of the difference between two sample means, the construction of confidence intervals for the difference between two population means, and in linear regression analysis.

If we take a random sample of n observations from a normal distribution, then the t-distribution with $\nu = n - 1$ degrees of freedom can be defined as the distribution of the location of the true mean, relative to the sample mean and divided by the sample standard deviation, after multiplying by the normalizing term $\sqrt{n}$. In this way, the t-distribution can be used to estimate how likely it is that the true mean lies in any given range.

Degree of freedom is the number of values in the final calculation of a statistic that are free to vary. Estimates of statistical parameters can be based upon different amounts of information or data. The number of independent pieces of information that go into the estimate of a parameter is called the degrees of freedom.

The t-distribution is symmetric and bell-shaped, like the normal distribution, but has heavier tails, meaning that it is more prone to producing values that fall far from its mean. F-distribution is also a *continuous probability distribution*. If a *random variable* x has an F-distribution with parameters $d_1$ and $d_2$, we write $x \sim F(d_1, d_2)$. This means that x has F-distribution with $d_1$ and $d_2$ degrees of freedom. It is actually a ratio of two independent chi-squares.

The chi-square or $\chi^2$-distribution with k degrees of freedom is the distribution of a sum of the squares of k independent standard normal random variables. It is one of the most widely used probability distributions in inferential statistics, especially in hypothesis testing.

The reader may refer to the write-up at the end of the chapter for some mathematical details on probability distributions.

## 1.5 Sampling

A sample is a part of a population, called the 'universe', or the 'parent population'. We consider only those populations which have a finite number of units. Sampling is the process or technique of selecting a sample. The population is the aggregate of the elements or the sampling units. Listing of the sampling units with identification according to certain specifications is called the 'sampling frame'. Appropriate sample selection and its allocation are crucial to design set up for carrying out the research.

The reference population may be populations of people who are residents of a geographical area, possess a particular attribute, may have certain disease, participators of a certain program, workers in a particular occupation, or people exposed to some intervention. It may be of interest to estimate prevalence of the disease that is the proportions of individuals suffering from the disease, total number of persons with a particular occupation, say labor, or percentage of illiterate girls of age group 6–10 years. The total or proportion obtained from sampled observations is taken as an estimate of the population total or proportion. If the expected value of the sample total or proportion is same as population total or proportion, then the estimate is called unbiased. Further, the variance of the sample total or proportion which is the variance of the sampled observations is called the sampling error. There can be many other sources of variability like non-response, incorrect response, and errors in data recording, editing, etc. These are called non-sampling errors. For biased estimators the measure of variability is the mean square error (MSE) which is given by

$$\text{MSE} = \text{variance} + (\text{bias})^2$$

where bias is the difference between the totals or proportions of sampled and population values.

### 1.5.1 Sampling procedures

Random sampling ensures a positive chance of selection to every unit in the population. Non-random or purposive sampling assigns more chance to certain units, and certain units do not have a chance to get selected. Sometimes purposive sampling is adopted due to some special reasons like including certain focused target groups. By a sampling procedure, we mean a unit-by-unit mechanism of drawing units from the population.

#### *1.5.1.1 Simple random sampling*

Simple random sampling guarantees that each member of the population has an equal chance of being selected at any draw. The common methods of simple random sampling are lottery and use of random numbers. Even the digits of currency notes could also be used as a substitute of random number table. The lottery method assigns identifiable numbers to the population; these numbers are then thoroughly mixed and a specified number is drawn at random without replacement to provide the desired sample size. Tables of random numbers are used by starting anywhere in the random number table and continue selecting numbers until the desired sample size is reached. The procedure is best explained through a simple example. If the population size is 50 and a simple random sample of size 10 is to be selected, then after assigning each one of these in to 50 identifiable units, a random number is drawn from a two digit random number table. If the selected number is less than 51, it is included in the sample. If the selected random number is more than 50, then divide the selected random number by 50 and select the remainder as the selected sampling unit. Suppose the selected random is 98, then after dividing it by 10, the remainder is 48. Thus the selected sampling unit is 48. The process is repeated until 10 units are selected. However, to ensure without replacement sample, no sampling unit is to be repeated.

#### *1.5.1.2 Stratified sampling*

In stratified sampling, the population is divided into homogeneous groups called strata according to certain common characteristic; then a random sample is drawn from each stratum. For example, a population might be divided according to geographical location like regions of a state, social classes, income groups, etc. After the sample of required size is selected, there is an important issue of allocation of sample to different strata.

Deep stratification or nested stratification (stratification within stratification) is a very useful tool, if appropriately used. The technique provides a sampling design which requires a smaller overall sample size and is intuitively more efficient than the conventional stratified design using only one stratification variable. Deep stratification automatically controls variability according to dis-aggregated groups and simple random sampling within each stratum leads to a near self-weighting design, which is easy to analyze and interpret.

#### *1.5.1.3 Systematic sampling*

In systematic sampling, the first unit is chosen at random and then other units for the sample are chosen in a systematic way with an interval. Continuing with the example of selecting a sample of size 10 out of a population of size 50, the first step is to divide the population size 50 by the sample size 10. The divider is 5. It is called the interval. Now a random number is drawn between 1 and 5. Let it be 3. Then it is the first selected unit in the sample. The remaining 9 units of the sample are systematically selected with an interval of 5. The sampling units are 3, 8, 13, 18, 23, 28, 33, 38, 43, and 48. When the sample size is not a multiple of the population size, some modification in selecting a systematic sample is required. For details on these, see for example Cochran (1977).

#### *1.5.1.4 Cluster sampling*

Concept-wise cluster sampling is exactly opposite to stratified sampling. In cluster sampling population is divided into non-overlapping groups called clusters, and then a random sample of clusters is drawn from the population clusters. The method is operationally convenient as clusters are usually formed of neighboring units. Cluster sampling is more efficient than simple random sampling if clusters contain non-homogeneous units. But it is difficult to ensure heterogeneity within groups and hence this sampling procedure is generally less efficient than simple random sampling.

World Health Organization (WHO) developed 30-cluster sampling design which is usually employed in immunization coverage evaluation surveys. We discuss this separately in Chapter 5.

#### *1.5.1.5 Multistage sampling*

Among the most useful sampling procedure is the multistage sampling. In large-scale surveys, the sample is mostly selected using different stages. For example in a state-level survey on adolescent girls, different stages of selection could be districts, blocks/talukas, villages, households and adolescent girls.

#### *1.5.1.6 Probability proportional to size*

In probability proportional to size (PPS) sampling, the probabilities to different units are assigned in proportion to their sizes. For instance, for selecting villages, size is taken as population of the villages; and for selecting individuals or households, size can be the yearly income. This is a case of unequal probability sampling procedure. We explain this through an example. Suppose a PPS sample of n villages is to be selected from a total of N villages. For the selection of n villages with probability proportional to population size, we need the population of all the N villages. Let the total population of the N villages be T. First step is to determine the sampling interval k which is T/n. Villages are then arranged from the least populated to maximum populated ones and these are numbered from 1 to N. The next step is to get the cumulative totals of all the ordered villages and draw a random number between 1 to k. Let the random number drawn between 1 to k be r. The first selected village is the one whose cumulative total is either equal to r or just above it. Add k to r which gives k + r. The next sample village is whose cumulative total is either equal to k + r or just above it. The process is repeated till a sample of size n villages is accomplished.

The above selection of villages ensures that villages with higher population have larger probability of selection. However, if we ensure selection of same number of households from each village, then the overall sample is a simple random sample.

For selection of households in a village, first a rough sketch of the village is to be prepared. Next step is to identify a centre and draw all lanes/by lanes from the centre. Select one of the lanes/ by lanes randomly. Let the selected lane be fifth. Walk from the centre to the end of the lane and count the steps (say 41). Select a random number between 1 and 41, say '14'. Walk again from the centre and stop at step '14' which is the random start. The house on your left is the randomly selected house. If the target is to select 10 pregnant women from each village, then as a first step enquire whether there is a pregnant woman in the house. If yes collect the information about the woman otherwise proceed to next house following right hand rule. Continue till 10 women are selected. This is to be followed in all the selected villages.

In India, village comprises of mohallas/tolas. The mohallas may be divided into SC, ST and others. Sample could be selected from each of these groups following the approach described above.

## 1.6 Analysis

After selecting the sample and collecting information from the target groups through questionnaires, focus group discussions (FGD) and in-depth interviews, the next step is to enter data in a computer suited to the software to be used for analyses. Questionnaires are the tools for quantitative data whereas FGD and in-depth interviews mostly provide qualitative data (see, Chapter 2). If SPSS is chosen to analyze quantitative data, commonly used tools for data entry are excel or SPSS spreadsheets. In the analysis of data, steps involved are data entry and management, data cleaning and validation, choice of analytical techniques for obtaining valid estimates and inferences, and choice of appropriate software. The analysis and tabulation plan should be consistent with the objectives. Most type of data analyses can be done using SAS, SPSS or R. Some type of analyses can also be done using epi info. We discuss some aspects of data entry and management, and data cleaning and validation later in Section 1.11.

## 1.7 Tests of hypothesis

Every research has an objective which could be translated into a research hypothesis which is an assumption about the unknown parameter. A hypothesis is called the null hypothesis if it specifies that the effect of interest is zero; this statistical null hypothesis is often the negation of the research hypothesis. On the other hand, an alternative or research hypothesis implies that the effect of interest is not zero.

For example, for testing the null hypothesis that anemia levels are same in adolescent girls and boys, one may take the alternate hypothesis that adolescent girls are more anemic than adolescent boys. If $p_b$ and $p_g$ are proportion of anemic boys and girls respectively, then the null hypothesis is

$$p_b = p_g$$

and the alternate hypothesis that anemia prevalence is higher in adolescent girls is

$$p_g > p_b$$

In the general setting, null hypothesis implies zero or no difference, that is, $H_0$: $p_1 = p_2$ whereas the alternate hypothesis may take any of the following forms:

$$H_1: p_1 \neq p_2 \text{ two tailed}$$
$$p_1 < p_2 \text{ or } p_1 > p_2 \text{ one tailed}$$

Following Table 1.1 indicates possible errors in drawing statistical inferences while testing the null hypothesis.

**Table 1.1** Possible errors in inference

| In Actual | Inference | |
|---|---|---|
| | Accept $H_o$ | Reject $H_o$ |
| $H_o$ True | Correct decision (Confidence level) | Type 1 error |
| $H_o$ False | Type 2 error | Correct decision (Power) |

Thus, Type 1 error = reject Ho when it is true; and Type 2 error = accept Ho when it is false. These two taken together is called the critical region. Further, the level of significance a is the probability of Type 1 error so that confidence level of the test is 1-α which is the probability of accepting null hypothesis when it is true. Further, β is the probability of Type 2 error and power of the test 1-β is the probability of rejecting null hypothesis when it is false.

The level of significance is generally fixed at 5 percent. When a difference is statistically significant at 5 percent level of significance, it means that the observed difference could have occurred by chance in only up to 5 percent of the occasions. If a corresponding hypothesis test is performed, the confidence level is the complement of respective level of significance, i.e. a 95 percent confidence interval reflects a significance level of 0.05.

The level of significance could be even 10 percent in case of exploratory or behavioral studies. In case of introduction of new drugs or an intervention dealing with human beings, the level of significance has to be fixed 0.1 percent or even lower to ensure safety.

## 1.8 Tests of significance

Among the commonly used analytical tools are t, F and $\chi^2$ tests of significance. First of these, t test can be for testing means from one or two normal populations. While two sample t tests are carried out to test the difference between means of two treatments (intervention vs. control), F test is often used in analysis of variance for testing more than two treatments. Another context in which F test is used to test the null hypothesis that two variances of two normal populations are equal.

The chi-square distribution is used in the common chi-square tests for goodness of fit of an observed distribution to a theoretical one, the independence of two criteria of classification of qualitative data, and in confidence interval estimation for a population standard deviation of a normal distribution from a sample standard deviation.

### 1.8.1 One sample t-test

Let $x_1, x_2, \ldots, x_n$ be n sample observations from a normal population. In testing the null hypothesis that the population mean is equal to a specified value $\mu_0$, one uses the statistic

$$t = d / (s/n^{1/2})$$

where $d = (\bar{x} - \mu_0)$; $\bar{x}$ is the sample mean and s is the *standard deviation* of the sampled observations. The value of t as computed above from sample observations is called the test statistic. If follows the t distribution with n – 1 degrees of freedom. The computed value is compared with the t-distribution values at n – 1 degrees of freedom. If the computed value is smaller than the table value for a given significance level, the null hypothesis is accepted. The t- distribution values are available in textbooks of Statistics which give t at different degrees of freedom and significance levels.

### 1.8.2 Independent two sample t-tests

*Equal or unequal sample sizes, equal variance*

Let $x_1, x_2, \ldots, x_{n1}$ be $n_1$ observations from a sample of size $n_1$ from a normal population with mean $\mu_1$ and variance $\sigma^2$ and $y_1, y_2, \ldots, y_{n2}$ be another independent sample of size $n_2$ from a normal population with mean $\mu_2$ and variance $\sigma^2$. This test is used only when it can be assumed that the two distributions have the same variance. The t statistic to test whether the means are equal ($\mu_1 = \mu_2$) can be calculated as follows:

$$t = d/s_{xy}\,(1/n_1 + 1/n_2)^{1/2}$$

where d is the difference of two sample means ($\overline{x} - \overline{y}$),

$$s_{xy} = [\{(n_1 - 1)\,s_x^{\,2} + (n_2 - 1)\,s_y^{\,2}\}/(n_1 + n_2 - 2)]^{1/2}$$

Here, $n_1 + n_2 - 2$ is the total number of degrees of freedom, which is used in significance testing.

**Example:** Table 1.2 is taken from Vir et al. (2008). It gives mean hemoglobin levels of school going adolescent girls according to age before and after12 months of weekly IFA intervention.

**Table 1.2** Mean hemoglobin levels (g/dL) in school going adolescent girls

| Age | Pre (n = 596) | Post (n = 573) |
|---|---|---|
| 11 | 10.7 | 11.7 |
| 12 | 10.8 | 11.8 |
| 13 | 10.9 | 11.8 |
| 14 | 11.0 | 11.8 |
| 15 | 11.0 | 11.9 |
| 16 | 11.0 | 11.9 |
| 17 | 10.3 | 12.1 |
| 18 | 11.0 | 11.6 |
| Average | 10.8 | 11.8 |

The average Hb levels improved from 10.8 to 11.8 g/dL. On applying independent two-sample t-test, the value of t is computed as 9.76 which is highly significant ($p < 0.01$). Here $p < 0.01$ means that computed value of t is greater than the table value for 1 percent level of significance.

*Equal or unequal sample sizes, unequal variances*

This test is used only when the two population variances are not assumed to be equal (the two sample sizes may or may not be equal) and hence must be estimated separately. We skip this case and refer the reader to any standard book in Statistics.

### 1.8.3 Paired t-test

This test is used when the samples are dependent; that is, when there is only one sample having repeated measures or when there are two samples that have been matched or 'paired'. This is an example of a paired difference test. The statistic t is given by

$$t = d / (s/n^{1/2})$$

Here d is the mean of all paired differences. The pairs are either one person's pre-test and post-test scores or between pairs of persons matched into meaningful groups (for instance drawn from the same family or age group). The s is the standard deviation of the paired differences. The degree of freedom (d.f.) is $n - 1$.

### 1.8.4 t-tests for proportions

The formulae given above get easily extended to testing the difference between two proportions. If $p_1$ and $p_2$ are the two proportions observed from two independent samples, with observations $n_1$ and $n_2$ respectively, then t statistic at $n_1 + n_2 - 2$ d.f. is given by

$$t = (p_1 - p_2)/[\{p_1 (1 - p_1)/n_1\} + \{p_2(1 - p_2)/ n_2\}]^{1/2}$$

This could be the case if anemia prevalence percentages are available for baseline and endline stages, and it is intended to test whether there is any change in anemia prevalence due to intervention. Thus if $p_1 = 0.964$, $p_2 = 0.729$, $n_1 = 280$ and $n_2 = 303$, then t is computed as 8.44.

Similarly, if $p_1$ and $p_2$, and $p_3$ and $p_4$ are respective prevalence percentages at pre- and post- intervention stages of two areas or districts, and it is intended to compare the changes between two areas, that is $p_1 - p_2$ versus $p_3 - p_4$ then t test statistic is given by

$$t = [(p_1 - p_2) - (p_3 - p_4)]/A$$

where $A = [\{p_1(1 - p_1)/n_1\} + \{p_2(1 - p_2)/n_2\}]^{1/2} + [\{p_3(1 - p_3)/n_3\} + \{p_4 (1 - p_4)/ n_4\}]^{1/2}$

For $p_1 = 0.833$, $p_2 = 0.649$, $p_3 = 0.987$ and $p_4 = 0.515$; $n_1 = 150$ and $n_2 = 241$ $n_3 = 151$ and $n_2 = 262$, the calculated value of t is 5.38.

### 1.8.5 F test

F test is in a sense a generalized form of t. While t tests are used to compare two means, F test compares several means through analysis of variance. Analysis of variance is simply dividing total variation into one or more assignable variations and un-assignable variations (termed as error components) and comparing the assignable variations against error.

**Example:** Testing the difference of anemia among scheduled castes, scheduled tribes and others.

Table below is a typical ANOVA Table displaying steps to compute F.

**Table 1.3** Components of ANOVA Table

| Source of variation | Degrees of freedom (d.f.) | Sum of squares (s.s) | Mean squares (s.s./d.f.) | F at k-1, k(n-1) d.f. |
|---|---|---|---|---|
| Assignable causes | K – 1 | $s_i^2$ | m.s.i | m.s.i / m.s.e |
| Between interventions (k) | | | | |
| Error | k(n – 1) | $s_e^2 = s_2 - s_i^2$ | m.s.e | |
| Total | nk – 1 | $s^2$ | | |

Here Table 1.3 is displayed for k interventions on n individuals, giving a total of nk observations. The k (>2) interventions can be like trying daily, weekly and fortnightly IFA administration to adolescent girls, or even comparing different grass-root-level NGOs implementing some information, education and counseling strategies. An interesting application of ANOVA appears later in Chapter 3 to test 1-, 2- and 3-days 24 hours recalls for assessing dietary intakes.

## 1.8.6 Chi-Square ($\chi^2$) test

We now discuss $\chi^2$ test for independence. It is applied when two categorical variables form a single population. By categorical data is meant any data set classified according to categories. For instance, in any 2 × 2 contingency table data can be classified into two categories – educational status and grades of anemia. It is used to determine whether there is a significant association between the two variables. For example it may be desired to test the association of education on infant-feeding practices.

The test procedure is appropriate when the variables under study are categorical and the expected frequency count for each cell of the contingency table is at least 5.

Suppose that attribute A has *r* levels, and attribute B has *c* levels. The test statistic $\chi^2$ is

$$\chi^2 = \Sigma [(O_{i,j} - E_{i,j})^2 / E_{i,j}]$$

where $O_{i,j}$ is the observed frequency count at level i of A and level j of B, and $E_{i,j}$ is the expected frequency at levels i and j. The $\chi^2$ is at (r – 1)(c – 1) d.f.

The expected frequency count E i,j for the cell i,j is given by

$$E_{i,j} = (n_i. \text{ x } n.j)/n$$

where n is the total sample size, and $n_i$. and n.j are row and column totals of ith row and jth column, respectively.

Like t-distribution, tables are also available in textbooks for F and chi-square distributions.

**Example:** In 2012, IASDS carried out a study *"Household Survey for the Assessment of Nutrition and Education Status"* in Purulia district of West Bengal for Welthungehilfe for its 'fight hunger first' initiative. In order to establish the association between undernutrition and social group affiliations, Chi-square test for goodness of fit was applied for all the three under-nutrition indicators to test the hypothesis that the 'prevalence of under-nutrition is independent of caste affiliation'. We use the following stunting data according to social groups for illustration. Table 1.4 gives observed stunting figures whereas Table 1.5 gives expected figures.

**Table 1.4** Grades of stunting by social groups (Observed)

| Social Group | Severe | Moderate | Normal | Total |
|---|---|---|---|---|
| SC | 208 | 44 | 200 | 452 |
| ST | 203 | 54 | 168 | 425 |
| OBC | 128 | 38 | 161 | 327 |
| General | 570 | 90 | 561 | 1221 |
| Total | 1109 | 226 | 1090 | 2425 |

**Table 1.5** Grades of stunting by social groups (Expected)

| Social Group | Severe | Moderate | Normal | Total |
|---|---|---|---|---|
| SC | 206.7085 | 42.12454 | 203.16696 | 452 |
| ST | 194.3608 | 39.60825 | 191.03095 | 425 |
| OBC | 149.5435 | 30.47505 | 146.9814 | 327 |
| General | 558.3872 | 113.7922 | 548.8206 | 1221 |
| Total | 1109 | 226 | 1090 | 2425 |

Calculated value of $\chi^2$ is 20.316. Comparing it with the table value 12.592 of $\chi^2$ at 6 degrees of freedom and 5 percent level of significance, the hypothesis is rejected indicating that 'stunting' is dependent on caste affiliation of children.

## 1.9 Non-parametric tests

Tests like t and F assume that parent population is normally distributed. But, $\chi^2$ test is an exception and does not depend upon normality or any other distribution. This is why it is called distribution free test. There are many other non-parametric tests like sign and run tests. Though nutrition data like growth and dietary intakes have non-normality, yet the use of non-parametric tests for their analysis and inference is not common.

## 1.10 Correlation and regression

Among other commonly used statistical tools are correlation and regression. Whereas correlation measures the extent of linear relationship between two variables, regression explores the type of relationship. In case of more than two variables, these are called multiple correlations and multiple regressions, respectively. Suppose we have n (paired) observations $(x_1, y_1), (x_2, y_2),\ldots, (x_n, y_n)$ on two variables, X and Y. The linear correlation coefficient between two variables X and Y with n observations each is given by

$$r = s_{XY} / s_X s_Y$$

where $s_{XY}$ is the covariance between X and Y and is given by

$$s_{XY} = \sum [x_i - \bar{x})] [y_i - \bar{y})]/n$$

$s_X$ and $s_Y$ are standard deviations of X and Y, respectively.

Depending upon the sign of $s_{XY}$ the value of r will be positive or negative. Further, the absolute value of r lies between 0 and 1. Thus $-1 \leq r \leq 1$. A value of r = 0 means no correlation while r = 1 means the two variable are perfectly correlated that too in the same direction. Similarly, r = – 1 means prefect negative correlation with the two variables moving in opposite directions.

Often, one is interested to test the hypothesis that the population correlation coefficient, say ρ, is equal to zero. Note that the observations $(x_1, y_1), (x_2, y_2), \ldots, (x_n, y_n)$ are a sample from a bivariate distribution of the variables X and Y. To test the hypothesis $\rho = 0$ against the alternative hypothesis $\rho \neq 0$, one employs a t-test. The test statistic for this test is given by

$$T = r\,(n-2)^{1/2} / (1-r^2)^{1/2}$$

where r is the correlation coefficient computed on the basis of the n observations, $(x_1, y_1), (x_2, y_2), \ldots, (x_n, y_n)$. The statistic T, under the hypothesis, follows a t-distribution with n – 2 degrees of freedom and we reject the hypothesis (of zero correlation) at $\alpha$ level of significance if the absolute value of T exceeds the table value of t-distribution for n – 2 degrees of freedom and $\alpha/2$ level.

In case of more than two variables, that is, between Y and k other variables jointly, the linear relationship is measured by multiple correlation coefficient, R, which is necessarily positive and takes values between 0 and 1. Its main utility is in the context of multiple regressions which we discuss now.

In practice, we are often interested in the relation between (say) two variables. For example, suppose a group of children (of about the same age) are given fixed amounts of nutritious food for a specified time. The body weight of each child is recorded before the nutrition program starts and again recorded after the specified time of nutrition intervention elapses. One can then obtain the values of change in body weight for each child. If the amount of nutritious food given to the ith child is $x_i$ and the change in body weight for the same child is yi , then we get paired observations, $(x_1, y_1), (x_2, y_2), \ldots, (x_n, y_n)$, where n is the number of children. If the amount of nutritious food, considered as a variable, is denoted by X and the change in body weight is denoted by Y, then while there is no functional relationship between X and Y , there exists some relationship between these two variables. If we treat X and Y as random variables, then we can postulate that (X, Y ) form a bivariate distribution. If this distribution is known exactly, one can compute the expected (or, average) value of Y for a given value of X. This expected value is called the regression of Y on X . For example, if (X, Y ) follow a bivariate normal distribution, then it is known that the expected value of Y for a given value of X is of the form $\alpha + \beta X$ , where $\alpha$ and $\beta$ are functions of the parameters in a bivariate normal distribution. In practice, however, the exact form of the distribution of (X, Y ) is often unknown and one has to approximate the relationship between these variables based on data recorded for the variables.

If we postulate that the variable Y is 'dependent' on X , then we say that Y is the dependent variable and, X , an 'independent' variable (or, the regressor). Suppose we have paired observations $(x_1, y_1), \ldots, (x_n, y_n)$ on the regressor X and the dependent variable Y , then the first step is to build a suitable 'model' which approximates the relationship between X and Y. In the case of a single regressor, some idea of a suitable model can be obtained by plotting the values of Y against those of X , such a plot being commonly called a scatter plot. The utility of the scatter plot is that it gives some idea about the degree of correlation and the regression trend.

One can postulate one of the following models:

$$y_i = \alpha + \beta x_i + e_i$$

$$y_i = \alpha + \beta x_i + \gamma x_i^2 + e_i$$

where $e_i$ is the error associated with the $i^{th}$ observation $y_i$, $x_i$ being assumed non-random. As is customary, we assume that the errors, $e_i$'s have zero mean and constant variance, say $\sigma^2$. This means that the expected value of $y_i$ (in the case of the first model above) is $\alpha + \beta x_i$. Thus, the error $e_i$ corresponding to the observation $y_i$ is actually the difference between the realization yi and its expectation. In order to estimate the unknown parameters, say $\alpha$ and $\beta$, one can employ the method of least squares in which estimates of $\alpha$, $\beta$ are obtained by minimizing the sum of squares of the errors, $\sum e_i^2$. It is known that least squares estimates are best linear *unbiased estimators* (BLUE) of the coefficients having minimum variance in the class of all linear unbiased estimators.

If it is hypothesized that a variable Y is dependent on k regressor variables $x_1, ..., x_k$ , then we have a multiple regression set up. We can then postulate a regression model of the type

$$y_i = \beta_0 + \beta_1 x_1 + \beta_2 x_2 + \cdots + \beta_k x_k + e_i$$

and fit this model based on the data on the dependent variable Y and each of the regressors, $x_1, ..., x_k$.

The next step in regression analysis is to test the adequacy of the fitted model. This is achieved by first dividing the total variation among the $y_i$ values as measured by the sum of squares between the $y_i$'s, $\sum(y_i - \bar{y})^2$ into two parts, one due to "regression" and the other called "deviation from regression". The first component is that portion of the total variation which is explained by the fitted model and the remaining portion is due to unexplained causes. The adequacy of the fitted model can then be tested by an F test, the test statistic being the ratio of the regression mean square (obtained by dividing the sum of squares due to regression by its degrees of freedom) to the deviation from regression mean square. A related method of determining the adequacy of the fitted regression model is provided by $R^2$, the coefficient of determination, which is given by

$R^2$ = Regression sum of squares/total sum of squares.

We have already discussed multiple correlation coefficient, R. Clearly, $0 \le R^2 \le 1$. Higher the value of $R^2$, better is the fit.

A major use of building a regression model is in 'prediction'. Suppose we have fitted a regression model based on n observations on the dependent variable Y and a single regressor X , the fitted model being

$$y = \hat{\alpha} + \hat{\beta}x,$$

where $\hat{\alpha}$ and $\hat{\beta}$ are the least squares estimators of $\alpha$ and $\beta$, respectively. Suppose it is desired to predict the value of the dependent variable Y at a (given) value, say $x_0$ of the regressor X. Then, the predicted value of Y at $x_0$ is simply

$$\hat{y} = \hat{\alpha} + \hat{\beta}x_0$$

It is to be noted that $x_0$ has to be within the range of X in the experiment, and it is not advisable to predict the value of Y at a value of X that is outside the range of X. This is because one can never be sure whether the fitted model is still valid outside the range of X; in other words, a regression model in general should not be used for extrapolation.

To sum up, regression analysis involves identifying the relationship between a dependent variable and one or more independent variables. The analysis involves two steps: first to explore a suitable model among competing models and then exploit the selected model for inferential purpose. A model of the relationship is assumed, and estimates of the parameter values are derived using least squares technique. This procedure is called fitting the regression equation. Various tests of significance are then employed to determine if the model is satisfactory. If the fitted model is satisfactory, the estimated regression equation can be used to predict the value of the dependent variable for given values of independent variables.

After the chosen model is fitted through least squares technique, it is used for drawing inference. It is done through ANOVA. The total variation in y is divided into two components: one due to the regression model (explained part) and the remaining variation which is unexplained. The regression part is tested against unexplained (called error) part through F test. Coefficient of determination $R^2$ is then determined which gives the variation explained due to regression relative to total variation. It indicates how well data fit the model and the extent to which the dependent variable is predictable.

There are a number of competing models. These are linear, curvilinear of polynomial family – quadratic, cubic etc., or even models involving inverse powers of x. All these are linear in parameters. Others are models which are nonlinear in parameters but can be linearized through some transformation. Power curve $y = \beta_0 x^{\beta}$ is nonlinear in $\beta$, but it is linear in log y. After log transformation on each side, it is given by $\log y = \log \beta_0 + \beta \log x$. Most other nonlinear models like logistic, Gompertz, modified exponential, etc., cannot be linearized through any transformation and need special techniques of fitting and inference. Of particular interest among these is the logistic regression for identifying risk factors in any causal factor analysis. For instance, one can determine risk factors along with their loading factors associated with undernutrition. We discuss this model separately in Chapter 3.

## 1.11 Current status of monitoring and evaluation studies

Though both monitoring and evaluation form very important components of any development project, these activities are sometimes carried out without any scientific flavor. For effective evaluation, comparison of key indicators in the pre- and post-stage of the project is essential. The pre-stage determination of key indicators has to be done through a baseline survey carried out in the project area. It can also be done in a control area having similar features as the project area. For making valid comparisons between findings of endline and baseline surveys, one has to ensure that these are comparable.

However, for some of the projects (even internationally funded), differences exist in the two stages in terms of sampling designs, coverage, sample size, questionnaire and analytical tools. Some projects have been implemented even without any valid baseline survey and baseline has been substituted by past data from other surveys. Some surveys give more emphasis to process indicators like purchases, infrastructure, staff, etc., rather than to outcome of the project. Any proper evaluation has to give maximum weight to the outcome indicator.

Specification of objectives and the formulation of relevant hypotheses form an important component of any development-related research program. Both these components must be clear, unambiguous and specific. An appropriate sampling design is then chosen keeping in view the extent of variability and nature of the characteristics to be studied and expected outcomes. Next step is to formulate questionnaires for eliciting information from the respondents through direct or indirect probing. The data collected through such a survey need to be properly checked for inconsistencies before its use for analyses.

Research studies sometimes lack in clarity of objectives and on the relevance of the hypotheses. Objectives are not clearly spelt out and are sometimes too many and ambiguous in nature. The hypotheses are either routine and traditional, or sometimes complex and consequently difficult to be tested. Choice of proper survey design including adequate sample size, clarity and coverage of questionnaires, data cleaning/handling and choice of analytical techniques for obtaining valid and efficient estimates are also among other matters of concern. These result in wasting precious funds employed for research programs. It also often ends up with invalid and misleading estimates, which may have strong policy implications.

While a proper and efficient sampling design is needed for obtaining efficient and valid estimates, the type and coverage of questionnaires is also a crucial deciding factor in obtaining quality data. Any ill-conceived questionnaire will lead to substantive non-response, incorrect and evasive responses. In many surveys, questionnaires are unduly lengthy and have questions not relevant to the study. Sometimes, these are too short to provide a satisfactory coverage. A lengthy questionnaire increases the cost of the survey and makes management and supervision work cumbersome and time consuming. It also creates problems in editing and cleaning of data and may result in a decrease in efficiency. A questionnaire with insufficient coverage is likely to be less efficient because of the failure to collect some vital information.

A questionnaire can be refined through training of interviewers, data editors/cleaners, and through test data analysis. Sufficient time should be given for field practice and the training should be evaluated. During field work there should be effective and quality monitoring. This allows for making amends for the ambiguity and inconsistencies. Effective training and pre-testing allows both the project handlers and the interviewers gain insight into the spirits underlying different questions. Even at data entry level, there should be data validation employing range check, valid value check as well as internal consistency checks. The follow-up checks and corrective measures improve not only the quality of data gathered but also making the resulting estimates much more relevant. However, this aspect is usually taken rather casually in many surveys conducted in our country.

## 1.12 Determination of sample size

### 1.12.1 Sample size for estimation of a parameter

Adequate sample size is very crucial to valid estimation and inference. Sample size has to be adequate to provide valid estimates and allow tests of statistical significance to be applied to the data collected. Even if a study is well conducted and analyzed, using an inadequate size will result in inadequate power and inferences which may be misleading (Pandey, 2009). However, sometimes there could be constraints of cost, time and the efforts prohibiting a larger sample size providing higher precision in estimates.

For determining the sample size, some knowledge or assumptions such as the prevalence of the characteristic to be studied, the variability between different sampling units, the desired level of statistical significance and the magnitude of sampling errors are all required. Some of these aspects are detailed below.

The formula by Cochran (1963) for calculating sample size n for estimating a parameter is as follows. The parameter of interest could be say nutritional status of children in a district.

$$n = (z_\alpha^2 pq) / d^2$$

where p = likely value of the parameter, q = 1 – p; d = permissible margin of error; and $z_\alpha$ = value of standard normal deviate corresponding to level of significance, α. If we take d = ep, then

$$n = z_\alpha^2 q / pe^2$$

where e = relative permissible margin in error.

Thus, n α 1/p; this implies that n is inversely proportional to p. We need a large sample size for lower values of p. This is the case with rare diseases which have very low prevalence. Similarly a smaller sample size may suffice for high prevalence.

Further, as n α $1/e^2$, which implies that n and e are also inversely proportional, for higher precision (that is lower relative margin of error) larger sample size may be required. In addition, as n α $z_\alpha^2$, larger sample size may be needed for higher confidence level.

Sample sizes for some typical values of p are given in Table 1.6 for α = 0.05 and 10 percent relative margin of error. The sample size is usually inflated to take care of the non-response and is multiplied by design effect, which is the ratio of variances of the sampling design used to that of simple random sampling (see, Section 5.6).

**Table 1.6** Sample size for a given proportion

| p | n |
|---|---|
| 0.90 | 45 |
| 0.70 | 171 |
| 0.50 | 400 |
| 0.10 | 3600 |
| 0.05 | 7600 |
| 0.005 | 80,000 |
| 0.0005 | 8,00,000 |

Usually, design effect is taken around 1.5. It is seen that sample sizes rapidly increase with the decline in expected prevalence rates. Such cases are found while determining sample sizes for infant mortality that is infant deaths per 1000 births and expected infant mortality around 50 gives p around 0.05, and maternal mortality: deaths per 100000 births and expected maternal mortality around 230 gives p as 0.023. The sample sizes for 10 percent relative margin of error are 7600 and 199600, respectively. If we multiply these sizes with a design effect 1.5, it raises the sample sizes to 11400 and 299400.

### 1.12.2 Sample size for comparative studies

As stated earlier, an intervention study involves comparison of baseline and endline indicator estimates. For instance, it may be desired to compare whether hemoglobin levels improved from baseline to endline because of intervention. Or else, interest may be to compare hemoglobin in a district where some intervention is planned with another (control) district where no intervention is planned. The information required in arriving at the sample size for two time point comparisons in different situations is as under:

When the interest is to compare baseline and endline proportions, the sample size is calculated using the formula

$$n = \{(z_\alpha + z_\beta)^2\}\{p_1(1 - p_1) + p_2(1 - p_2)\}/d^2$$

where $d = p_1 - p_2$ is the difference to be tested, and za is the standard normal deviate corresponding to selected significance level and confidence interval. Normally, level of significance is taken as 0.05 and the confidence interval as 95 percent. In this case $z_\alpha = 1.96 \approx 2$. The value is easily seen from standard normal deviate tables in any standard book in Statistics. Similarly, $z_\beta$ is the desired statistical power which can also be seen from standard normal deviate tables for a given power. If it is desired to have a power of 80 percent, then $z_\beta = 0.842$.

Suppose it is intended to determine sample size for estimating the change in severe anemia levels among schoolchildren from pre- to post-intervention periods. If it is assumed that pre- and post-intervention expected prevalence are 0.15 and 0.10 respectively, then for $\alpha = 0.05$ and 80 percent of power of test the sample size is worked out as approximately 703. This sample size can be inflated to take account for non-response and design effect.

The second case of interest is to compare proportions in a district where some intervention is planned with another (control) district where no intervention is planned. In this case the comparison is between difference in proportions for group 1 and the difference in proportions for group 2. With usual notations (subscript b for baseline and e for endline)

Difference in proportion for group 1 = $p_{b1} - p_{e1}$

Difference in proportion for group 2 = $p_{b2} - p_{e2}$

With usual notations, the sample size is calculated using the formula

$$n = \{(z_\alpha + z_\beta)^2\}\{p_{b1}(1 - p_{b1}) + p_{b2}(1 - p_{b2}) + p_{e1}(1 - p_{e1}) + p_{e2}(1 - p_{e2})\}/d^2$$

where $d = (p_{b1} - p_{e1}) - (p_{b2} - p_{e2})$.

**Example:** if $p_{b1} = 0.28$, $p_{b2} = 0.20$, $p_{e1} = 0.26$, $p_{e2} = 0.22$; then $d = 0.04$ so that $d^2 = 0.0016$. Further, $z_\alpha \approx 2$ for 5 percent significance level and $z_\beta =$ 0.842

for a power of 80 percent. The term $\{p_{b1} (1 - p_{b1}) + p_{b2} (1 - p_{b2}) + p_{e1} (1 - p_{e1}) + p_{e2} (1 - p_{e2})\} = 0.7256$. Substituting these in the formula gives n = 366. The sample size has to be inflated to take account for non-response and design effect.

## 1.13 Evidence reviews

Evidence-based decision making has emerged as a critical ingredient for effective programs and policies. Though it has always been important in clinical medical practice, it has also assumed significance for public health programming. While high-quality research should form the basis for generating evidence, the type and mode of research are most relevant to program decision making. During 2006–08 evidence reviews (2007) were conducted by selected experts for Vistaar project of IntraHealth International – USAID. Objectives of these reviews were to foster knowledge sharing, facilitate consensus and collaboration around evidence-based models and approaches, generate lessons learned and recommendations that will lead to results when implemented at scale, document evidence and experiences on and around operational issues, identify knowledge gaps for demonstration and learning, identify areas for refinement or experimentation, and identify capacity building areas. The projects included in these reviews covered wide-ranging topics. These were delay of marriage and first birth, complementary feeding, anemia prevention and treatment, village health committees, newborn care and skilled birth.

The process adopted for these reviews included involving wide group of experts and stakeholders. Its focus was on effectiveness, efficiency and expandability, using high standards of evidence, look for models that can be adopted at scale within government programs and include gender and equity focus. One core consideration from statistical point of view was to assess quality of evaluation/ methodology. Majority of the projects under evidence reviews failed on this count because of inadequacy of sample size, inappropriate or non-inclusion of baseline or doing the impact assessments by project staff instead of an external agency.

## 1.14 Inadequacy of sample size and its implications

A close look into the research studies reveals that sample size is sometimes arbitrarily decided, without taking into consideration the extent and nature of the variability of the character being studied. Even when adequate sample size is taken, there is an attempt to present analysis by sub-groups in terms of related socio-economic, demographic, housing or household characteristics. This leads to decomposition of sample size according to these sub-groups. It should be noted that while a smaller sample size leads to invalid estimates with unduly large standard errors, a larger sample involves avoidable wasteful expenditure. It is worthwhile to highlight some of the observations on these issues by Nigam (2004) and Nigam and Singh (2011).

Reporting of indicators in most of the large scale surveys is usually done by sub-groups like caste, religion, gender, age group, grades of nutritional status, grades of anemia, etc. In most situations, sample size for some of these sub-groups is grossly inadequate. Examples of this are found in the reportings of NNMB, National Family Health Survey (NFHS), Reproductive Child Health (RCH), and District Level Household Surveys (DLHS) and others. The sample size is usually determined for all the groups keeping in mind the precision, complexity of the design and expected non-response. Any temptation to the reporting by sub-groups makes such estimates highly imprecise. It may be a better practice to give interval estimates (confidence interval) instead of point estimates. However, the best alternative is to develop small area estimates for the sub-groups. Small area estimation is described later in Chapter 13. Several examples of these types of dis-aggregated reporting are described in Nigam (2004) and Nigam and Singh (2011). For instance, in NFHS-2, nutritional status was reported only for 77 children in Hill Region, for 57 children of ST and for 65 children of self-employed parents. The reporting has further division according to grades of nutritional status. The reported prevalence of undernutrition ranged from 40 to 60 per cent for below-2sd and 16–30 percent for below-3sd in these groups. Similarly, any anemia among children is reported for 72 children in Hills, 73 in Bundelkhand and for 33 children of ST, with further division according to grades of anemia (severe, mild, etc.). The reported prevalence of any anemia ranged 73–80 percent and 5–13 per cent for severe anemia. One easily notices that sample sizes are not adequate for any of these sub-group estimates.

## 1.15 Food and nutrition security

Nutrition and food security are closely related concepts, though one is distinct from the other in some respects. Human body needs various types of nutrients and their shortage causes nutrition insecurity. Inadequate and imbalanced food consumption is the main reason for prevalence of nutritional insecurity. Nutritional security is attained when an individual is able to derive all the essential nutrients in required amount by consuming an adequate and balanced diet which includes foodstuffs such as cereals, pulses, milk, meat, fruits and vegetables.

Nutritional insecurity leads to undernutrition which is a condition of health disorder that develops due to lack of enough and proper diet. Nutritional need of an individual of a given age and sex composition is not fixed, but there are inter- and intra-individual variations in nutritional need. Calorie need of an individual depends on his/her age, sex, bodyweight, and climatic conditions; it also varies over a large range depending on the activity status.

A definition of food security is given by the World Food Summit organized by FAO in 1996: "Food security exists when all people, at all times, have physical and economic access to sufficient, safe and nutritious food to meet their dietary needs and food preferences for an active and healthy life". In practice, food preferences in this definition may mean food that is culturally acceptable by a community rather than person-specific preferences.

From this perspective, food security may be viewed as a necessary but not sufficient condition for nutritional security as non-food factors such as safe drinking water, good sanitation, pollution and prevalence of diseases are also crucial to nutritional security.

Integrated Child Development Services (ICDS) is the world's largest community-based program aimed at enhancing the health, nutrition and learning opportunities of below-6 children, adolescent girls and pregnant and lactating mothers. Prevention and management of severely undernourished children are important components of the ICDS and Integrated Management of Children Illness strategy. WHO also emphasizes on the management of severely undernourished children. When launched in 1975, the ICDS targeted at the poorest and most deprived children. The ICDS program aims for fulfilling the rights of young children to survival, development, protection and participation. It also serves as the crucial link between disadvantaged communities and the primary healthcare and education systems.

The scheme aims at reduction in mortality (infant, child and maternal), morbidity and undernutrition among children by improving their nutrition and health status, reduction in school drop-out rates, laying the foundation for proper psychological, physical and social development, enhancement of mother's capability to look after the development needs of their children and effective policy implementation and coordination. Under ICDS, a package of services including supplementary nutrition, immunization health check-up and referral services are being provided to children below-6 years of age, expectant and nursing mothers and adolescent girls. Non-formal pre-school education is imparted to children in the age group 3–6 years and nutrition and health education to women (15–45 years).

Besides ICDS, mid-day meal program for school children also aims at food and nutrition security. The mid-day meal program intends to improve enrolment and retention.

## 1.16 Dis-aggregated analysis

Normally research studies are planned to provide aggregated results but many times dis-aggregated results are desired for identifying the target groups and areas requiring special focus. Though in most cases dis-aggregated analyses may be inappropriate because of inadequate sample size as discussed earlier in Section 1.14, it can sometimes be more revealing. We have stated in Section 1.3.3 that sometimes the analysis of trends and patterns reflects some important features of data. Here we describe their utility through two examples.

**Example:** The current focus on preventing undernutrition is on children under-2 years of age. This is based on the past analysis in terms of age groups. The analysis of underweight data of a nutritional status study by IASDS (1995) through bar diagram for age groups of unequal widths 0–6, >6–11, 12–23, 24–35 and 36–59 months indicated maximum underweight in children occurring between 12 and 24 months. This analysis is likely to be erroneous because of unequal class intervals of age.

An alternative analysis of data on prevalence was undertaken by single months (Vir and Nigam, 2001) and was more revealing. It showed that the maximum underweight is attained at 11 months with the plateau beginning at 12 months itself (Fig 1.5), instead of 24 months, as shown above.

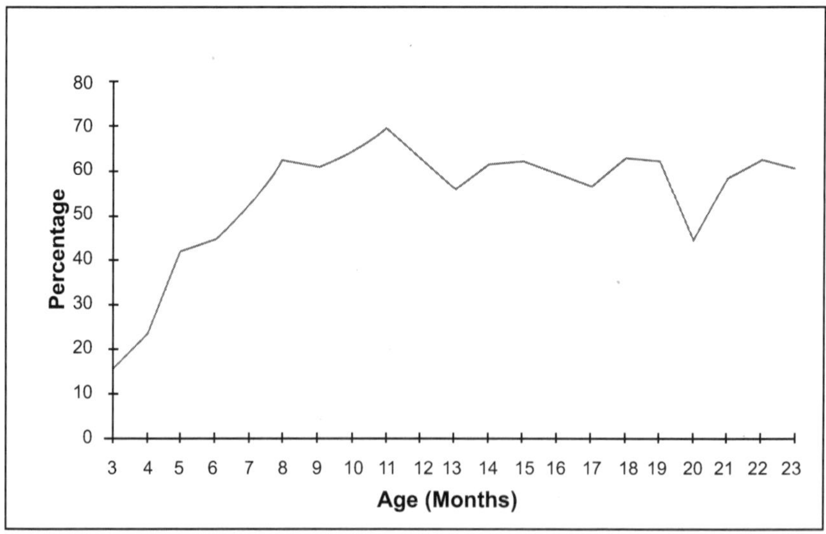


**Figure 1.5** Month wise pattern of underweight

This was further substantiated through a fitted quadratic regression (Nigam, 2001) to the prevalence of underweight data (Fig 1.6).

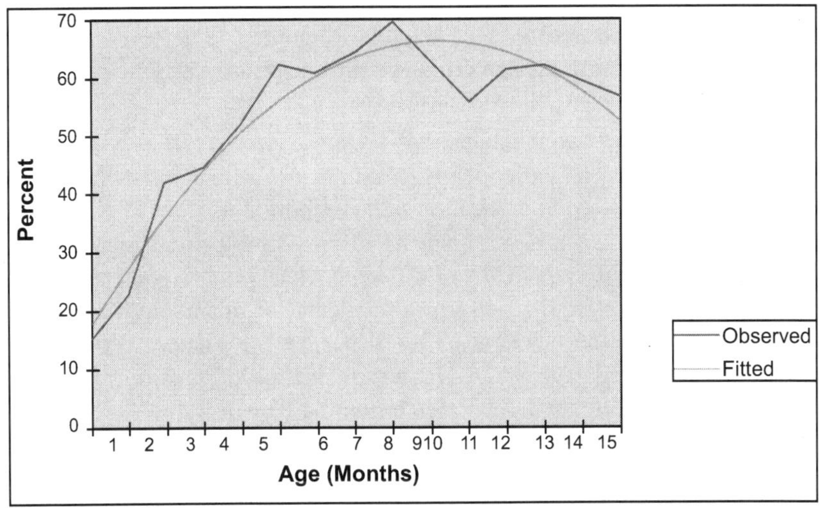


**Figure 1.6** Fitted quadratic regression on month wise underweight pattern

The maximum of the fitted curve was around 12 months. The above finding has important implications. The analysis has indicated that undernutrition sets in early in life and accelerates during 8–11 months. Maximum undernutrition prevalence is attained around one year followed by a plateau at 12–35 months. Some other data sets also indicate that maximum undernutrition is attained at 11 12 months with very little rise up to 24 months, followed by a plateau up to 35 months.

The explanation of the acceleration of undernutrition around 8–11 months is that causative factors like breastfeeding and complementary feeding practices, hygiene, and diseases like diarrhea and Acute Respiratory Infections (ARI) operate crucially during this period of child's growth. This age is therefore the right age for intervention programs for prevention of undernutrition. As maximum undernutrition is attained only during the plateau at 12–35 months, it is the right age for controlling undernutrition.

Any sampling, which is done ignoring the patterns as above, is bound to be less precise. It is therefore imperative to lay maximum focus during 8–11 months for preventing undernutrition. In almost every nutrition survey this is not done. For instance, if the derived sample size is 400, this is uniformly distributed over age; say up to 5 years, ignoring the pattern of undernutrition over age. It is illogical to uniformly distribute the sample size when there is a plateau during 12–35 months, with hardly any variation in the extent of undernutrition. While very few samples may suffice for this age group, much larger size is needed for 8–11 months when there is more variation. An increased sample size for the age group would also ensure carrying out critical in-depth analysis like associated risk factors.

**Example:** District-wise analysis of underweight data of IASDS (1995) also provides pattern of underweight children in UP in 17 districts of UP. The map showing the geographical pattern is reported in DWCD publication (1999) which gives an in-depth analysis of IASDS Nutrition Survey, 1995 data. It also appeared later in Vir and Nigam (2001) and Nigam and Singh (2011). On mapping the district-wise prevalence of underweight incidence of <50 per cent, 50–69 per cent and ≥70 per cent, a distinct geographical pattern was observed (Fig. 1.7). Highest incidence of undernutrition was observed in the waterlogged Terai area bordering Nepal, followed by Central belt comprising the entire tract of Gangetic plains, and the lowest underweight percentages were observed in the Vindhyachal ranges which also include the dry Bundelkhand region.

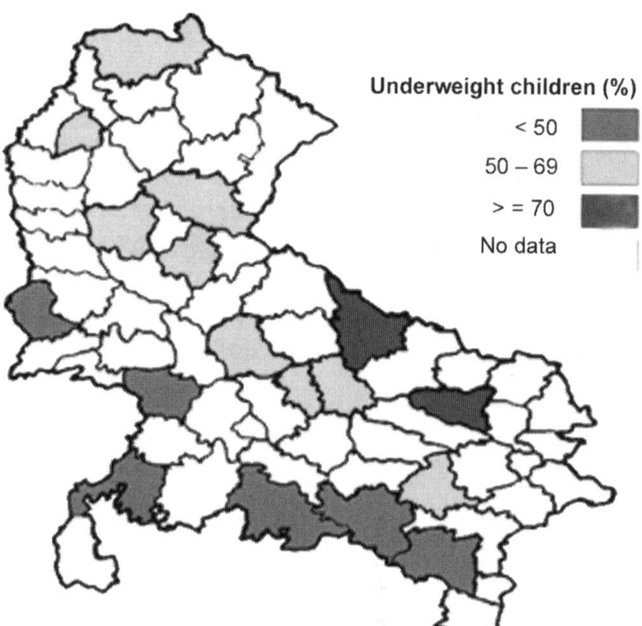


**Figure 1.7** Geographical pattern of underweight

This distribution of underweight in the state was not in concurrence with the common belief that the highest incidence of undernutrition in the state was in the poorer socio-economic region of Bundelkhand. Higher incidence of undernutrition was in fact noted in the waterlogged eastern region and in the wet Gangetic belt. This can be attributed to possibly higher occurrence of diarrhoea, infection and worm infestation which adversely affect the nutritional status of children.

## 1.17 Recent survey and analytical techniques

We now discuss ways for controlling errors, bridging data gaps, data reduction and improving the quality of data. These are applicable at different stages, viz. at handling of data, sample selection and estimation. Every survey encounters the problem of missing data or data with inconsistencies. The problem of missing data occurs when some, or all of the responses, are not collected for a sample element, or when some responses are deleted because they fail to satisfy certain edit checks. Inconsistencies in data may also occur due to a variety of reasons, such as errors in tabulation, data entry or even in copying from a secondary source. In all such cases, it is a norm to treat it as missing data and handle it accordingly. Whereas total non-response, i.e. when all of the responses on a unit are not available, is handled by some form of weighting adjustment techniques, item non-responses are taken care of by imputation.

Imputation is a technique to handle non-responses by replacing each missing value with a real value. A number of imputation procedures are now available for assigning values for missing responses. These are deductive imputation, overall and class-mean imputations, random imputation, hot-deck imputation and imputation based upon regression.

Data reduction can be achieved by a technique called principal components. It uses an orthogonal transformation to convert a set of observations of possibly correlated variables into a set of values of linearly uncorrelated variables called principal components. The number of principal components is less than or equal to the number of original variables. This technique is discussed in Chapter 9.

There are several diseases which prevail in community clusters. A hotspot is an area of high response or an elevated cluster for an event. Temporal, spatial and space-time scan statistics are now commonly used for disease cluster detection and evaluation for many diseases including cancer, granulocytic ehrlichiosis, sclerosis, diabetes, and giardiasis. A very interesting study was reported by Google which allows detection of influenza epidemics by using online web search queries, which are submitted by millions of users around the world each day. Among children, cluster-forming diseases are Japanese encephalitis, Bitot's spots and polio. Severe undernutrition also is pocketed in tribal areas. These are all discussed in Chapter 10.

Almost all surveys have few questions which attract multiple responses. A new method to analyze such responses is described in Chapter 11. The method is superior to the conventional method being used at present.

In many surveys, the intention is to seek information on sensitive characteristics. It is useful to employ the randomized response technique in such cases. The technique ensures confidentiality to the respondent and has become popular in recent years. Detailed applications of this technique are discussed in Chapter 12.

One of the areas of data gaps is related to micro-level planning, which requires estimates of different activities for 'smaller' areas having inadequate sample size. This is achieved by using small area estimation technique which is discussed in details in Chapter 13.

Two other techniques need special, though brief, mention. Re-sampling inference is a technique which aims at finding the standard error of variance estimates of non-linear statistics, such as ratios, regression coefficient, index numbers, etc. Some other applications are the standard errors of statistics such as median (height or weight), inflation rate, wholesale price index number and the like.

Common re-sampling procedures under this technique are jack-knifing, balanced repeated replications and bootstrap. The technique involved in these procedures involves replicated samples although replicates here are not real but only pseudo-replicates. Often these are generated using Monte Carlo simulations. Monte Carlo methods are a broad class of *computational algorithms* that rely on repeated *random* sampling to obtain numerical results. Repeated simulations are carried out in order to obtain the distribution of an unknown parameter. They are often used when it is difficult or impossible to obtain a closed-form expression, or infeasible to apply a *deterministic algorithm*. Monte Carlo methods are mainly used in three distinct problem classes: *optimization, numerical integration* and generation of draws from a *probability distribution*.

Another technique is for estimating the proportion of population possessing rare attributes. For instance, in problems concerning AIDS, it may be necessary to estimate the number of homosexuals or call girls. As there is no sampling frame of these individuals, 'snow-ball' and 'inverse' sampling can be used for getting a sample of desired size. The idea is somehow to locate one such individual and then get to the others through a chain of such contacts and stop the sampling when a predetermined number is obtained. Its utility is discussed in the context of locating maternal deaths in Chapter 3.

## 1.18 Some mathematical details on probability distributions

A discrete random variable is a real-valued function on a discrete sample space $\Omega$. Note that a discrete sample space has either a finite number or a countably infinite number of points (i.e., the points can be arranged in a sequence). Suppose a discrete random variable (r.v.) takes values $x_1$ , $x_2$, .... We denote the probability that X takes the value $x_j$ as P [X = $x_j$ ]. The function $f(x_j) = P[X = x_j]$, j= 1, 2, . . . defined for the values $x_1$ , $x_2$, . . .. is called the probability mass function or probability distribution of X .

We now describe some important discrete random variables. Let a random variable X assume only two values, 1 and 0, with respective probabilities p and q = 1 – p. This means that P [X = 1] = p and P [X = 0] = 1 – p, where $0 \leq p \leq 1$. The above two statements can be written as

$$P[X = x] = p^x (1 - p)^{1-x}, x = 0, 1.$$

This random variable is called Bernoulli or, equivalently, the above probabilistic statement is called the Bernoulli distribution.

Consider next the following experiment: each trial of the experiment results in one of the two outcomes, "success" or "failure" (or, 'Yes' or 'No'), the probability of success being p. Consider n such independent trials, the probability of success p remaining the same for all the trials. Define X to be the number of successes in n such trials. Clearly, X can take any of the values 0, 1, . . . , n. The probability distribution of X is then given by

$$P[X = j] = \binom{n}{j} p^j (1 - p)^{n-j}, j = 0, 1, ..., n$$

This is known as the binomial distribution. Here, for integers a, b, $a \geq b$ and $\binom{a}{b}$ (read as a choose b) is defined as {a (a – 1)(a – 2)....(a – b+1)}/ {b (b – 1)(b – 2).... 1}, and $\binom{a}{0} = 1 = \binom{a}{a}$.

Let X be a discrete random variable taking a finite number of values, $x_1$, $x_2$, ..., $x_n$ with probabilities $f(x_1)$, $f(x_2)$, ..., $f(x_n)$, respectively. Then we define the expected value (or, expectation or mean) of X as

$E(X) = x_1 f(x_1) + x_2 f(x_2) + \cdots + x_n f(x_n) = \sum n\, x_j f(x_j) = \mu_X$, say.

Next, suppose a discrete random variable assumes an infinity of values $x_1$, $x_2$, ... with respective probabilities $f(x_1)$, $f(x_2)$, .... Then the expectation of X is given by

$E(X) = x_1 f(x_1) + x_2 f(x_2) + \cdots = \sum^{\infty} x_j f(x_j) = \mu_X$, provided the above sum converges. The variance of X is given by

$Var(X) = E(X - \mu X)^2 = \sum^n (x_j - \mu_X)_2 f(x_j) = E(X^2) - \mu x^2$

Among the continuous random variable (or, continuous distributions), the most important and most studied one is the Normal distribution. If the random variable X has a Normal distribution, then its probability density function is given by

$$f(x) = \frac{1}{\sigma\sqrt{2\pi}} \exp\left\{-\frac{(x-\mu)^2}{2\sigma^2}\right\}, -\infty < x < \infty$$

where exp(·) is the exponential function. A Normal distribution is characterized by two parameters $\mu$ and $\sigma$. The parameter $\mu$ is the mean of the distribution (and, also equals the median and mode of the distribution) while $\sigma$ is the standard deviation. A normal distribution with mean 0 and standard deviation 1 is called the standard normal distribution, denoted by N (0, 1). A $N(\mu, \sigma^2)$ distribution is symmetric about its mean ($\mu$), which is also the median and mode of the distribution.

Another important distribution is the chi-square ($\chi^2$) distribution. Let $x_1$, $x_2$, ..., $x_n$ be independent N(0,1) random variables. Then $\sum^n x_i^2$ follows a chi-square ($\chi^2$) distribution with n degrees of freedom. It is characterized by the parameter (degrees of freedom) n. If U follows a $\chi^2$ distribution with n degrees of freedom, then the probability distribution of U is given by

$$f(u) = \{1/2^{n-2}\Gamma(n/2)\}\exp(-u/2)u^{n/2-1}, \text{ if } u \geq 0$$
$$= 0, \text{ if } u < 0,$$

where $\Gamma(\cdot)$ is the complete gamma function. The mean and variance of U are given respectively, by n and 2n. The $\chi^2$ distribution is skewed (un-symmetric), but becomes closer to the normal distribution (which is symmetric about its mean) as n increases.

An important continuous distribution is the t-distribution. Let X be a random variable having a standard normal distribution (i.e., a N (0, 1) distribution) and Y be a random variable having a $\chi^2$ distribution with n degrees of freedom. Furthermore, let X and Y be independently distributed of each other. Then the random variable $Z = x/\sqrt{(y/n)}$ follows a t distribution with n degrees of freedom. The integer n is the only parameter of a t distribution. The t distribution is symmetric about zero (the mean of the t distribution) and the variance of random variable having a t distribution with $n \geq 2$ degrees of freedom is $n/(n-2)$. The t distribution rapidly approaches the standard normal distribution as n increases.

Another important continuous distribution is the F distribution. Suppose U and V are independent $\chi^2$ random variables with respective degrees of freedom $n_1$ and $n_2$. Then $W = (U/n_1)/(V/n_2)$ follows an F distribution with $n_1$, $n_2$ degrees of freedom (written as $F\ n_1, n_2$). The integers $n_1$ and $n_2$ characterize an F distribution. It is to be noted that the order $n_1$, $n_2$ is important, because from the definition it is clear that the random variables $F\ n_1, n_2$ and $1/F\ n_2, n_1$ have identical distributions. We shall see later that each of the t, $\chi^2$ and F distributions play an important role in testing of hypothesis problems.

# 2
# Qualitative methods

## 2.1 Focus group discussions

A focus group discussion (FGD) is a mode of probing on a certain topic with a small group of people in participatory manner. Objective of the FGD is to gain detailed information on a specific issue, which often concerns ideas, concepts and perceptions of a group of individuals. In FGD, about 10–12 group members discuss the topic amongst themselves with the support of a facilitator who guides the discussion. There is an exchange of ideas between the participants, and the process provides collective information to the initiator of the discussion.

FGD is a tool to gather qualitative information for research. It could be for formative research to devise well-defined questions for a larger survey, or else, it could be to evaluate and/or monitor the progress or results of a program in a participatory way to understand (and resolve) certain problems that may arise during a program. In some cases, it could also be for sensitization towards some impending program. To explore sensitive topics depending on the objective and the time available, sometimes one FGD may suffice; in other cases more than one session might be needed.

Core components of any FGD are team preparation, discussion context, sensitive listening, sensitive questioning, judging responses, recording the discussion and self-critical review. Before proceeding for FGD, it is essential to review the status of preparedness on these components.

While organizing FGD the first step is the sensitization of group members to be involved in the FGD. The facilitator should first define clearly the purpose of conducting the FGD. Objective, date, time and location together with the participants should then be discussed. This is important as women and men have different time schedules. The facilitator should ensure that there are right participants who are knowledgeable about the subject and can discuss the topic freely. A circle or U-pattern setting is advisable for FGD, as everyone should to be able to see everyone.

The facilitator should first introduce himself and state the objective of the meeting. He should then let the participants introduce themselves. Participants should agree on some basic rules for discussion, like it being participatory, with one person speaking at a time and raising hand for interruption or for raising questions. Facilitator's teammates should take notes. Preferably use of a recorder is also recommended. However, the use of recorder should be with the permission of the participants. When the topic under discussion is of sensitive type, it is advisable not to record or write down anything during the discussion. It can instead be done afterwards.

The facilitator should be a part of the group. He should be active, showing interest, enthusiasm, and sincerity and be an attentive listener. However, his role should be limited to get the discussion started, to redirect questions, to rephrase an answer or to summarize. He should avoid a question and answer session with the individual participants and ensure that the discussion is not dominated or monopolized by only one or two persons. He should also get those members involved who are hesitant and have a tendency to keep quiet. He should redirect questions in order to ensure a lively communication between all participants.

At the end of each topic, the facilitator should summarize the discussion. This should also be done at the end of the discussion and important issues should be highlighted. The facilitator should ask if the participants agree with what was summarized.

## 2.2 In-depth interviews

Like focus group discussions, in-depth interviews explore the aspects of what people think and feel about a program being implemented, about their experiences and their perception about the success or otherwise of the program. An in-depth interview is a face-to-face conversation with an individual conducted by trained staff and usually collects specific information about one person.

It involves discrete probing and prompting without influencing respondent answers. It provides a history of behavior, highlights individual versus group concerns, reveals divergent experiences and outlier attitudes, provides a shortcut to community norms and develops other research tools. The following example will clarify the procedure and the type of analysis that can be used for handling FGD and in-depth interview responses.

**Example:** Institute of Applied Statistics and Development Studies (IASDS) conducted baseline and impact assessment surveys in Madhya Pradesh, Uttarakhand and Chhattisgarh in 2004 and 2005 for WFP for assessing the nutritional impact of mid morning snacks (MMS) fortified with iron and vitamin A in addition to mid-day meal (MDM) provided to primary school children. We take the data from tribal areas of Chhattisgarh where the study was conducted in two blocks each of Jashpur and Raigarh districts.

After one year of the baseline survey, the selected children were assessed on whether the MMS aided in improving their attendance, attention span, health and nutritional status and active learning capacity.

The general perceptions/observations of principals/teachers/parents on impact of feeding program (both MDM and MMS) and their recommendations on the program were analyzed. While information about principals/teachers is based upon in-depth interviews, that of parents was based upon FGD. The qualitative data were handled manually. At the baseline stage the probing was whether there was any improvement in the attendance, attention span, health & nutrition status and active learning capacity of children after joining the school and at the endline probing was done whether there was any change because of taking the mid morning snack.

The responses were coded in terms of suitable scale points (qualifiers) as given in Table 2.1.

**Table 2.1** Qualifiers for qualitative assessment

| Proportion of respondents | Qualifiers used |
|---|---|
| ≤20% | Very few (1+) |
| 21–40% | Few (2+) |
| 41–60% | Some/nearly half (3+) |
| 61–80% | Majority/most (4+) |
| >80% | Almost all/all (5+) |

Table 2.2 summarizes the coded responses of principals, teachers and parents for each of attendance, attention span, health & nutritional status and active learning capacity of children. It is realized that at the time of endline, there was all-round improvement in the scores in the two districts under all the categories, viz. attendance, attention span and health & nutritional status, and active learning capacity. Scores of Jashpur were generally higher than those of Raigarh.

**Table 2.2** Attendance, attention span, health & nutritional status and active learning capacity

| **Indicator** | **Principals** | | **Teachers** | | **Parents** | |
|---|---|---|---|---|---|---|
| **Baseline** | **Jashpur** | **Raigarh** | **Jashpur** | **Raigarh** | **Jashpur** | **Raigarh** |
| | | | **Attendance** | | | |
| Increased | 4+ | 3+ | 4+ | 4+ | 4+ | 4+ |
| As earlier | 2+ | 3+ | 2+ | 2+ | 2+ | 2+ |
| Decreased | 1+ | 1+ | 1+ | 1+ | 1+ | 1+ |

*Contd...*

*Contd...*

| Indicator | Principals | | Teachers | | Parents | |
|---|---|---|---|---|---|---|
| **Baseline** | **Jashpur** | **Raigarh** | **Jashpur** | **Raigarh** | **Jashpur** | **Raigarh** |
| | | | **Attention span** | | | |
| Increased | 4+ | 3+ | 3+ | 3+ | 2+ | 2+ |
| As earlier | 2+ | 3+ | 2+ | 3+ | 4+ | 4+ |
| Decreased | 1+ | 1+ | 1+ | 1+ | 1+ | 1+ |
| | | | **Health & nutritional status** | | | |
| Increased | 2+ | 3+ | 3+ | 3+ | 2+ | 3+ |
| As earlier | 4+ | 3+ | 3+ | 3+ | 4+ | 3+ |
| Decreased | 1+ | 1+ | 1+ | 1+ | 1+ | 1+ |
| | | | **Active learning capacity** | | | |
| Increased | 2+ | 2+ | 2+ | 3+ | 2+ | 2+ |
| As earlier | 3+ | 3+ | 3+ | 3+ | 4+ | 4+ |
| Decreased | 1+ | 1+ | 1+ | 1+ | 1+ | 1+ |
| **Indicator** | **Principal** | | **Teacher** | | **Parents** | |
| **Endline** | **Jashpur** | **Raigarh** | **Jashpur** | **Raigarh** | **Jashpur** | **Raigarh** |
| Attendance | | | | | | |
| Increased | 5+ | 5+ | 5+ | 5+ | 3+ | 3+ |
| As earlier | 1+ | 1+ | 1+ | 1+ | 2+ | 3+ |
| Decreased | 1+ | 1+ | 1+ | 1+ | 1+ | 1+ |
| Attention span | | | | | | |
| Increased | 5+ | 4+ | 5+ | 3+ | 3+ | 5+ |
| As earlier | 1+ | 2+ | 1+ | 2+ | 3+ | 1+ |
| Decreased | 1+ | 1+ | 1+ | 1+ | 1+ | 1+ |
| | | | **Health & nutritional status** | | | |
| Increased | 5+ | 5+ | 5+ | 5+ | 2+ | 1+ |
| As earlier | 1+ | 1+ | 1+ | 1+ | 4+ | 5+ |
| Decreased | 1+ | 1+ | 1+ | 1+ | 1+ | 1+ |
| | | | Active learning capacity | | | |
| Increased | 5+ | 4+ | 5+ | 4+ | 2+ | 1+ |
| As earlier | 1+ | 1+ | 1+ | 2+ | 4+ | 5+ |
| Decreased | 1+ | 1+ | 1+ | 1+ | 1+ | 1+ |

Some of the important recommendations made by principals/teachers/parents were increasing the allocation for MDM from Rs. 1 to Rs. 2 per child, increasing the quantity of food stuffs in MDM, changing the menu for MDM like puri, subzi (rather than rice pulao on most days), giving the responsibility of feeding program including storage to principal instead of pradhan, and even replacing MDM with ready to eat foods. They showed preference for biscuit of MMS, (which had been supplied in the area). Whereas the principals and teachers claimed that MDM distribution was satisfactory, the parents expressed exactly opposite views.

## 2.3 Process evaluation

Process evaluation is the assessment of the program process. It analyzes the effectiveness of program operations, implementation, and service delivery. It also attempts to identify the constraints. Process evaluation of an ongoing program is called monitoring of the program which can both be quantitative and qualitative. Process evaluations document the process of a program's implementation. The focus of a process evaluation is on the types and quantities of services delivered, the beneficiaries of those services, the resources used to deliver the services, the practical problems encountered, and the ways such problems were resolved.

Process evaluations are often used by managers as benchmarks to measure success, for example: whether the distribution of fortified food or IFA is reaching 80 percent of the intended beneficiaries. These benchmarks may be set by program managers, and sometimes by donors. Monitoring progress sometimes implies both outcome and process evaluations. As outcome evaluation is part of the type of assessments discussed in Chapter 1, we describe here only process evaluation. These evaluations help stakeholders see how a program outcome or impact was achieved.

Process evaluation can assess the capacity of an organization on promised outcomes by examining processes of program, management and infrastructure together. It can attempt to answer what specific interventions were put into place by the program; how they were placed; and whether the interventions worked or not. The idea is to judge reasons for the success or failure of the interventions. The process evaluation also probes about the problems encountered in delivering the program. In particularly it focuses upon whether there was adequate support to the program and was there continuity in timely flow of enough resources from the beginning to end. It assesses how well the program was managed. Other components of the evaluation include whether staff was trained and well educated for facilitating the program processes from beginning to end.

### 2.3.1 Utility of process evaluation

Process evaluation is like carrying out an analysis of strengths and weaknesses of program implementation. There is always a chain of cause and effect and the analysis as above is the right tool to find out whether the right resources were deployed from the beginning till end to get to the expected outcomes. Information from process evaluation is useful for understanding how program impact and outcome were achieved. It is a good learning experience for program replication. Thus process and outcome evaluations are complementary to each other. Even with good outcomes, it is necessary to analyze how they were achieved. Such an analysis should reveal about the type and manner of human resources involvement in getting good outcomes and also the **true costs** of the program.

## 2.4 Sensory evaluation

Sensory evaluation is a scientific discipline that analyses and measures human responses to the composition of say food and drink, e.g. appearance, touch, odor, texture, temperature and taste. In schools it provides an ideal opportunity for students to evaluate and give feedback on their dishes. The dishes could be either those from mid-day meal or even a comparison between cooked meals and ready to eat panjiri or biscuits. Many more examples can be thought of. There could be a case of evolving a hybrid variety of basmati rice, but the new variety must have the same flavor, taste and texture. A genetically modified maize variety can also be fortified but the taste and texture should not change. Some other such experimentation is in the product development area of home science and nutrition. Examples of this are developing health or energy drinks which may be fortified with vitamins, minerals and micronutrients. All these call for sensory evaluations. A good source of sensory evaluation is the book by Lawless and Heymann (2010).

Sensory evaluation can be used to (i) compare similarities/differences in a range of dishes/products; (ii) evaluate a range of existing dishes/food products; (iii) analyze food samples for improvements; (iv) gauge responses to a dish/product, e.g. acceptable vs. unacceptable; (v) explore specific characteristics of an ingredient or dish/food product; and (vi) check whether a final dish/food product meets its original specification; and provide objective and subjective feedback data to enable informed decisions to be made.

Sensory evaluation applies statistical principles for the purposes of evaluating products using any or more of the components like appearance, touch, odor, texture, temperature and taste. It requires panels of judges, on whom the products are tested, and recording the responses made by them. The responses are usually in the form of scores in say 10-point scale. By applying statistical techniques to the results, it is possible to make inferences and insights about the products under test. One of the common methods to analyze such data with multiple scores on different characteristics of the product is done by ranking method. Scores are combined to form a single composite index. This is done by adding all the ranks to get the aggregate rank. In this method all indicators are implicitly assigned equal weights, which may not always be appropriate. But determining differential weights for different characteristics like appearance, touch, odor, texture, temperature and taste could be very tricky. Reader may refer to appropriate literature for these.

**Example:** Consider the example of developing a juice using combinations of whey and fruits. Whey is a thin and watery by-product of cheese-making process. It is formed when curds /cheese separate out of milk. It is excellent source of protein, vitamins, minerals and lactose and hence can be an important addition to anyone's diet. Whey protein is a popular protein supplement for fitness primarily because of its high concentration in the branched chain amino acids (BCAAs), leucine, isoleucine, and valine. But still, in spite of surplus nutritive values, it is generally wasted.

BCAAs are needed for the maintenance of muscle tissue and appear to preserve muscle stores of glycogen, the storage form of glucose and may help prevent muscle protein breakdown during exercise. Whey also has immune-boosting benefits. One of the ways to avoid whey wastage is to develop squash by using whey. It can also prevent the environmental pollution which is caused because of it being drained into gutters.

Generally, squashes lag far behind in terms of nutritional values. Addition of whey to the squashes can help in increasing their nutritive values by improvising mineral profile. Commonly available fruit juices relate to the low pH which is generally unsuitable as thirst quenchers. Further, the cola beverages which contain phosphoric acid and often caffeine may increase the fragility of bones in children and adolescents.

On the other hand, whey beverages with higher pH are physiologically more acceptable as thirst quencher and when fortified with minerals and micronutrients may have immense nutritive value. Squashes are quite popular in general households and are liked by children, adolescents, girls and elderly. After incorporating whey in the squashes, a better option fulfilling their nutritional demands will be available to the public.

There is a lot of scope for the variations that can be tried on the whey-based squash like those involving: color, different combinations of fruits, trying different ratio of fruits and other ingredients in the formula, or developing a formula for diseases like diabetics, hypertension, etc.

Suppose for the development of the formula for the squash whey, water, sugar and two fruits ($x_1$ and $x_2$) are taken as the ingredients. Now several variations in the ingredients can be done, some of these could be as:

**Table 3.3** Some typical combinations of ingredients

| whey | water | $x_1$ | $x_2$ |
|---|---|---|---|
| 1 | 0 | 1 | 0 |
| 1 | 0 | 0 | 1 |
| 1 | 0 | ½ | ½ |
| 1 | 0 | ¾ | ¼ |
| 1 | 0 | ¼ | ¾ |
| ½ | ½ | 1 | 0 |
| ½ | ½ | 0 | 1 |
| ½ | ½ | ½ | ½ |
| ½ | ½ | ¾ | ¼ |
| ½ | ½ | ¼ | ¾ |

Each of the developed products from above combinations has to be evaluated by a panel of judges for sensory evaluation. It may be of interest to explore which blend is optimal in some way of objective-based judgments like taste, flavor, color, nutritive content, morbidity prevention and control, presentation, etc.

Most of the times, the ingredients and their combinations are decided by the experimenters on the basis of their personal judgment. The best combination is chosen among one of those tried in the experiment. A better alternative is to analyze this data by using the methodology of experiments with mixtures. This analysis which is similar to the usual regression modeling allows picking the optimal combination of ingredients. The aggregate index of the scores by judges for different characteristics as above will provide the dependent variable for regression modeling. The optimal combination may not necessarily be one among those tried in the experiment. For experiments with mixtures the reader is referred to Cornell (2002).

# 3

# Maternal and infant survival

## 3.1 Introduction

India has more than one-fifth of global maternal and child deaths, but also has one-fifth of births worldwide. Large numbers of women die each year of causes related to pregnancy and childbirth. India has the highest number of neonatal deaths each year, which is nearly one-third of the neonatal deaths globally. Many of these deaths could be averted with universal skilled attendance and access to emergency care. Though India has made progress in improving the overall health status of its population, it is far from satisfactory. The slow pace of decline of infant and child mortality on one hand and maternal mortality on the other hand is a cause of concern.

Improvements of maternal and newborn health are major millennium development goals (MDG), with a target to reduce maternal mortality by three-fourths and the mortality rate among children under-5 by two-thirds. Some of the major causes associated with maternal deaths are complications in delivery in all its stages: pre-intra-and-post. While pre-delivery complications are related to neglect during pregnancy, intra-delivery complications are due to lack of appropriate care and inappropriate facilities during delivery. Post-delivery complications arise due to neglect after delivery. These issues are discussed later in Section 3.8.

For safe motherhood and infant survival, essential components are sustainable and qualitative improvement in the health and nutritional status of pregnant and lactating women and infants by enhancing their access to health care services, health information and supplementary food. Increased coverage rates of appropriate health behaviors are crucial to safe motherhood and infant survival. These have a strong association with mortality reduction among pregnant and lactating women and their infants. Changes in health behaviors can be brought about by enhancing the capacity of community-based organizations (CBOs), non-government organizations (NGOs) and government functionaries. For sustained behavior change, the help of these organizations is necessary to sustain the promotion of health practices and improved nutrition.

## 3.2 Maternal mortality

The maternal mortality ratio is obtained by dividing the number of maternal deaths in a population during a given time interval by the number of live births occurring in the same period. It indicates the risk of maternal death relative to the frequency of childbearing. A related measure, the maternal mortality rate is the average annual number of maternal deaths in a population divided by the average number of women of reproductive age that is 15–49 years during the period. Thus, the maternal mortality rate reflects not only the risk of maternal death per pregnancy or per birth, but also the level of fertility in a population. General fertility rate is the number of live births per 1,000 women aged 15–49 in a given year.

The maternal mortality rate is the annual number of female deaths between ages 15–49 per 100,000 live births from any cause related to or aggravated by pregnancy or its management. A maternal death is the death of a woman while pregnant or within 42 days of termination of pregnancy, irrespective of the duration and the site of the pregnancy. The deaths due to accidental or incidental causes are not included in the category of maternal death.

The maternal mortality ratio (MMR) is the most widely used measure of maternal deaths. It measures obstetric risk, which is the risk of dying once a woman is pregnant. It omits the risk of being pregnant. Maternal mortality is a general indicator of the overall health of a population, of the status of women in society, and also of the functioning of the health system. As a consequence, high MMR values indicate wider problems of health status, gender inequalities, and health services. Though MMR is useful for advocacy purposes, it throws no light on the causes of high maternal mortality or the interventions required for reducing maternal deaths.

Maternal deaths are of two categories: direct and indirect obstetric deaths. Direct obstetric deaths result from obstetric complications of the pregnant state (pregnancy, labor, and puerperium), from interventions, omissions, incorrect treatment, or from a chain of events resulting from any of the above. Puerperium is the period of adjustment after childbirth during which the mother's reproductive system returns to its normal prepregnant state. Indirect obstetric deaths result from previous existing disease or disease that developed during pregnancy and which was not due to direct obstetric causes, but which was aggravated by physiologic effects of pregnancy.

## 3.3 Infant and child mortality

Infant mortality is the number deaths before the first birthday. Infant mortality rate (IMR) is such deaths among 1000 live births. Infant mortality is, therefore, the probability of dying before the first birthday. Child mortality or under-5 mortality refers to the death of infants and children under the age of five. The rate of each of these is to be taken out of 1000 live births. Sample Registration System (SRS) is a large-scale demographic survey for providing reliable annual estimates of birth rate, death rate and other fertility and morality indicators at the national and lower levels. The SRS sample is replaced every 10 years based on the latest census frame.

Infant mortality is the death of a child less than one year of age. Child mortality is the death of a child before the child's fifth birthday. National statistics tend to group these two mortality rates together. Globally, ten million infants and children die each year before their fifth birthday, and most of these deaths occur in developing nations. Infant mortality is detrimental to society's potential physical, social, and human capital.

Infant and under-5 mortality rates are key indicators for assessing the health status of communities, and also of districts and countries. These indicators are used internationally as sensitive indicators and reflect the level of mortality, health status, and health care of population. They also indicate the effectiveness of preventive care and the attention paid to maternal and child health particularly prenatal cares. IMR is an indicator not only of the health status of infants but also of whole population, their socio-economic conditions and the availability, access and utilization, and effectiveness of health services. It is not only an indicator by which the health status of a population can be judged, but also an important statistics for planning and evaluating health interventions.

According to the Annual Health Survey (AHS), 2011–12, IMR in the state of Uttar Pradesh was 71 (68 in AHS: 2012-13) and neonatal mortality rate (NMR) was 50. According to the Office of Registrar General (RGI), Government of India (2012), in 2012 the under-5 mortality rate in India was 52 per 1000 live births. The sample size for AHS has been arrived for estimation of IMR at district level with desired margin of error, whereas under SRS it is for estimation of IMR at state level. The results by two sources usually differ in most cases. For similar reasons, different estimates from NFHS and DLHS also vary.

On the basis of birth weight, new born is characterized as normal (≥2500 gm), low birth weight (<2500 gm), very low birth weight (<1500 gm) and extremely low birth weight (<1000 gm). The newborns with birth weight <1500 gm are at maximum risk. It can be the outcome of pre-term delivery or prematurity or both. Premature low birth weight births are at greater risk as nearly half of the neonatal deaths occur in such babies (Sherif, 2004). Lower the birth weight, higher are the chances of mortality. Low birth weight is an important cause for clinical complications and almost 60 percent of neonatal deaths occur due to birth asphyxia and infections.

Low birth weight (lbw) accounts for 60–80 percent of the infant mortality rate in developing countries whereas lowest mortality rates occur among infants weighing 3.0–3.5 kg. For infants born below 2.5 kg, the mortality rate rapidly increases with decreasing weight, and most of the infants weighing up to 1.0 kg die. As compared to normal birth weight infants, those with low weight are almost 40 times more likely to die in the neonatal period. Further, for infants with very low birth weight, the relative risk of neonatal death is almost 200 times greater. Infant mortality due to low birth weight is usually a direct cause arising from other medical complications such as preterm birth, poor maternal nutritional status, lack of prenatal care, maternal sickness during pregnancy, and unhygienic home environments (Andrews et al., 2008). Along with birth weight, period of gestation makes up the two most important predictors of an infant's chances of survival and their overall health (MacDorman and Mathews, 2009).

At present, there is no focused program or policy to manage lbw children. Even in the urban areas, most hospitals and nursing homes are ill equipped to manage such newborns and as a result such children are prone to get infected and develop complications.

### 3.3.1 Causes of infant mortality

Generally the most common cause of infant mortality worldwide had been dehydration from diarrhea, a preventable disease. A variety of programs to control this problem have decreased the rate of children dying from dehydration. Many factors contribute to infant mortality such as the mother's level of education, environmental conditions, hygiene and medical infrastructure. Improving sanitation and hygiene, access to clean drinking water, immunization against infectious diseases, and other public health measures could help reduce high rates of infant mortality.

Leading causes of congenital infant mortality are malformations, *sudden infant death syndrome*, maternal complications during pregnancy, and accidents and injuries. Environmental and social barriers prevent access to basic medical resources and thus contribute to an increasing infant mortality rate: 99 percent of infant deaths occur in developing countries, and 86 percent of these deaths are due to *infections*, *premature births*, complications during delivery, and perinatal *asphyxia* and birth injuries (Andrews et al., 2008). Greatest percentage reduction of infant mortality occurs in countries that already have low rates of infant mortality (Bishai et al., 2007). Common causes are preventable with low-cost measures. The determinants of low birth weight include socio-economic, psychological, behavioral and environmental factors (Osel, 2008). According to a *Save the Children* paper (2001), children from the poorest households in India are three times more likely to die before their fifth birthday than those from the richest households.

## 3.4 Current status of MMR estimates

According to RGI (2013), MMR figures in India were 230, 213, 212 and 178 in the years 2008, 2009, 2010 and 2012 respectively showing declining trend. It was very high in northeastern states and relatively much lower in southern states. Table 3.1 gives levels of MMR by regions, in the years 2010 and 2012.

**Table 3.1** Levels of MMR by regions, 2010–12

| Regions | MMR | |
|---|---|---|
| | **2010** | **2012** |
| India | 212 | 178 |
| EAG states and Assam | 308 | 257 |
| Southern states | 127 | 105 |
| Others | 149 | 127 |

In Empowered Action Group (EAG) states and Assam almost 24 women per lakh of women in age group 15–49 died due to maternal causes whereas in southern states number of maternal deaths was only 6. There are 8 EAG states. These are Bihar, Jharkhand, MP, Chhattisgarh, Orissa, Rajasthan, UP and Uttarakhand. All these states lag far behind others in containing population growth and need area-specific programmes for improvements. Table 3.2 gives maximum and minimum MMR values in these states during two time periods 2007–2009 and 2010–2012.

**Table 3.2** Maximum and minimum MMRs during 2007–2009 and 2010–2012

| | 2007–09 | | | | 2010–12 | | | |
|---|---|---|---|---|---|---|---|---|
| | Minimum | | Maximum | | Minimum | | Maximum | |
| EAG and Assam | Odisha | 258 | Assam | 390 | Bihar | 219 | Assam | 328 |
| Southern | Kerala | 81 | Karnataka | 178 | Kerala | 66 | Karnataka | 144 |
| Others | Maharashtra | 104 | Punjab | 172 | Maharashtra | 87 | Punjab | 155 |

AHS gives top 100 districts in order of IMR and then 57 common districts and top 25 administrative divisions in order of MMR featuring in these 100 districts. Assam, Madhya Pradesh, Rajasthan and Uttar Pradesh feature in these 57 districts. These lists are given in Table 3.3.

**Table 3.3** gives 57 common districts featuring in top 100 districts in order of IMR and top 25 administrative divisions in order of MMR

| S. No. | State | List of 57 common districts featuring in top 100 districts in order of Infant Mortality Rate and top 25 administrative divisions in order of Maternal Mortality Ratio | S. No. | State | List of 57 common districts featuring in top 100 districts in order of Infant Mortality Rate and top 25 administrative divisions in order of Maternal Mortality Ratio |
|---|---|---|---|---|---|
| 1 | Assam | Kokrajhar | 30 | Uttar Pradesh | Pratapgarh |
| 2 | Assam | Marigaon | 31 | Uttar Pradesh | Maharajganj |
| 3 | Assam | Dhubri | 32 | Uttar Pradesh | Shahjahanpur |
| 4 | Assam | Darrang | 33 | Uttar Pradesh | Basti |
| 5 | Assam | Karimganj | 34 | Uttar Pradesh | Kaushambi |
| 6 | Assam | Sonitpur | 35 | Uttar Pradesh | Kushinagar |
| 7 | Assam | Nagaon | 36 | Uttar Pradesh | Ghazipur |
| 8 | Madhya Pradesh | Panna | 37 | Uttar Pradesh | Sitapur |
| 9 | Madhya Pradesh | Satna | 38 | Uttar Pradesh | Chandauli |
| 10 | Madhya Pradesh | Damoh | 39 | Uttar Pradesh | Hardoi |
| 11 | Madhya Pradesh | Shahdol | 40 | Uttar Pradesh | Lakhimpur Kheri |
| 12 | Madhya Pradesh | Rewa | 41 | Uttar Pradesh | Azamgarh |
| 13 | Madhya Pradesh | Chhatarpur | 42 | Uttar Pradesh | Bareilly |
| 14 | Madhya Pradesh | Dindori | 43 | Uttar Pradesh | Varanasi |
| 15 | Madhya Pradesh | Sidhi | 44 | Uttar Pradesh | Jaunpur |
| 16 | Madhya Pradesh | Sagar | 45 | Uttar Pradesh | Saharanpur |
| 17 | Madhya Pradesh | Umaria | 46 | Uttar Pradesh | Mau |
| 18 | Madhya Pradesh | Tikamgarh | 47 | Uttar Pradesh | Deoria |
| 19 | Rajasthan | Bhilwara | 48 | Uttar Pradesh | Pilibhit |
| 20 | Rajasthan | Dungarpur | 49 | Uttar Pradesh | Etah |
| 21 | Rajasthan | Rajsamand | 50 | Uttar Pradesh | Ambedkar Nagar |
| 22 | Rajasthan | Jhalawar | 51 | Uttar Pradesh | Ballia |
| 23 | Rajasthan | Bundi | 52 | Uttar Pradesh | Gonda |
| 24 | Uttar Pradesh | Shrawasti | 53 | Uttar Pradesh | Barabanki |
| 25 | Uttar Pradesh | Faizabad | 54 | Uttar Pradesh | Aligarh |
| 26 | Uttar Pradesh | Balrampur | 55 | Uttar Pradesh | Jyotiba Phule Nagar |
| 27 | Uttar Pradesh | Budaun | 56 | Uttar Pradesh | Bahraich |
| 28 | Uttar Pradesh | Siddharthnagar | 57 | Uttar Pradesh | Sant Kabir Nagar |
| 29 | Uttar Pradesh | Allahabad | | | |

## 3.5 Estimating maternal mortality

Estimation of MMR is one of the most difficult problems. A major problem for estimation of MMR is the requirement of huge sample size. We noted in Section 1.12.1 that the sample size requirement is around 3 lakhs births. At the current birth rates in our country, to track such huge number of births a population of size exceeding 1 crore is required. Another problem is lack of reliable data on causes associated with maternal deaths on such huge scale and accurate classification of maternal death. We would elaborate on both these aspects in the present and forthcoming sections.

It is desirable to have the estimates of MMR along with the associated causes at state levels. The availability of such information would be of immense help for the planning of appropriate and effective strategies to reduce the maternal deaths in the country. NFHS–2 in 1992–1993 was the first to provide the national level estimate of MMR as 424 per 100,000 live births for the period 2 years preceding the survey. But regional or state level estimates could not be produced because of sample size constraints. RGI has been producing estimates of MMR for India and its states. These estimates have, however, large standard errors and for small states the estimates are not good enough because of the inadequate sample size.

Several indirect methods have been proposed for estimation of maternal mortality. Graham et al. (1989) developed sisterhood method which makes use of the data collected from female respondents in a sample survey on the number of ever married sisters they had, the number who were not currently alive, and the number who died while pregnant, during childbirth or within 6 weeks after delivery. The sisterhood method requires lower sample size than the direct method because women generally have several sisters who could have been exposed to the risk of maternal mortality. The limitation with sisterhood method is that it generally underestimates maternal mortality because of omission of events in the survey (Stanton et al., 2000). Mari Bhat et al. (1995) developed an indirect procedure of estimating maternal mortality from sex differentials in mortality at reproductive ages. Sisterhood method was also used by them to provide levels and differentials in maternal mortality in rural India. The estimate of MMR was estimated as 638 per hundred thousand live births in rural areas of India during 1982–86. This estimate was derived from SRS data on sex differentials in mortality in the reproductive age. Mari Bhat (2002) updated these estimates for India and its major states for the period 1987–96. These indirect methods used for estimating MMR have their own limitations. Inaccuracy in maternal deaths occurs when a maternal death is inaccurately classified to causes not used for the purpose of identifying maternal deaths and underreporting of maternal deaths due to misclassification or because the death was not reported.

Pal et al. (2002) conducted a study in Rural North–24 Praganas to derive estimates of MMR and study its related causes to ascertain the epidemiological factors which were associated with maternal deaths. The complexities involved in measuring maternal mortality were discussed by WHO, UNICEF and United Nations Population Fund (UNFPA) in 2009. The document also gives the rationale for the development of 1995 estimates of maternal mortality along with a description of the process through which this was accomplished. It gives an analysis and interpretation of the results and compares them to the 1990 estimates developed by WHO and UNICEF. The document also describes the difficulties that such comparisons involve. It also presents a review of progress in reducing maternal mortality over the past few years. The document also suggests the interventions needed to achieve sustained reductions in the coming few years.

### 3.5.1 Factors associated with maternal mortality

Past studies have shown that there was no significant decline in MMR over time indicating an urgent public health concern. The complications of pregnancies and the births continue to be the leading causes of deaths and disability among women of reproductive age. The health problems of mothers and newborns arise due to a variety of reasons like undernutrition, poverty, illiteracy, unhygienic living conditions, infections and unregulated fertility. Poor infrastructure and inefficient public health services are also major causes for low inadequate obstetric care.

### 3.5.2 Constraints in estimation of MMR

A document from WHO (2006a) provides a good account of data limitations in computing MMR. It gives guidelines for their generation, interpretation and analysis of MMR for global monitoring. Maternal deaths are difficult to investigate not only because of their rarity on a population basis, but also due to factors like reluctance to report abortion-related deaths, problems of memory recall, or lack of medical attribution. No single source or data collection method is therefore adequate for investigating all aspects of maternal mortality in all settings (WHO, 2006a). Ironically, only few developing countries provide reliable population estimates.

A major problem with health services data relates to the selectivity of the service-using population. Without detailed knowledge of the use of health-related services by the catchment population, it is difficult to assess whether the maternal mortality ratio under- or over-estimates the level for the general population. This is particularly so because the general population also includes non-users of the service. In addition to these confoundings, health services information has inaccuracies in routine registers and omission of deaths occurring outside maternity wards.

Population-based surveys are the primary source of information for calculating the maternal mortality ratio in many developing countries. These types of surveys are either reproductive age mortality surveys or part of a general health-oriented household survey. While the first type seeks to identify all female deaths in the reproductive period, using a combination of approaches, such as cross-sectional household surveys, continuous population surveillance, hospital and health centre records, and key informants (WHO, 1987), the second type relies on asking questions about maternal deaths in a household during a recent interval of time, say one to two years. Both these types of methods provide reasonable estimates but are time consuming and costly because they require large sample sizes to obtain single point estimates with sufficiently narrow confidence intervals to enable monitoring of time trends.

The sisterhood method overcomes large sample size requirements to some extent by interviewing adult respondents about the survival of all their sisters. The indirect method (Graham et al. 1989) involves fewer questions to respondents but provides a pooled estimate that relates statistically to a point around 10–12 years prior to the survey. The direct method (Stanton et al. 2000) provides a more current estimate at about 3–4 years prior to the survey, but requires more questions and is more costly and time consuming. Because of the imprecision in these estimates, modeling and other methods have also been developed (WHO, UNICEF and UNFPA, 2003; AbouZahr et al., 2001; AbouZahr and Wardlaw, 2004). But these may have their own limitations like appropriate model explorations and replicability of their findings in other data sets.

Maternal mortality ratios are only a broad indication of the level of maternal mortality, rather than a precise measure, because of the underlying limitations in most measurement methods. The use of confidence interval instead of an imprecise point estimate is to some extent a better alternative to monitor trends. Data sources and collection methods used for estimating MMR have very different strengths and weaknesses and yield estimates of varying reliability. Because of such complexities surveys to estimate maternal mortality usually take place in about 5–10 years.

In view of the discussions as above, it is difficult to interpret the reduction in MMR values over time. Graham et al. (1996) argued that that observed differences do not necessarily indicate improved maternal health status. Non-sampling errors such as changes in the accuracy of reporting or of classification over time or between districts or populations (Stanton et al., 2000) are one of the major reasons. Changes in the definition of a maternal death between ICD-9 and ICD-10 (WHO, 2004) have also to be taken into account while interpreting trends in MMR. Presentation of the maternal mortality ratio should state which version it used. For instance, for ICD-10, it should be specified which of the three categories: direct and indirect maternal deaths up to 42 days postpartum, late maternal deaths, pregnancy-related deaths were used for the classification of the maternal death.

### 3.5.3 The IRMS study

The Institute for Research in Medical Statistics (IRMS) – now the National Institute of Medical Statistics (NIMS) – carried out a pilot study in 2002 for deriving estimates of maternal mortality ratio in India and some of its states. The study also aimed at identifying major causes of maternal deaths. Some of its major findings are now presented.

The objective of the pilot study was to develop survey tools and instruments to estimate the level of MMR and ascertain the related causes of maternal deaths. It also proposed to try out various options of data collection and examine the feasibility of these options in varying field conditions. The pilot study was designed in five states of India namely Uttar Pradesh, Karnataka, Uttaranchal, Maharashtra and Delhi.

The study provides an analytical view of various approaches of data collection based on the field study. Specifically it aims to capture maternal deaths as compared to house-to-house survey and the estimates of MMR in above five states along with their standard errors and confidence intervals.

#### *3.5.3.1 Sample size*

As per RGI, during late nineties, the estimate of MMR in India varied from 400 to 407 per lakh live births during the period of the study. Assuming MMR of 400 per hundred thousand live births, a sample of 3.8 lakhs live births was calculated to provide an estimate of MMR at all India level with 95 percent confidence level and less than 5 percent margin of error. Assuming a birth rate of 28.5 per thousand population, this would amount to covering about 1.30 crore population. The birth rate is the total number of births per 1,000 of a population in a year.

#### *3.5.3.2 Selection of health centre*

The total sample was allocated to different states taking into account the state specific MMR, birth rate, primary health centres (PHCs)/urban centres, births and associated relative margin of error. This allocation was supposed to provide results at state level with different precisions. For bigger states like U.P., Bihar, M.P. and Rajasthan, the relative margin of error was less than 5 per cent whereas for smaller states – Haryana, Punjab, J&K, Himachal Pradesh – it was around 18–21 per cent. For the northeast states the relative margin of errors were less than 10 per cent and for the remaining states the relative margins of error were about 20 per cent. In arriving at these, a population of 30,000 was assumed under a PHC though it could be more than 40,000 in many cases. For instance, Delhi had health centres with the population in excess of 50,000 instead of 30,000. Therefore, the precision of the estimates was expected to be much higher than assumed.

The selected PHC was visited for collection of data on births and maternal deaths. Within selected PHCs, method of snowball sampling (Section 1.17) was carried out for identifying the maternal deaths as the rare event. For the enumeration of live births, house-to-house survey was done in addition to using snowball sampling. The reference period for maternal deaths and live births was three years preceding the survey. The causes of maternal deaths were assessed by verbal autopsy.

#### *3.5.3.3 Methodology for data collection*

The pilot study was conducted in five states, namely, Uttar Pradesh, Maharashtra, Karnataka, Uttaranchal and Delhi. These states were selected representing high MMR, medium and low MMR states. One district from each of these states was covered and from the selected districts, two PHCs from rural area and one centre from urban area were taken.

Snowball sampling was used to identify households where a maternal death occurred through some key informants in the village. Each of these households was then asked to name some other households where maternal deaths occurred, and so on. By this method of snowball sampling, all the maternal deaths were covered by contacting few related households. Some details of the procedure can be found in the paper by Singh et al. (2007).

Five different types of tools were used to collect the data for births and maternal deaths. These were schedules for PHC, sub-centre, house-to-house survey, snowballing and verbal autopsy. Listing of combined households with births and maternal deaths was done. Pre-testing was done for testing the tools in one slum area each in Delhi and Kanpur district covering a population about 15000 and in one rural PHC in Mathura district. Based upon the pre-testing, the survey instruments were modified by adding some new characteristics like information on place of delivery, parity, age of the mother during delivery, caste and literacy of the mother. Additions were also made on socio-economic variables, birth planning and health beliefs in the verbal autopsy questionnaire.

The house-to-house survey was expected to under-enumerate maternal deaths. This could be mainly because the information on maternal deaths being suppressed by some households for fear or otherwise. This could be overcome by resorting to snowball sampling. A better coverage was expected by strengthening the house-to-house reporting through snowballing.

#### *3.5.3.4 Process of pilot study*

The study was carried out in eight rural PHCs in the selected states and one urban slum each in Delhi and Kanpur in Uttar Pradesh. In each area of the pilot study, house-to-house survey approach was followed for the collection of information on births on the modified scheduled for household that included additional variables like religion, caste, family size, income, education, birth planning, place of delivery, delivery conducted by whom and maternal deaths. For capturing the maternal deaths, the house-to-house survey was supplemented by snowballing approach for the completeness of maternal deaths. Different teams were employed for carrying out the fieldwork, one for carrying out the house-to-house survey and the other for snowballing.

#### *3.5.3.5 Results*

Results included the demographic profile with estimates of MMR and its standard error with confidence interval for the states/districts based on PHC covered for MMR study. The overall relative standard error of the estimate of MMR was close to 10 per cent as assumed. The relative standard error for the states covered ranged from 28 to 45 per cent.

The maternal deaths during the last 3 years per 1 lakh births were obtained both by snowballing and house-to-house survey. Number of maternal deaths in case of snowballing was higher as expected. This is because snowballing captures maternal deaths missed in the house-to-house survey. Such omissions were over 10 percent. The estimates of MMR and birth rate for the states, though based on small samples, provided estimates comparable with those from other prevalent sources.

#### *3.5.3.6 Profile of maternal deaths*

The results included the profile of maternal deaths which is discussed now. About 24 percent of the deaths were observed to be during antenatal period, about 70 percent deaths in postnatal period and the remaining during delivery. More than 60 percent of the maternal deaths occurred in SC, ST and OBC households. A vast majority of the maternal deaths occurred among families with low socio-economic standard and among illiterate women living in unhygienic conditions. This is evident from the following details. Over 35 percent of households had no electricity, for one-third of households drinking water source was hand pump, and around one-third of households each had either no draining system or had open and stagnant or open and running drainage in front of the house. Further, there was no toilet facility in 93.7 percent households, and 70.8 percent households were living in kutcha or semi-pucca houses. Over 65 percent households were nuclear, over 85 percent women were housewives, and over 58 percent women were illiterate. Over 52 percent of households did not have a separate kitchen in their houses. These factors appear to be main causes of maternal deaths. However, logistic regression may be appropriate tool to not only determine causal factors but also their loading factors.

Some other maternal death related reasons as revealed through the survey are now discussed. More than 50 percent of the respondents reported that the health facility was 4–5 km away from their houses and no transport facilities were available in about 14 percent of the cases. More than 55 percent reported that due to inadequate facility of transport, they could not take proper treatment which resulted in about 15 percent dying on the way. In the hilly area of Uttarakhand, health facility was 40 km away from the village and there was no transport facility available in the village. In one-third of maternal death cases, women did not receive antenatal care which included tetanus toxoid vaccination. Forty seven percent did not consume IFA tablets during ante-partum period. Thus both bad transport system and ineffective health facility lead to inadequate obstetric care.

About 48 percent deliveries were conducted at home by untrained dais. About 69 percent of maternal deaths occurred during postnatal period. It was observed that about 59 percent of the women died in hospital and 16 percent died on the way. This could be due to the late referral of women to hospital by untrained dais. About 59 percent woman stayed in the hospital for one to two days before the death. It indicates that after the delivery conducted at home by untrained dai woman got infected and rushed to the hospital and died within one or two days.

The main causes of deaths were observed as post-partum hemorrhage (17%), and septicemia and anemia (13% each). It was observed that 7.5 percent of the maternal deaths reported to be due to retained placenta and about 8.6 percent due to non-obstetric reasons. Another interesting finding was that 50 percent of maternal deaths occurred before the age of 25 years of which 15 percent had parity one and about 43 percent with parity three or more. The majority of maternal deaths occurred to women who were relatively young and case of first delivery.

## 3.6 Major causes of complications in delivery

It was pointed out in Section 3.1 that some of the major causes associated with maternal deaths are pre-intra-and-post complications in delivery. Some of these causes as well as their timing are also discussed in the preceding section. The purpose of this section is to assess further the current status on these factors. The findings when viewed in conjunction with those in the preceding section present a grim view of the current scenario. It was also stated earlier that Madhya Pradesh is one of the poor performing states in terms of maternal and infant mortality. The current status of this state on the critical factors leading to complications in pregnancy and delivery related factors is now discussed. This is done on the basis of an assessment study conducted by IASDS for CARE India's Maternal and Infant Survival Project (MISP) in 2005 in Madhya Pradesh.

MISP was implemented in Madhya Pradesh, a state that is generally classified as one of the most disadvantaged states in India. The findings of the study on the current scenario of complications during pregnancy and delivery and after also gives a fairly good idea about these critical factors in other poor performing states as well.

The findings are based upon the baseline survey done in Hoshangabad, Seoni Malwa, Sohagpur and Piparia blocks in district Hoshangabad, and block Timarni in district Harda. The focus of the quantitative assessment was to assess the practices on critical factors during pregnancy, delivery and thereafter.

An important feature of antenatal care is the provision of at least one health check up before the end of the first trimester. It was found that amongst all those who had health check-ups, only one-third had it in the first 3 months. Services provided during checkups were only giving medicines, examination of tongues, eyes and nails and giving dietary suggestions. Many other important checkups were missed out. There were very few home visits by Anganwadi worker, ANM and CBO during pregnancy and advice given confined only to TT injections, IFA tablets, nutritious food and rest, and not to carry heavy weights.

When probed why they did not want to have ANC, about 60 percent of them thought that the checkups were unnecessary. Only about one-tenth of them were weighed during pregnancy. Only three-fourth of the respondents had received the tetanus injections. Among these, one-fourth had received only a single dose. Among the respondents who had not received the tetanus injection, nearly 36 percent thought that it was not necessary.

One of the major reasons for complications during pregnancy is related to low hemoglobin status resulting in anemia. During pregnancy, though the woman should consume 100 tablets of IFA, only half of respondents even received the tablets.

Forty-three percent mentioned that they faced some complications during pregnancy. An analyses of complications revealed that the percent of respondents facing problems in the first trimester was about one-third of those facing a complication in the third trimester. The most commonly mentioned complications were excessive weakness, dizziness and giddiness (25%), difficulty seeing at nights (18%), pain in stomach (15%), fever (14%) and excessive swelling of hands/feet (13%). Nearly half among these did nothing, 35 percent went to a doctor and 11 percent to a government health facility.

An analysis of the intra-natal period revealed that 83 percent of deliveries were conducted at home and in nearly half of cases, Dai/TBA was the one who helped. In all home delivery cases, the chord was cut by Dai/TBA but 29 percent among them had come only for cutting the cord and were not present from the beginning of labour. Only half of them washed hands with soap. The usage of new or boiled blade or a blade from the birth kit was widespread to cut the cord. There was also widespread use of new thread for the purpose. As regards the clean surface for delivery, it was ensured in two-third of home deliveries. But in very few cases disposable delivery kit was used at the time of delivery.

Thirteen percent home delivery cases mentioned facing one or the other problem during delivery. The problem faced were too much pain (42%), labour longer than 12 hours (24%), rupture of bag of water (12%), placenta not delivered (10%), excessive bleeding, convulsions and others (4% each). Nearly 15 percent of the respondents mentioned facing problems/ complications immediately after delivery. The most commonly mentioned problems were pain in stomach (31%), fever with chill (29%) and bleeding (10%).

Home visits by ANM, Anganwadi worker and CBO in the first week after delivery were very few. Though women with children up to 6 months are eligible for receiving supplementary nutrition from the Anganwadi centre only 29 percent received it. Nearly 62 percent of them mentioned sharing it, mostly with children in the family.

Nearly 27 percent mothers made an advance arrangement with the service providers for their impending delivery. Among the mothers who did not deliver at home were asked how far the place where they went for delivery was and whether any transport arrangement was made in advance. About 22 percent of mothers took less than half an hour to reach the place of delivery, 15 percent took between half to 1 hour, 26 percent took 1–2 hours and 17 percent, 3 or more than 3 hours. Prior transport arrangement was made in half of the cases where the delivery was not conducted at home. In nearly half of cases where delivery was not conducted at home, husband was the one who accompanied the pregnant women to the place of delivery. In about 31 percent cases, someone from the woman's maternal family accompanied her. However, in 38 percent of the cases, the escort arrangement was not planned. Further, only 37 percent of the respondents mentioned that they had saved some money. Nearly 37 percent of the respondents saved more than Rs. 500 and 19 percent of them saved more than Rs. 1000.

One of the reasons for poor maternal health is believed to be non-usage of family planning methods, resulting in frequent pregnancies. Forty one percent of mothers wanted to have more children and among these, 43 percent wanted to have them in near future. Only a very small percentage of mothers not wanting to have child in near future, were using a family planning method.

## 3.7 Strategies to prevent maternal mortality

### 3.7.1 Skilled birth attendants

The presence of a skilled birth attendant (SBA) at delivery is one of the most important factors in averting maternal and neonatal mortality and morbidity. Trained traditional birth attendants (TBAs) cannot, in most cases, save women's lives effectively because they are unable to treat pregnancy and delivery complications (Carlough, 2005). According to Graham et al. (2001), skilled attendants at the time of deliveries can reduce maternal mortality by 13–33 percent.

In India, ANMs do not fulfill the international definition of a skilled birth attendant, as they are not mandated to provide the 6 elements of basic emergency obstetric care. According to the recent Indian government guidelines, there are 3 skills which they cannot perform: manual removal of placenta, manual vacuum delivery and manual vacuum aspiration of early pregnancy bleeding. In order to improve maternal and child health, the Government of India has expanded the scope of practice for ANM, Lady Health Visitor (LHV) and Staff Nurse (SN) to allow them to use certain drugs for basic emergency obstetric care and to perform simple procedures like active management of third stage of labor (AMTSL), use of partograph to improve labor monitoring, use of antibiotics for management of infection, management of eclampsia before referral and initial management of post-partum hemorrhage. As per Government of India Guidelines (2005), implementation of this strategy means empowering the ANM, LHV and SN not to only manage normal deliveries but also provide basic emergency care and initial management of complications during childbirth.

First effort in this direction was made in 2005 in Jharkhand under ACCESS Program, CEDPA/WRAI with the support from the Government of Jharkhand. It aimed to reduce maternal and neonatal mortality and morbidity through skilled birth attendants in 3 blocks of Dumka district. The program included a comprehensive 12-week competency-based training program in practice areas and supportive supervision for the newly trained ANMs.

### 3.7.2 Deoghar project

A program was launched in 2007 in Deoghar district under IntraHealth International's Vistaar Project funded by USAID. The project was scaled up for intervention in all 24 districts of the state in 2009. The project also established a Management Information System (MIS) to capture process-level data during 2008–2012 in 14 of these districts. The two programs Dumka and Deogarh were different. The ACCESS program in Dumka was an operations research (OR) project while Vistaar's was a technical assistance program. Dumka followed a 12-week curriculum while Vistaar followed Government of India's 3 weeks schedule. Dumka's OR project had a community mobilization component while Vistaar did not have that and instead had a supportive supervision component.

At the time of launching of Vistaar project, MMR in Jharkhand was very high, close to 400 per 100,000 live births with only 11 percent institutional deliveries reported in the rural areas of the state (NFHS-3, Jharkhand Factsheet). Only 21 per cent of births in the rural areas were reported to be assisted by a doctor, nurse, LHV, ANM or other trained health personnel. The coverage of Sections 3.7.2.1, 3.7.2.2 and 3.7.3 are based upon the Technical Brief Document by Vistaar in 2012.

#### *3.7.2.1 Key strategies*

Key strategies under the program were:

(i) *Strengthening district facilities to conduct quality, competency-based maternal and newborn care training:* Training requires a clinical practice site where quality maternal and newborn care services are offered consistent to practices to be taught (such as basic infection prevention practices, use of partograph, essential drugs, etc). Training centres/sites (government funded) were strengthened to conduct quality competency-based training. These facilities were strengthened to provide back-up support for emergency obstetric and newborn care (EmONC).

(ii) *Train and prepare ANMs to fulfill the community-based midwifery care role:* Training was designed to ensure that trainees gained the knowledge and skills for the expanded skills as defined in the government guidelines in 2005 for antenatal care and skilled attendance at birth by ANMs and LHVs. It included basic midwifery skills and competency-based training on newborn care at the community level.

(iii) *Develop supportive supervision systems:* The program sought to build existing mechanisms within the government health care system to support the ANMs placed in the community. These efforts were intended to ensure that ANMs had adequate supplies, drugs and kits from the PHCs, a strong referral link between the ANMs and referral hospital for emergency obstetric and newborn care (EmONC), and supervisors skilled in providing supportive supervision.

(iv) *Increase community awareness and demand for SBAs through a birth preparedness and complication readiness campaign:* The program was designed to promote birth preparedness and complication readiness through existing community health education mechanisms to encourage the use of a range of ANM services, including antenatal care, childbirth, postnatal care and post-partum care.

#### *3.7.2.2 Monitoring and evaluation*

Baseline survey was done in 2008, followed by an endline in 2012 in Deoghar district. Additionally, the endline survey included a cross-sectional study in the district of Hazaribagh to capture progress in a scale-up district, where the intervention started later than in Deoghar. A slightly different training model was used in this district, and intervention was the second longest and number of ANMs trained as SBAs was the second highest (after Deoghar).

The baseline survey was conducted with ANMs before their SBA training, while the endline survey was conducted with ANMs trained as SBAs to assess their knowledge, attitude and practices with regard to skilled birth care. In addition, also included were MOs to assess the supervisory support mechanism and HSCs (health service centres) where the trained SBAs worked to assess the capacity of these facilities to provide quality delivery services and to review the stock and supply status, with specific reference to supplies needed for delivery care.

An analysis was done on data from ANMs of HSCs. A qualitative study was also conducted in Hazaribagh and Deoghar districts to validate successful trends indicated from Project MIS data and to better understand the factors underlying its success.

#### 3.7.2.3 *Improvement in the performance of ANMs*

The joint efforts of the project and the Department of Health & Family Welfare in Jharkhand have resulted in an increase in the number of births with a skilled attendant at lower-level facilities (i.e., HSCs) and improved quality of care. The Project MIS and surveys both indicate that interventions led to improved performance of ANMs in conducting deliveries.

In Deoghar, there was a marked increase in the reported number of births attended by ANMs at the HSC level. The average (mean) number of deliveries conducted by ANMs at HSCs over a period of 6 months preceding the endline survey was reported to be 33, which is significantly higher than the average of less than 9 deliveries conducted by ANMs at these centres at baseline. Home deliveries conducted by the ANMs also increased from 7 to 11.

Both knowledge and practice of the partograph improved, with 78 percent ANMs reporting using the partograph to monitor labour in over 75 percent of the deliveries conducted by them. At endline, the knowledge regarding AMTSL was double the level at baseline. Over 90 percent of the ANMs interviewed at endline were aware of the use of Oxytocin/Misoprostol as the most important step of AMTSL to prevent postpartum hemorrhage (PPH). More significantly, 86 percent of ANMs interviewed at endline reported using AMTSL in all the deliveries conducted by them.

Higher percentage of ANMs could list the elements of essential newborn care, including prevention and/or management of neonatal hypothermia and hyperthermia (89% at endline against 39% at baseline), keeping the baby's cord clean (40% against 17%), early and exclusive breastfeeding (75% against 61%), colostrum feeding (68% against 49%) and cleaning of air passage (70% against 68%). Higher number of mothers initiated breastfeeding within 1 hour and higher number of newborns were dried and wrapped appropriately to reduce hypothermia.

There was higher awareness of the complications during pregnancy, labour, and the postnatal period than at baseline. All of the ANMs interviewed at endline were aware that post-partum care needs to be provided within 24 hours of delivery and a significantly higher percentage of ANMs at endline were aware of what should be included in post-partum check-ups compared to baseline.

Percentages of ANMs at endline who were aware that postpartum check-ups included examining the mother for PPH (70%), ensuring that the uterus is contracted (36%), measuring the mother's blood pressure (74%), providing breastfeeding advice (81%), checking for any bleeding from the newborn's cord (46%), and keeping the baby warm (88%) improved. Knowledge on these was almost negligible at the baseline stage.

The project resulted in significant improvements not only in the supply side of the effort to improve maternal and newborn care, but also increased the number of SBA-attended births at HSCs which are located closer to the communities. These findings show simple, proven and low cost interventions that the government system can scale up to improve SBA performance. However, to assess the sustainability of the SBA training efforts, there is a need to carry out current status surveys in the two intervention districts at regular intervals of 2–3 years.

## 3.8 Preventing infant deaths

We now discuss the issue of preventing infant deaths. It is known that most infant deaths occur during neonatal period which is the first 28 days of life. Deaths of children aged 29 days to one year are classified as postneonatal mortality. A newborn is called a neonate during the neonatal period. This is further classified into early neonatal period, 0–7 days and late neonatal period, 8–28 days. Main cause of neonatal death is inadequate access and utilization of basic medical care during pregnancy and after delivery.

IMR includes neonatal as well as postneonatal mortality. Early neonatal mortality is associated with maternal health and access to care around the time of delivery, where as postneonatal mortality is associated with socio-economic conditions, preventive and curative health services. As neonatal mortality accounts for substantial proportion of infant mortality, it needs to be given special attention. The factors responsible for the deaths of neonates are entirely different from the factors affecting child health below 1 year of age. Neonatal carc is not available to most neonates in developing countries because hospitals are inaccessible and costly, and neonatal care providers, particularly in the villages, (either from within the family or the community) have very low level of knowledge/ awareness on such care.

As discussed earlier, low birth weight (lbw) is an important contributor to neonatal mortality. Nearly one-third of all neonates born in major hospitals of India every year are of low birth weight. Further, about 82 percent neonatal deaths occur among lbw which is the highest in the world (Bisai et al., 2006). According to Pandey and Vir (2011), burden of neonatal deaths in India is primarily from northern states (Bihar, Uttar Pradesh, Rajasthan, Madhya Pradesh and Rajasthan) contributing to more than half of all neonatal deaths and Bengal.

As neonatal mortality rate (NMR) contributes significantly to IMR, controlling neonatal deaths is crucial to preventing infant deaths. Reduction in MMR by way of safe motherhood is also a critical factor towards controlling neonatal deaths. There had been a secular decline in IMR until 1996, and thereafter there was stagnation in IMR. The decline in IMR was on account of the decline in postneonatal mortality. The future decline is anticipated due to decline in neonatal mortality. As the neonatal mortality is largely governed by the maternal causes, there is a need to monitor maternal mortality ratio in the population.

Due to the demographic diversity in Indian states, infant mortality rates vary considerably in different states. Kerala has the lowest IMR, whereas states like Madhya Pradesh, Orissa and Uttar Pradesh have recorded five to six times higher figures. In Uttar Pradesh, the IMR was 83 infant deaths per 1000 live births in 2002, which was nearly five times that of Kerala. In the year 1997, NMR in Uttar Pradesh was 51.1, which is 60 percent of the IMR, and postneonatal mortality (PNMR) was 34.4, which is 40 percent of the IMR.

Although IMR varies across different states, a decline has been observed in the percentage over past decades. However, the decline has not been rapid for the past few years, and the stagnation in the declining of IMR is of serious concern. As IMR is one of the key indicators of development, it also reflects stagnation in socio-economic development of the state. There is an urgent need to explore the reasons for such stagnation so that appropriate intervention strategies can be adopted to fulfill India's population goals.

Table 3.4 gives top 100 districts in order of IMR sorted in alphabetical order of states as per AHS, India (2011–12). It can be seen that Assam, Bihar, Madhya Pradesh, Orissa, Rajasthan and U.P. are poor performing states in that order. Among the 100 districts 7 are from Assam, 3 from Bihar, 30 from Madhya Pradesh, 8 from Orissa, 9 from Rajasthan and the remaining 53 from U.P.

## 3.9 Trends in infant mortality

To explore the possible factors leading to high infant mortality, it may be worthwhile to examine past and present trends in the IMR. India's figures have been among the worst in the world. UNICEF (2010) reported that around 5,000 children under the age of 5 died in 2010 every day in India; nearly half of all children in India were undernourished.

NFHS-1 and NFHS-2 reported IMR as 99.9 and 86.7, respectively. It was 57 according to NFHS-3. As per the SRS bulletin of 2013, the IMR of Uttar Pradesh has fallen by four points, from 57 per 1,000 live births in 2011 to 53 per 1,000 live births in 2012. The IMR of India is 42, down from 57 in 2005 and U.P. with 53 is still amongst the top three states with highest IMRs, after Madhya Pradesh (56), Assam (55) and Orissa (53).

**Table 3.4** Gives top 100 districts in order of IMR sorted in alphabetical order of states

| S. no. | State | List of top 100 districts in order of IMR sorted on alphabetical order of states | S. no. | State | List of top 100 districts in order of IMR sorted on alphabetical order of states | S. no. | State | List of top 100 districts in order of IMR sorted on alphabetical order of states |
|---|---|---|---|---|---|---|---|---|
| 1 | Assam | Kokrajhar | 24 | Madhya Pradesh | Sidhi | 47 | Orissa | Balangir |
| 2 | Assam | Dhubri | 25 | Madhya Pradesh | Ratlam | 48 | Orissa | Rayagada |
| 3 | Assam | Darrang | 26 | Madhya Pradesh | Jhabua | 49 | Rajasthan | Karauli |
| 4 | Assam | Marigaon | 27 | Madhya Pradesh | Barwani | 50 | Rajasthan | Sawai Madhopur |
| 5 | Assam | Nagaon | 28 | Madhya Pradesh | East Nimar | 51 | Rajasthan | Barmer |
| 6 | Assam | Sonitpur | 29 | Madhya Pradesh | Vidisha | 52 | Rajasthan | Jalor |
| 7 | Assam | Karimganj | 30 | Madhya Pradesh | Sehore | 53 | Rajasthan | Bundi |
| 8 | Bihar | Sitamarhi | 31 | Madhya Pradesh | Raisen | 54 | Rajasthan | Bhilwara |
| 9 | Bihar | Madhepura | 32 | Madhya Pradesh | Betul | 55 | Rajasthan | Rajsamand |
| 10 | Bihar | Khagaria | 33 | Madhya Pradesh | Hoshangabad | 56 | Rajasthan | Dungarpur |
| 11 | Madhya Pradesh | Sheopur | 34 | Madhya Pradesh | Katni | 57 | Rajasthan | Jhalawar |
| 12 | Madhya Pradesh | Datia | 35 | Madhya Pradesh | Narsimhapur | 58 | Uttar Pradesh | Saharanpur |
| 13 | Madhya Pradesh | Shivpuri | 36 | Madhya Pradesh | Dindori | 59 | Uttar Pradesh | Jyotiba Phule Nagar |
| 14 | Madhya Pradesh | Guna | 37 | Madhya Pradesh | Mandla | 60 | Uttar Pradesh | Bulandshahr |
| 15 | Madhya Pradesh | Tikamgarh | 38 | Madhya Pradesh | Chhindwara | 61 | Uttar Pradesh | Aligarh |
| 16 | Madhya Pradesh | Chhatarpur | 39 | Madhya Pradesh | Seoni | 62 | Uttar Pradesh | Etah |
| 17 | Madhya Pradesh | Panna | 40 | Madhya Pradesh | Balaghat | 63 | Uttar Pradesh | Budaun |
| 18 | Madhya Pradesh | Sagar | 41 | Orissa | Bargarh | 64 | Uttar Pradesh | Bareilly |
| 19 | Madhya Pradesh | Damoh | 42 | Orissa | Dhenkanal | 65 | Uttar Pradesh | Pilibhit |
| 20 | Madhya Pradesh | Satna | 43 | Orissa | Nayagarh | 66 | Uttar Pradesh | Shahjahanpur |
| 21 | Madhya Pradesh | Rewa | 44 | Orissa | Khordha | 67 | Uttar Pradesh | Lakhimpur Kheri |
| 22 | Madhya Pradesh | Umaria | 45 | Orissa | Puri | 68 | Uttar Pradesh | Sitapur |
| 23 | Madhya Pradesh | Shahdol | 46 | Orissa | Kandhamal | 69 | Uttar Pradesh | Hardoi |

*Contd...*

*Contd...*

| S. no. | State | List of top 100 districts in order of IMR sorted on alphabetical order of states | S. no. | State | List of top 100 districts in order of IMR sorted on alphabetical order of states | S. no. | State | List of top 100 districts in order of IMR sorted on alphabetical order of states |
|---|---|---|---|---|---|---|---|---|
| 70 | Uttar Pradesh | Farrukhabad | 81 | Uttar Pradesh | Bahraich | 92 | Uttar Pradesh | Mau |
| 71 | Uttar Pradesh | Kannauj | 82 | Uttar Pradesh | Shrawasti | 93 | Uttar Pradesh | Ballia |
| 72 | Uttar Pradesh | Jalaun | 83 | Uttar Pradesh | Balrampur | 94 | Uttar Pradesh | Jaunpur |
| 73 | Uttar Pradesh | Lalitpur | 84 | Uttar Pradesh | Gonda | 95 | Uttar Pradesh | Ghazipur |
| 74 | Uttar Pradesh | Chitrakoot | 85 | Uttar Pradesh | Siddharthnagar | 96 | Uttar Pradesh | Chandauli |
| 75 | Uttar Pradesh | Pratapgarh | 86 | Uttar Pradesh | Basti | 97 | Uttar Pradesh | Varanasi |
| 76 | Uttar Pradesh | Kaushambi | 87 | Uttar Pradesh | Sant Kabir Nagar | 98 | Uttar Pradesh | Sant Ravidas Nagar Bhadohi |
| 77 | Uttar Pradesh | Allahabad | 88 | Uttar Pradesh | Maharajganj | 99 | Uttar Pradesh | Mirzapur |
| 78 | Uttar Pradesh | Barabanki | 89 | Uttar Pradesh | Kushinagar | 100 | Uttarakhand | Hardwar |
| 79 | Uttar Pradesh | Faizabad | 90 | Uttar Pradesh | Deoria | | | |
| 80 | Uttar Pradesh | Ambedkar Nagar | 91 | Uttar Pradesh | Azamgarh | | | |

However, U.P. and Orissa are the only two states in the country to register a fall of four points, the highest, in the last year. IMR for the country has reduced by two points – from 44 to 42 per 1,000 live births. While Assam has registered no fall, Delhi, Gujarat, Karnataka, Madhya Pradesh and Rajasthan all have registered a fall of three points in their IMR. Infant mortality rate in India has declined by 30 percent over the past 10 years.

The most significant improvements have occurred in the states of Tamil Nadu, West Bengal and Maharashtra which had percentage declines in IMR as 46, 37, and 35, respectively. Orissa and Karnataka also had fairly good percentage declines as 33 and 29, respectively. Kerala continues to be the best performing state with an IMR of just 12. These data are encouraging, though it is still much higher than the MDG target of 28 per 1,000 live births by 2015.

Infant mortality declined by only 23 percent in a decade in urban areas across India, as opposed to a 27 percent decline in rural areas. Two states, Karnataka and Assam, showed an increase in neonatal deaths in urban areas, while urban Delhi remained unchanged for the past 10 years. Delhi is the only major state that has seen a worsening of IMR, particularly in rural areas. This is attributed to large settlements of slum-dwellers in the rural periphery of Delhi and the lack of civic amenities and poor living conditions. Other poor performing states are Rajasthan (59), Assam (61), Uttar Pradesh (63), Orissa (65), and Madhya Pradesh (67).

The positive impact of programs like the Janani Suraksha Yojana that encourages institutional deliveries was clearly seen in the decline in neonatal deaths in rural Chhattisgarh and Orissa, both being economically backward states.

### 3.9.1 IMR in UP: past trends

It may be interesting to study the trends in IMR in the state of Uttar Pradesh. The state is a very poor performer in terms of both maternal and infant mortality as seen from Tables 3.1 and 3.4. It is expected that the scenario will not be much different in other poor performing states.

Though the IMR drastically declined from 167 in 1971 to 83 in 2002 in the state of UP, it was still at elevated levels. Table 3.5 gives the estimates of IMR for UP in some selected years. During the decade 1971–80, the percentage decline in IMR was 4.8, and during 1981–90 it was 34. But during 1991–2000, there was a reversal of trend as the decline percentage was only 13.4. However, during 2002–11 the decline percentage again picked up to a 31.4. The maximum reduction in infant mortality is achieved post 2000. The IMR declined by 31 points between 2000 and 2012.

It may be interesting to investigate the reasons behind it.

**Table 3.5** IMR over years (1971–2002) in UP

| Year | IMR |
|---|---|
| 1971 | 167 |
| 1980 | 159 |
| 1981 | 150 |
| 1990 | 99 |
| 1991 | 97 |
| 2000 | 84 |
| 2001 | 84 |
| 2002 | 83 |
| 2005 NFHS-3 | 72.7 |
| 2011 | 57 |
| 2012 | 53 |

### 3.9.2 The NMR factor

The disproportionate decline in post-neonatal as compared to neonatal mortality is the major cause of sluggish decline in IMR. The neonatal mortality had a percentage share of 54 in the IMR during the period 1971–1979 (Table 3.6), while the remaining 46 percent was due to the post-neonatal mortality. The neonatal mortality as percentage of IMR, however, registered upward trends during the following periods: 60 percent during 1980–1989 and 62 percent during 1990–1997.

The AHS estimates for IMR are 70 and 68 in 2011 and 2012, respectively. The AHS estimate of NMR in 2011 is 50. If we go by these figures, then postneonatal mortality rate (PNMR) in 2011 is 20. In percentage terms these are 71.4 for NMR and 29.6 for PNMR. These figures indicate that declines in PNMR are at a faster rate than in NMR. The scenario is not much different at the country level. Thus there is an urgent need to focus on neonatal mortality for any further reduction in IMR.

It is observed that there is a considerable decline in IMR during 2002 to 2012. The IMR has declined from 83 to 53 (Table 3.5). The analysis of Table 3.6 indicates that there is further scope of reducing IMR by concentrating in the decline of NMR.

**Table 3.6** NMR and PNMR as percentage of IMR

| Year | NMR | PNMR | Year | NMR | PNMR |
|---|---|---|---|---|---|
| 1971 | 59 | 41 | 1985 | 61 | 38 |
| 1972 | 47 | 53 | 1986 | 59 | 41 |
| 1973 | 53 | 47 | 1987 | 56 | 44 |
| 1974 | 55 | 45 | 1988 | 56 | 44 |
| 1975 | 51 | 49 | 1989 | 58 | 42 |
| 1976 | 58 | 42 | Average | 60 | 40 |
| 1977 | 54 | 46 | 1990 | 66 | 34 |
| 1978 | 56 | 44 | 1991 | 66 | 34 |
| 1979 | 56 | 43 | 1992 | 59 | 41 |
| Average | 54 | 46 | 1993 | 61 | 38 |
| 1980 | 58 | 43 | 1994 | 61 | 39 |
| 1981 | 64 | 36 | 1995 | 60 | 40 |
| 1982 | 64 | 36 | 1996 | 60 | 40 |
| 1983 | 67 | 33 | 1997 | 60 | 40 |
| 1984 | 61 | 39 | Average | 62 | 38 |

### 3.9.3 Health and welfare programs

Various family-welfare-oriented programs were launched from time to time since early eighties with a view to improve maternal and child health care practices. The National Health Policy (NHP) of India launched in 1983 had the objective to provide universal and comprehensive primary health services to the population. It included (a) maternal and child health care, including family planning; (b) immunization against infectious disease; (c) promotion of food supply and proper nutrition; (d) adequate supply of safe water and basic sanitation. The quality of the health service delivery remained poor, with limited funding for health, unresponsive health care staff and absentee doctors, etc. It was not until 1990s when funding increased and the revival of the programs like Child Survival and Safe Motherhood (CSSM) and Reproductive and Child Health Program (RCH) brought the desired funding and catalytic effect to revive the PHC system in the country.

The health system was further strengthened with the launch of National Population Policy (NPP) in 2000, and strengthening of NHP in 2002 to ensure equitable access to health services, and increased allocation of resources to PHC. The NHP-2002 also focused upon strengthening the decentralized public health system by establishing new infrastructure in deficient areas and upgrading existing institutions.

National Rural Health Mission (NRHM) was launched in 2005. NRHM is an umbrella health program aimed to bring fundamental architectural corrections in the Indian public health system; also envisages a synergistic primary health care approach for decentralized health management at the village and district level. It can be said that NRHM brought the necessary political will, funding and desired direction to revive the system and the PHC system in India has witnessed a major shift in since NRHM.

The PHC definitely gets the credit for bringing the health services to the rural people, which were largely focused for urban areas, till mid-70s. The involvement of individuals, families and communities in the promotion of their own health and development is an essential component of PHC. The community participation includes formation of Village Health and Sanitation Committee (VHSC) decentralization and involvement of Panchayati Raj Institutions at various levels (from village to district level) for ownership of public health service delivery within their domain.

The NRHM has made efforts to converge with different health related sectors through District Health Society, Village Health and Sanitation Committee, Anganwadi Centres and the collaboration with non-governmental and civil organizations, to supplement and strengthen health service delivery.

The recruitment of Accredited Social Health Activist (ASHA) to act as interface between the community and health services is based upon those evidences and is also a revival of VHGs with the lessons learned from the implementation experiences from that scheme.

The RCH I focused on strengthening facility-based newborn care and the RCH II provided provision of ENC, irrespective of the place of delivery – home or facility. The functioning primary health care facility and the availability of skilled attendance at birth and EmOC have a huge potential to improve ENC and reduce neonatal deaths. The quality of facilities at urban and rural health centres still need major improvement as the SBA training does not adequately cover skills for newborn care, roll-out is slow, and there is shortage of necessary equipment at the facilities.

The Gadchiroli trial (Bang et al., 1999) has shown the usefulness of HBNC and following this, the government has been implementing community- and home-based postnatal care (to both mothers and babies) through ASHAs, in selected districts of the 5 states. However, there are concerns regarding the impact, when an initiative is scaled up at a larger level. The capability of ASHA's to provide quality newborn care is yet to be investigated. The quality of newborn services delivered in the community and home are difficult to evaluate, particularly in the absence of effective mechanisms for monitoring and supportive supervision in the field.

Sick Newborn Care Units (SNCU) and Newborn Corners are being established at district hospitals and CHC/PHC's, respectively, to provide quality care for the newborn babies referred from the community and sub-centres. The Purulia model of SNCU has shown that how quality neonatal care can be given in a resource-constrained environment and without high-tech equipments.

The Integrated Management of Neonatal and Childhood Illnesses (IMNCI) approach encompasses a range of interventions to prevent and manage major childhood illnesses. The strategy includes components of provision for both community- and facility-based care such as improved case management through up-gradation of skill; strengthening health care infrastructure; and improved household practices and community involvement. The IMNCI is currently being implemented in 193 districts and more than 70,000 personnel have been trained.

Universalization of ICDS, convergence of mid-day meal scheme with rural and urban development, and establishment of Nutrition Rehabilitation Centres (NRC) for the management of severely undernourished children were some other programs which aimed at enhancing health care.

Though Janani Suraksha Yojna (JSY) focused upon directly on the reduction of maternal mortality, it had indirect benefits on child survival and care. These additional benefits are yet to be evaluated but it has been considered as one of the success stories. JSY has clearly increased the proportion of institutional deliveries in poor performing states of India. The transport mechanism used in the JSY scheme paved the way for developing an effective referral mechanism in India. The transport used for JSY is also being used for the referral of sick children by several states of the country.

The ARI and diarrhea are the two leading causes of child mortality and morbidity in the country. Though diarrhoea guideline has been revised, orientation trainings have not rolled out. Zinc tablets to all cases of diarrhoea are expected to be delivered through same mechanism. Similar is the story of prophylaxis programs for iron and vitamin A, as the coverage with both of these micronutrients has been low.

All of the above initiatives, particularly those launched in late nineties and after, contributed in their own way in controlling IMR in the entire country. Other possible contributor is the intense involvement of major international and national agencies. These agencies have launched numerous maternal and infant survival programs which have generated increased awareness on safe maternal and newborn health practices which include hygiene and sanitation among others. It is hoped that both maternal and infant mortality would see accelerated declines in coming years. These aspects are discussed further in Section 3.11.

## 3.10 Estimating infant mortality

The issues relating to the complexities involved in estimating MMR have been discussed in earlier sections. The problems involved in the estimation of IMR are also of similar nature though these are of smaller magnitude. First is the problem of sample size requirement. Assuming an expected IMR of around 40 per thousand live births, the required sample size for 10 percent relative margin of error and with design effect 1.5 is 14400 live births. To get such births, a total population of approximately 5 lakhs is to be tracked. This is an extremely difficult task if IMR estimates are required for district or even for smaller states and union territories. The complexities are similar to those of estimating MMR particularly in terms of getting good quality and reliable data on infant deaths and the associated factors.

## 3.11 Status of neonatal care

Effective neonatal care practices have a direct bearing on neonatal deaths. The first 45 days of the baby's life are very crucial. Traditionally also the newborn is handled with greater care during this period. It may be interesting to examine the current practices of neonatal care. Some of these practices have already discussed in Section 3.6 in respect of MISP project in Madhya Pradesh. A more detailed analysis of the current practices of neonatal care in Uttar Pradesh is presented in this section.

Maternal and childcare practices are very poor in Uttar Pradesh. Various factors contributing to the slow decline in IMR revolve mostly around poor knowledge and attitude of the community towards neonatal care and also around the lower social, cultural and health status of women. It is necessary to conduct studies that would throw light on the basic problems. Though immunization is expected to reduce post-neonatal mortality, for further reduction in infant mortality, neonatal mortality must be lowered. In this direction, few efforts particularly on home-based neonatal care have been made by Bang et al. (1999) in Gadchirolli district of Maharashtra and by Saksham project during 2003–07 in Shivgarh of U.P.

Before we discuss Gadchiroli and Shivgarh trials, it may be worthwhile to describe a study on knowledge, attitude, practice and behavior of the community for newborn care. The GTZ supported SRIJAN study was carried out by Vatsalya in 2003 in Uttar Pradesh. The study involved 4954 families with a population of 39023 in 13 districts of UP, spread all over Eastern, Central and Bundelkhand regions of the state. The analysis of this study throws light on some new features and characteristics, which would have to be addressed to achieve success similar to that was observed in the Gadchiroli and Shivgarh interventions.

A female animator selected from the community conducted the survey regarding the neonate care. The survey also involved observation of the delivery process and follow up of newborns till the 28$^{th}$ day of birth at home. One supervisor was also selected to help the animator for each area. The animator and supervisor were trained to take histories of pregnant women, observe the process of labor and newborns and to record findings. The trainings included live delivery observation and exposure visits in government hospitals.

In all, 624 pregnant women who were in the third trimester of their pregnancy were followed for observation of birth process, and newborn care for 28 days (on day 1, 2, 3, 5, 7, 14, 21, 28 of childbirth and on any other day when required). The animators were provided digital thermometer and weighing machine to record temperature and weight of the newborn. They monitored the newborns for a time period of 28 days after birth or until the mother left the village or the newborn died. Verbal autopsy was also done for 89 cases of death within 28 days of childbirth.

The findings revealed that ANC was very poor among the women. Only 33 percent of the mothers reported of ANC check up. Even out of those who went for ANC check up, only 28 percent reported of having three check-ups. Further, 36 percent had their first dose of TT vaccine as late as in 6 months. Majority of women (80%) consumed less food during pregnancy.

Of the 567 birth process observed, 86 percent were home deliveries of which 70 percent were performed by untrained *dai* or elderly women/ neighbors. The various reasons reported by the women for not opting institutional deliveries was: (i) ill behavior of the staff at facility, (ii) distance from primary health centre, and (iii) unavailability of money and transport.

At the time of birth process, observations were made on aspects of newborn care, like place of delivery; bathing the newborn, breast-feeding practices, cord care etc. These practices have direct or indirect bearing on neonatal mortality. The room should be warm enough but only 45 percent of the respondents made any effort to warm the room; 29 percent used mud stoves, 8 percent fire and 8 percent opted for other methods like dung cakes. Over three-fourth of newborn were given bath before third day. About 69 percent of neonates were given bath after birth. Almost all babies who were bathed received bath within 24 hours of birth. However, nearly 38 percent of them did not use warm water for bathing during winters also. Fifty percent of the babies were bathed in open area. Over 18 percent were wiped dry immediately after birth while 60 percent were dried after placenta was removed. Over 19 percent were kept warm by keeping baby in skin contact. About 53 percent of the mothers did not use any clothes for wrapping the newborn after bath. But the data show practice of not covering the newborn's head as nearly 50 percent of the babies were wrapped keeping the head open. Similarly, 50 percent of the respondents did not use warm clothes for the neonate in winters. Weighing of the child at birth was rare. Only 29 percent of children were weighed after the delivery. Among these only 32 percent were weighed within 7 days of birth. Out of the 50 percent neonates who were weighed, nearly 49 percent were lbw with weight less than 2.5 kg.

Among 96 percent of the mothers, the cord was tied with thread. The mothers were asked if the tying material was boiled or not and only 31 percent of them replied in affirmative. The lowest percentage was reported in Bundelkhand region (26%). Out of 31 percent, who boiled it, only 27 percent adhered to the norms and boiled the thread for over 15 minutes. Majority (88%) of the mothers reported of tying the cord at one place. Nearly 30 percent amongst them reported of cord bleeding. It was surprising to find that in 30 percent of cases two different persons were involved in birthing and cutting the cord. Although most of them mentioned about new blade being used to cut the cord still materials like old blade, knife was used (8%).

In majority of cases, the first breastfeed was given after more than 8 hours, the reasons for delay being mostly physiological or were related to social custom. There were no colostrums feeding in more than half cases. Instead they were fed cow's milk, jaggery and water. Only 8 percent mentioned that they had not fed anything else apart from breast milk in the first 6 months of the child. Average age of initiation of complementary feeding for less than 1 year children was 6.6 months, while that for children aged 12–23 months was 8 months. Nearly three-fourth of children aged between 7 months to <1 year age were initiated to complementary feeding. Although 91 percent of mothers reported that after birth child was kept with them, only 11 percent of them put the neonate to breast. Thus the practice of immediate breastfeeding was rarely followed. About 64 percent of the neonates were deprived of colostrums feeding. Nearly 85 percent of the neonates were given pre-lacteal feed which was mostly cow's milk (32%). Honey was the second choice for feeding the neonate (21%).

As regards, complications in neonates, fever, itching, cough, and jaundice were more commonly mentioned problems in neonates. In majority of the cases, the mothers either took the child to a private hospital in the village or to a private doctor. The facility of PHC/sub-centres was used only in 3 percent of cases. More than one-fifth of the index children had suffered from loose motions in last 14 days. The usage of oral rehydration supplements (ORS) was abysmally low. Only 5 percent respondents mentioned using ORS. The incidence of high fever accompanied by rapid or difficult breathing in past 2 weeks was reported to be at 20 percent.

It was important to assess the relation between the knowledge, attitude, practice and behavior of the community in regard to neonatal care and the causes of neonatal deaths. Verbal autopsy can provide some leads on this. The verbal autopsy was conducted for 100 neonates. The village animators who were involved in KAPB study conducted the verbal autopsies also. Out of 100 births, only 39 were female and 61 were males. There were only 89 live births and the remaining 11 were stillbirths; 2 were macerated (confirmed stillbirths) and 9 were fresh deaths. During focus group discussion, it was evident that the stillbirths are grossly under reported because community has a tendency to hide such births.

Out of 89 live births, timing (day) of death could be ascertained only for 81 deaths. Out of these, 69 deaths occurred within one week, 9 during the second week and remaining 3 neonates died in the late neonatal period of 16–28 days. Over 85 percent deaths occurred during the first week, whereas 96.3 percent of total deaths occurred up to second week. This suggests that intervention on preventing deaths must take place during first week, and even during starting days of the first week. Such a strategy may also be helpful in preventing neonatal deaths in subsequent weeks because of its carry over effects.

Among the causes of neonatal deaths, asphyxia/birth injury was the most prominent one accounting for 41 deaths. Other major causes identified were sepsis (septicaemia – 2, tetanus – 3, pneumonia – 7), and respiratory distress syndrome (7). The cause of death on 1st day was either birth asphyxia or prematurity. In some cases findings suggested more than one factor (hypothermia and prematurity) responsible for death. There were also many associated findings with birth asphyxia. Six percent of birth asphyxia cases were in breech presentation. Prematurity in 6 percent and hypothermia in 3 percent cases were associated with birth asphyxia. Further, 22 percent cases showed prolonged labor, out of which 15 percent showed meconium-stained liquor. Hypothermia alone was responsible for death in only one case, though it was contributory factor in prematurity, pneumonia and birth asphyxia.

The next important cause of death was sepsis (22 cases). Out of 22 deaths, 10 cases were of pneumonia, 5 were of tetanus and 7 of septicemia. Though tetanus can be prevented by adopting safe delivery practices and universal immunization of pregnant women, it still accounted for 6 percent of neonatal deaths. Prematurity was also a reason in many neonatal deaths whereas deaths due to diarrhea were reported in mid neonatal period.

Efforts to reduce mortality through proper care of neonates are likely to be very rewarding. These should focus around important determinants (health and nutritional, socioeconomic, environmental, behavioral determinants). Focus should be to provide affordable, cost-effective and culturally appropriate solutions to the communities who need it most. However, due to wide regional variations each state/region must evolve its own program primarily focusing on the major determinants in that area/state. It should be borne in mind that majority of newborn babies require only basic primary care, which is both feasible and affordable.

Some important issues that need to be addressed in U.P. are now discussed. Eighty five percent of deliveries in rural area took place at home. Majority of home deliveries was performed with no assistance/ help of traditional birth attendants. Community women had maximum faith over the family or neighborhood elderly women for delivery rather than ANMs or doctors because they remained available for full package of multiplicity of services even after delivery. ANM covers 5–7 villages and often lives outside the assigned area. She is often not available to conduct deliveries or to attend to the sick neonates who may need immediate attention, day or night.

For reduction in the neonatal mortality among deliveries at home, there is a need to impart skills in conducting safe deliveries to all the possible grass-root providers including home-based attendants. This approach can be seen as add on to the SBA strategy in Section 3.7. Home-based care and community involvement becomes the most important issue to be addressed. It is necessary to identify stakeholders (mothers / mothers-in-law / elderly person/ neighbors) in the community who are likely to be available at the time of delivery. A community chosen health worker capable of antenatal care and midwifery can transform the neonatal health scenario.

In Uttar Pradesh, an important cause of maternal and neonate complications is tetanus. The community should be advocated that two doses of TT vaccine given one month apart during early pregnancy is nearly 100 percent effective in preventing tetanus among newborns and mothers. The first TT dose should be administered in the 4th or 5th month and second after a month's gap.

Ideally 2 hours of rest and sleep at daytime is recommended for the pregnant women. Rest during daytime is important particularly for the young anemic women eating less during pregnancy. There were various reasons supporting this practice but the most common was the wrong notion of "problem of obstruction during delivery" due to increased weight of the child. Importance of additional diet during pregnancy and proper rest should be emphasized and the pregnant, lactating women and the family members should be told about iron and iodine deficiency and its causative as well as preventable factors. Proper diet and prevention from anemia as well as iodine deficiency could prevent low birth weight, which is an important predisposing factor in large number of neonatal mortality.

Other factors like environment at the time of delivery, newborn care, etc., also affect neonatal mortality directly or indirectly. For keeping the room warm for the neonate, mud stoves, fire and dung cakes were normally used. But many of those who warmed the room did so with the purpose of getting rid of the bad air and evil spirit and not for warming the room. This practice has a hazardous impact as rooms with poor ventilation will lead to suffocation (room filled with smoke) and in turn to asphyxia.

The findings revealed that poor practices were widely prevalent relating to giving bath to the neonate and keeping him warm. All these practices could cause hypothermia and ultimately result in neonatal death. So there is an intense need of disseminating information about correct practices. The mothers and other family members should be made aware about Kangaroo Care for keeping the baby warm. In a newborn the head is larger than the rest of the body; hence, they have a big surface area. As a result maximum heat loss takes place from head so it is important to cover the head of newborns.

The newborn are dressed properly only after "Chathi", a ritual performed on sixth day of birth.

Cord bleeding might lead to anemia in newborns and presence of such bleeding may further encourage infections. Hence the cord should be tied at two places after milking. Preferably same person should be involved in birthing and cutting the cord. If the cord cutter is not present at the time of delivery, the time gap could lead to infections or other problems. The problem is that cord cutter is considered to be untouchable or someone who is looked down upon. Hence it should be advocated that cord cutting is not an inferior work and one person should be performing both the task.

Another harmful practice observed was application of various materials on the cord of the newborn. This might lead to cord infection or sepsis. Ideally the umbilical cord should be tied within 30 minutes so that baby could be cleaned and wrapped immediately but this practice was followed by half of the mothers. Rest of them tied the cord within 1–6 hours. This is sufficient time to expose the newborn to hypothermia especially in winter months. An unhygienic environment exposes them to the risk of septicemia, pneumonia and diarrhea. Systemic bacterial infections are the biggest killers of newborn infants. These infections manifest clinically as septicemia, pneumonia, meningitis, diarrhoea and tetanus neonatorum. The trained health worker and the family/community members should be advocated that all a newborn need is a clean and warm room, to be dried immediately, to be observed for breathing, and to be given to the mother for warmth and breast-feeding.

Proper thermal protection is important to ensure safety of newborn. Effective basic resuscitation can revive more than three-fourth of newborns with birth asphyxia. Regardless of the cause of birth asphyxia, the most important initial step should be ventilation. The main aim is to ensure oxygenation and to initiate spontaneous breathing. Every birth attendant must be trained in resuscitation and must have resuscitation equipment and supplies in perfect condition. If the newborn does not cry or breathe at all, or is gasping within 30 seconds of birth, and after being dried, the essential steps of resuscitation should be taken immediately. The important steps in resuscitation are prevention of heat loss, opening the airway and positive pressure ventilation that starts within the first minute of life. Prevention of heat loss is critical. Each newborn should be dried first and then covered with a dry towel. Drying provides sufficient stimulation of breathing in mildly depressed newborn and no further stimulation is required. Slapping the newborn, soaking it in cold water, sprinkling it with water, stimulating the anus, using the onion juice, cooking the placenta and milking the cord are a few examples of ineffective and harmful practices still in use. Resuscitation is also needed more often if the newborn is preterm and/or growth retarded. The lower the gestational age, the more difficulties the newborn may have in starting breathing spontaneously. Preterm newborns often take longer than term infants to start breathing spontaneously and their breathing may be difficult. These newborns are more likely to require referral to a special care unit. Health care institution should introduce basic newborn resuscitation first. Basic resuscitation should also become part of the pre-service training of health care providers trained in midwifery. Few steps should also be told to the family members and the community people as they are the ones that perform delivery most of the times.

Besides the direct causes of newborn deaths, 60–80 percent of newborn deaths occurred among the lbw infants and more than half among these had very low birth weight. The priority agenda for the programs, therefore, should be management of (i) lbw, (ii) sepsis and (iii) asphyxia.

The mother is the best source of warmth, affection, food and protection from infection. Whenever a newborn is put to the breast of mother, he gets warmth from the mother's body i.e. skin-to-skin transfer of heat which helps in preventing hypothermia. Although great emphasis is being laid on colostrums and breast feeding but the low percentage shows that the message is not properly being disseminated. Colostrum was normally considered to be yellowish and impure milk and therefore the newborn was not breastfed for first 3 days. The early use of prelacteal feed may cause infections like diarrhea which could ultimately lead to neonatal death. In the wake of consequences, it is imperative to explain the importance of avoiding these feeds and encouraging feeding of colostrums. Ideally a newborn should be breast fed after every three hours or when it is required.

Although standard advice is to admit every ill neonate to hospital, hospitals with facilities for neonatal care are inaccessible and cost prohibitive for rural and urban slum populations. Until such time that institutional deliveries are possible, all home deliveries should be attended by trained personnel. Regular visits by these persons should be done throughout the 28 days. Early identification and referral of newborns with health problems is also important.

Community mobilization is particularly important because of the unique traditional/ cultural practices associated with maternal and newborn health. It is essential from the beginning to mobilize and involve community leaders and representative of local government agencies, women's groups, and local NGO. At the community level, promotion of the essential newborn care package is the highest priority. This will involve educating and encouraging families and training birth attendants and community health workers. Enabling caretakers to identify health problems in newborn and seek early and appropriate care is another priority.

## 3.12 Effective neonatal care projects

Two important neonatal care projects described earlier are now discussed in details in this section. These are Gadchiroli and Shivgarh projects.

### 3.12.1 Gadchiroli project

Ideally it is a sound decision to admit every ill neonate to hospital, but hospitals with facilities for neonatal care are not only costly but are also inaccessible for rural populations. Traditional beliefs and practical difficulties also prohibit many parents to move ill neonates from home. This is the main reason why most neonatal deaths occur at home. Because of problems in timely transporting sick neonates to hospitals, those who arrive are generally seriously ill. This scenario suggests about the alternative to provide neonatal care, especially managing sepsis (pneumonia, septicaemia, and meningitis) at home.

Management of children with pneumonia, diarrhoea, or malaria by health workers is the main strategy of several child-survival programmes and of the Integrated Management of Childhood Illnesses programme. This strategy, however, has not been used for management of sepsis in neonates. Earlier efforts by Bang and coworkers in management of pneumonia in neonates with oral co-trimoxazole given by village health workers resulted in 20 percent reduction in neonatal mortality. This success led them to believe that management of neonatal sepsis at home was possible.

Realising that neonatal care is not available to most neonates in developing countries because hospitals are inaccessible and costly, Bang et al. (1999) developed a package of home-based neonatal care, including management of sepsis, and tested it in the field, with the hypothesis that it would reduce the neonatal mortality rate by at least 25 percent in 3 years.

There were 39 intervention and 47 control villages in tribal district, Gadchiroli, about 1000 km from the state capital, Mumbai. Baseline data were collected during 1993–95, followed by the introduction of neonatal care in the intervention villages 1995–98. Village health workers trained in neonatal care made home visits and managed birth asphyxia, premature birth or low birth weight, hypothermia, and breastfeeding problems. They diagnosed and treated neonatal sepsis. They were provided assistance by trained traditional birth attendants. Health education and fortnightly supervisory visits were also arranged. All births and deaths in the intervention and the control area during the period 1993–98 were recorded to estimate mortality rates.

Intervention and control areas were similar at the time of baseline in terms of population characteristics and mortality rates. Baseline neonatal mortality rate in the intervention and the control areas was 62 and 58 per 1000 live births, respectively. In the third year of intervention 93 percent of neonates received home-based care. Neonatal, infant, and perinatal mortality rates in the intervention area (net percentage reduction) compared with the control area, were 25.5 (62.2%), 38.8 (45.7%), and 47.8 (71.0%), respectively ($p<0.001$). Case fatality in neonatal sepsis declined from 16.6 percent (163 cases) before treatment, to 2.8 percent (71 cases) after treatment by village health workers ($p<0.01$).

Home-based neonatal care, including management of sepsis was not only acceptable, feasible and highly cost effective; it reduced neonatal and infant mortality by nearly 50 percent among the undernourished, illiterate, rural study population.

Reasons for the high acceptance of home-based care in Bang et al. study were: the huge unmet need of neonatal care in villages, involvement of traditional birth attendants, health education, good quality of care, availability of care at home by a village health worker resident in the village, successful management of sepsis, the faith of rural people in injections, and good motivation, training, supervision and performance-linked remuneration for the village health workers. Along with this, effective monitoring by qualified doctors for validation and taking remedial measures was also a contributing factor towards the success of such management.

To apply any strategy in a population, it is necessary to assess the social, cultural and economical background of the population on the neonatal care practices. Collecting a baseline data can help to attain this objective. The strategy by Bang et al. was applied to a limited area within a district, which was also compact and contiguous having near similar neonatal care practices before start of the project. Its success/replication and adaptation over a wider range of population need to be reaffirmed.

### 3.12.2 Shivgarh project

Another very important contribution on reduction in infant and neonatal mortality came from the Saksham Project by using non-medical homemade care. It was implemented during 2003–2007 by a collaborative research work of the John Hopkins University, USA, and King George's Medical University (KGMU), Lucknow. This project was a community-based program in rural India to promote newborn care practices through community mobilization and behavior change communications. It was implemented in 299 villages in Shivgarh Block, Raebareli District, Uttar Pradesh, covering 117,000 people. Many of the results in the project are available in Kumar et al. (2008).

A positive impact on reducing neonatal mortality was noted by focusing on community mobilization and home visits during pregnancy and neonatal period to promote optimal newborn care prevention practices including care seeking for illness.

The Shivgarh study which was a community-based cluster randomized controlled trial investigated impact of community health workers through home visits and community mobilization to prevent newborn mortality. Workers offered neither referral nor treatment services and only educated families about essential newborn care including prevention of hypothermia. Community perceptions of the cause of neonatal death – predominantly evil spirits – were found to be very different than a clinical model. Perceived cause of neonatal deaths was the single most important determinant of preventive behaviors and care/care seeking for newborns. The majority of newborns in the study catchment area were given some form of medication and care was predominantly sought from the unqualified medical practitioners (40–50%), government doctors (10–15%) and self (20–25%).

The intervention involved 7 days of training and a cadre of predominantly male community health workers, who identified pregnant women and educated them in essential newborn care. Two antenatal and two postnatal visits were conducted, with the first postnatal visit on day one and the second on day three or four. There was one community health worker per 3500 and one supervisor for every seven workers. An early analysis of the intervention data suggested a 50 percent reduction in NMR.

To summarize, the project has a sustainable robust community health system approach which provides convincing scientific evidence that communities do have the potential to save newborn lives if they are given the right tools and respect. Vaccines and behavior change management are two scientifically proven interventions for prevention of preventable diseases. Water and hygiene are very important risk factors for neonatal and maternal mortality particularly deaths due to infection, e.g. neonatal sepsis, pneumonia, diarrhea, maternal infection etc. We need to ensure that the visits by community health workers are made during the most critical period where the newborns are at highest risk. We need to focus on strengthening the quality of services in facilities and focus on evidence-based care at the most critical time within the first hour and the first day.

# 4
# Undernutrition

## 4.1 Types of undernutrition

The nutritional status of women and young children is one of the most important indicators not only for judging their health status, but also is indicative of development. It is closely related to food security, level of poverty, status of women, growth rate of population and access of the population to health, education, safe drinking water, environmental sanitation, hygiene and other social services. Nutritional status gives the status of an individual in terms of nutritional deficiency or excesses. It can be assessed by measurement of anthropometric aspects like weight, and height according to age and dietary intakes. It also involves clinical assessments for clinical signs of deficiency and also biochemical measures of blood.

The term malnutrition implies undernutrition as well as overnutrition or obesity. If there is inadequate or excess protein or calorie intake, it may lead to protein energy (calorie) malnutrition (PEM); undernutrition if inadequate intake, otherwise, overnutrition or obesity. However, undernutrition is no longer considered as an outcome of food deficiency or a health problem but as a multi-dimensional problem inter-facing all efforts of developing human resources. Besides protein–energy undernutrition, other forms of undernutrition are vitamin A and iodine deficiency disorders, and nutritional anemia. Each one of these is discussed in Chapters 4 and 6.

Undernutrition is widely prevalent in India among children below 5 years. The nutritional status of Indian women is also poor. Undernutrition in expectant mothers has a significant impact on the health of the infants. In order to improve the survival status and development of children and women, it is essential to find out the nutritional status of young children and women.

At present, there is very little micro-level information available on nutritional status of young children and women in our country. NFHS-1 carried out in 1992–93 provides only state-level analysis on nutritional status of young children less than 4 years of age. NFHS-2 was carried out in 1998–99, giving nutritional status of young children under 3 years of age and also of women in the age group 15–45. In between these, on a request from UNICEF, in 1995, IASDS also carried out nutrition survey in 17 districts of Uttar Pradesh which also included two districts of Uttarakhand. It gave the regional and district profiles of nutritional status of children up to 5 years and women in the age group 15–45. National Institute of Nutrition (NIN) and IASDS carried out a comprehensive nutritional status study jointly in 2002 under the overall framework of the project – nutrition profile of community in all the districts of Uttar Pradesh (including Uttarakhand). NFHS-3 was carried out in 2005–06. In addition to the indicators covered in NFHS-2, NFHS-3 provides information on several new and emerging issues such as perinatal mortality, male involvement in the use of health and family welfare services, adolescent reproductive health, high risk sexual behavior, family life education, safe injections, and knowledge about tuberculosis. A major new component of NFHS-3 was blood testing for HIV prevalence and behavior-related information among adult men and women. In addition to interviewing ever-married women age 15–49, NFHS-3 included never married women age 15–49 and both ever-married and never married men age 15–54 as eligible respondents.

## 4.2 Nutritional status of children

### 4.2.1 Commonly used indicators of undernutrition

Measurement of growth of children is an important and widely used method for the assessment of the nutritional status of communities. The extent of protein energy undernutrition is reflected by anthropometric indicators based upon age, height and weight of children and adults in comparison to established standards. Anthropometric measurements, viz. height and weight, are taken using standard equipment like anthropometer rod/infantometer and lever actuated weighing scale, by adopting standard procedures. Clinical examination is also done to examine the presence of the clinical signs of nutritional deficiency disorders.

Nutritional status of children can be gauged from weight-for-age, height-for-age and weight-for-height indicators. Each of the three indices provides different information about nutritional status. Weight-for-age is a composite measure which reflects both chronic and acute undernutrition. The height-for-age index measures linear growth retardation or stunting among children is a measure of long-term effects of undernutrition. Stunting indicates chronic undernutrition which often leads to recurrent diarrhea. It is typically associated with poor feeding practices, inadequate food intake and poor environmental conditions. The weight-for-height measure is an index reflecting body mass in relation to body length. The weight-for-height measure indicates the prevalence of acute undernutrition and is the only index which does not depend upon accurate age reporting. The most serious nutritional problem therefore is that of wasting which reflects the extent of acute undernutrition.

### 4.2.2 Use of reference population and standards

The observed growth performance is evaluated against a standard which is considered to best represent normal growth. National Centre for Health Statistics (NCHS), in collaboration with an expert working group of WHO, developed the growth standards using anthropometric indicators of nutritional status in late 1975, which were till recently being used to assess children's growth. This reference was considered inadequate as it was based on data from a limited sample of bottle-fed children belonging to United States of America (USA). Recently, on the basis of a multi-country study involving more than 8000 children from Brazil, Ghana, India, Norway, Oman and USA, WHO (2006b) developed new growth standards for children aged below 5 years of age for assessing their nutritional status all over world by taking single age (month-wise) and gender as reference parameters. These standards, which are considered as norm for growth and development of breastfed children, proved to be a significant improvement over the existing NCHS growth reference, as for the first time they provide us with the evidence and guidance regarding how every child in the world should grow.

Since the nutritionists have also recommended breastfeeding as the optimal source of nutrition during infancy, tools to assess the growth by fixing breastfed child as the norm brings about coherence between the proposed guidelines and global infant-feeding practices. The new WHO child growth standards thus tend to confirm that children, if given, the optimum start in life, have the potential to develop within the same range of height and weight, no matter where they are born and which country they belong to. The average growth is similar across large populations; although, individual differences may occur among children. The new standards also indicate that differences in children's growth are more influenced by nutrition, feeding practices, environment and health care than genetics or ethnicity alone.

The children in the study were selected, keeping in mind certain criterion of optimal environment for proper growth of infants. Some of these were as follows: selecting infants whose mothers did not smoke, following recommended infant and young child feeding practices, providing good healthcare and other similar factors associated with good health outcomes.

### 4.2.3 Cut-offs for assessing undernutrition

Prevalence of undernutrition in children is described in terms of the percentage of individuals below a specific cut-off, such as certain percent of the median or standard deviation (sd) in terms of z scores of the reference population. The z score of a given age for weight-for-age is given by z = (observed weight– median weight of the reference population) / sd, where sd is the standard deviation of median of the reference population.

Classifications like Gomez's and Indian Association of Pediatricians (IAP) are on the basis of cut-off points as percentage of median (standard) weight-for-age. Gomez's classification (1956) of undernutrition was proposed on the basis of prognostication studies from hospitalization. Three grades of undernutrition were: (i) Normal: >90% of standard weight-for-age; (ii) Grade I: 90-75%; mild undernutrition; (iii) Grade II: 75-60%; moderate undernutrition; and (iv) Grade III : <60%; severe undernutrition.

Similarly, the Nutrition Sub-Committee of the Indian Academy of Pediatrics in 1972 proposed the IAP classification of undernutrition (1972): (i) Normal: >80% of standard weight-for-age; (ii) Grade I: 71–80%; (iii) Grade II: 61–70%; (iv) Grade III: 51–60%; and (v) Grade IV: <50%. Usually Grades III and IV are referred to as severe undernutrition. Both Gomez's and IAP classification classify severe undernutrition as below 60% of median (standard) weight-for-age.

The third classification is based upon the standard deviation (sd). According to these cut-off points, prevalence of moderate and severe levels of undernutrition is defined as the proportion of children below –2sd of the median value (which is the same as a z-score of below –2) of the NCHS reference population. Children who are more than 2sd below the reference median are termed underweight. Children who are more than 2sd below the reference median are considered short for their age or stunted. Children who are more than 2sd below the reference median are too thin or wasted.

The recommended cut-off point for severe undernutrition is –3sd (z-score of –3). Severe undernutrition leads to significantly higher risk of death among young children. These classifications are now widely used to analyze and present data from NNMB surveys and by other major stakeholders like WHO, WFP, UNICEF, USAID among others. Even, NFHS, the largest national surveys in India, which form the basis for planning by policy makers and program implementers, present nutritional status data in terms of sd classifications only.

In the new WHO growth standards, besides developing standards for weight-for-age, length/height-for-age and weight-for-length/height indicators, a new indicator BMI-for-age is also proposed for the children up to age 5. On referring to these new standards, parents, doctors, policy makers and child advocates will meet with better chances of knowing the time slot at which the nutrition and healthcare needs of children are not being met. All types of undernutrition viz. undernutrition (weight-for-age, length/height-for-age and weight-for-length/height), overweight and obesity and other growth related conditions can then be detected and addressed at an early stage.

The z scores based upon WHO growth standards together with tools developed are given at http://www.who.int/childgrowth/standards/en/. Tables based upon these for children up to 5 years of age for each of the indicators weight-for-age, height/length-for-age and weight-for-height/length are given for meaningful combinations at the end of the book. Also given are Tables for each of boys and girls for BMI-for-age.

To illustrate the use of these Tables, let us consider the case of a boy aged 49 months, for height-for-age indicator. Table 4.1 gives the following z-scores for height in cm.

**Table 4.1** Typical values of age and height for age in New Growth standards

| Age in months | –3sd | –2sd | –1sd | median | 1sd | 2sd | 3sd |
|---|---|---|---|---|---|---|---|
| 49 | 91.2 | 95.4 | 99.7 | 103.9 | 108.1 | 112.4 | 116.6 |

If the observed height for a boy aged 49 months is 95.2 cm, then a comparison from Table 4.1 suggests that boy is between –2sd and –3sd cut-offs; if the observed height is 90.8 cm, then the boy falls below –3sd cut-off and is severely undernourished (stunted). Alternatively, one can compute z-score. For the first case

$$z = (95.2 - 103.9) / 4.2 = -8.7/4.2 < -2$$

and for the second case

$$z = (90.8 - 103.9) / 4.2 = -13.1/4.2 < -3$$

Here $$sd = 103.9 - 99.7 = 4.2$$

It may be interesting to compare the estimates of undernutrition or overnutrition based upon new growth standards and current estimates based upon earlier NCHS reference. For a good discussion on these, readers should refer to Shah and Sachdev (2011).

According to Adhikari et al. (2015), the prevalence rate of underweight of under-2 year children in India is 38.7 percent with severe cases being 14.9 percent. In fact the prevalence of underweight has increased from 37.2 percent during the period of NFHS-2 to 38.7 percent during the period of NFHS-3.

Further, prevalence of underweight is higher in rural areas. It is also highest among the tribal children and among the poorest people. Stunting prevalence rates increase with increase in age and the highest prevalence rate is by two years of age. About a third of under-2 years children are observed to be stunted by 2 months of age. The data of NFHS-2 and NFHS-3 for stunting among under-2 years indicates a substantial decrease which is statistically significant, a decrease from 49.5 percent in 1998–99 to 40.2 percent in

2005–6. The differentials show that prevalence of stunting is higher in rural areas and is highest among the SC/ST children and among the poorest people.

According to all (IASDS, 1995, NFHS-1, NFHS-2 and NFHS-3) studies, rural areas had higher percentage of children suffering from undernutrition. In the IASDS and NFHS-1 studies, male children happened to be more undernourished than female children in terms of weight-for-age and height-for-age indicators. However, this finding is different from NFHS-2, where the females have higher prevalence of undernutrition. As per NFHS-3, prevalence of underweight under 3 years children was 40.4 percent and those of stunting and wasting were 44.9 and 22.9 percent, respectively. The joint NIN and IASDS (2002) study showed no difference by gender.

According to IASDS, 1995 study in Uttar Pradesh, about one-half of the children under 5 years of age were underweight. Over 59 percent were stunted and 20 percent wasted. The percentage of severely undernourished children (3sd below reference median) was also high: 22 percent were underweight and 31 percent stunted.

Of all the regions, Eastern region had highest prevalence of undernutrition on the basis of all three measures. On the other hand, children of Bundelkhand region had better nutritional status in comparison to other regions. The NFHS-2 study, for children under age 3 years, however, reported Central and Bundelkhand regions as those with maximum undernutrition.

IASDS study also assessed prevalence of undernutrition among children in seventeen selected districts. Out of these, almost all the districts of the Eastern region showed greater undernutrition among children. Basti (75 per cent underweight, 79 per cent stunted and 25 per cent wasted) and Bahraich (73 per cent underweight, 73 per cent stunted and 29 per cent wasted) districts were the worst affected. Lowest percentage of undernourished children was found in Etawah district of the Western region on the basis of all three measures. Interestingly, in Lucknow also, which is the state capital, undernutrition among children was higher than the state figures in terms of all the three indicators.

### 4.2.4 Efforts to control undernutrition

Many agencies such as UNICEF, WFP, USAID, CARE, etc., are engaged in child care and intervention projects of which management of severely undernourished children is a key factor. As stated earlier, ICDS is a nationwide community-based program enhancing the health, nutrition and learning opportunities of infants, young children and their mothers.

In spite of such intensive and mammoth efforts as above, there seem to be clear indications of these being not effective. This is evident from recurrent events of deaths of children reported from different pockets of the country due to undernutrition. The government has advanced a number of diseases like diarrhea, pneumonia, low birthweight, etc., as the cause of death. Indeed, clinically, it is rarely the case when the cause of death can be medically diagnosed as the undernutrition. It is the undernutrition which is responsible for diseases, and diseases, in turn give rise to undernutrition.

### 4.2.5 Misclassification

A major problem was that IAP and sd classifications had different nutritional assessments. A recent study by Nigam (2003) showed that –3sd cut-off is same as 67 percent of median (standard) weight-for-age. Thus there is a difference in IAP and –3sd cut-offs (60% in IAP and 67% in –3 sd). A comparison between the two cut-offs made in another study by Nigam (2005) using district level results from the joint study of NIN and IASDS (2002) showed considerable gaps in reporting severe undernutrition under field conditions.

Percentages of children left out by IAP classification were very high across all the districts. Interestingly, while in terms of percentage cut-offs, there is only a difference of 7 percent between two classifications, the percentage of children left out exceeds 50 and is even 100 in one district. The reason for this is the underlying asymmetry in the distribution of severe undernutrition.

In terms of program implications, the above findings show that at the state level, 61.1 percent of severely undernourished children were left out in Uttar Pradesh and 72.4 percent in Uttarakhand. At the regional level, in Uttar Pradesh, these left out percentages are: 58.1 in Western region, 59.9 in Central region, 67 in Eastern region and 53.4 in Bundelkhand region. In numbers, in UP alone out of about 6 million estimated severely undernourished children; over 3.5 million such children are likely to be left out.

In intervention projects, severely undernourished children are targeted and monitored. As ICDS used IAP classifications for growth monitoring and identifying severely undernourished children, it is not difficult to realize the gravity and magnitude of the problem with regard to left out severely children at the national level. This was perhaps one important reason why in spite of massive efforts undernutrition was not declining in the country. However, fortunately the situation is likely to change due to the introduction of new growth standards of WHO, which use only sd classification for assessing undernutrition.

### 4.2.6 Associated risk factors of undernutrition in children

#### 4.2.6.1 Logistic regression

Logistic regression is a very useful tool to identify risk factors associated with undernutrition. The analysis provides relative importance (factor loads or odds ratios) of different factors. Besides identifying risk factors associated with undernutrition, logistic regression can be usefully exploited in many other areas as well. One of these could be risk factors associated with transmission of HIV infection like extra marital sex without condoms with a single or multiple partners, homosexuality and anal sex, oral sex, drug addiction and blood transfusion. Other areas could be risk factors associated with diseases like tuberculosis, cancer, and even problems related to heart.

First study to identify determinants of nutritional status of young children in India using NFHS-1 data is by Rajaretnam and Jyoti (2000). Analysis of the data showed that children above 2 years become less underweight but more and more stunted. Children born to young mothers (below 18 years), of higher birth orders (4+), and those with a birth interval of less than 2 years are at higher risk of being severely undernourished. Low birthweight babies are also at a greater risk of being severely under nourished. A more comprehensive study is reported in DWCD, UP, 1999 part of which also appeared later in Vir and Nigam (2001). The most recent study is by Mishra et al. (2015) who utilized NFHS-3 data. We first describe the logistic regression model and then give some detailed results from the DWCD, 1999, and from Mishra et al. (2015) publications.

The multivariate logistic model with binary outcomes has the form

$$y = [1/(1+e^{-(\Sigma\beta ixi)}] + e, i = 0,1,\ldots,k$$

where y is the dependent variable, $\beta_0$ is a constant, $\beta_1,\ldots, \beta_k$ are regression coefficients for the independent variables $x_1,\ldots, x_k$. All the variables are usually dichotomised and coded as 0 or 1. Statistical analysis can be performed using standard software like SAS, SPSS, R, etc.

Before carrying out the multivariate logistic regression analysis, univariate analysis should be performed on each of the dependent variables to check whether they are individually affecting the dependent variable. Variables found significant in univariate analysis are used for multivariate binary logistic regression analysis. Table 4.2 displays some typical values appearing in the analysis. Columns 2–4 give β, Exp (β) and 95 percent confidence interval (C.I.) for Exp (β). The value Exp (β) is the factor loading for the corresponding variable (mother's literacy in this case) and next column gives the 95 percent confidence interval for the factor loading. Any value of

Exp (β) exceeding one is important as for example, the value 1.67 for Exp (β) reflects that children of illiterate mothers are 1.67 times more likely to become underweight.

**Table 4.2** Typical layout of logistic regression results

| Variables | | Underweight | |
|---|---|---|---|
| | β | Exp(β) | 95% C.I. for Exp(β) |
| **Mother literacy (code)** | | | |
| Illiterate (1) | 0.51 | 1.67 | 1.43-1.95 |

In the DWCD, 1999 study, univariate analyses of risk factors revealed that child's age, age at introduction of complementary feeding, prevalence of diarrhea, measles and ARI during the last 15 days, level of education of the mother, mother's BMI, care taken by the mother during the last 3 months of pregnancy, type of house and toilet have associations of varying degrees with the nutritional status of children. The associated relative risks of these factors were further examined by the multivariate logistic regression analysis. The analyses were done for each of the indicators – underweight, stunting and wasting. The analyses were done for undernutrition (less than −2sd times reference median) and severe undernutrition (less than −3sd times reference median). The following Table 4.3 gives details of the variables chosen along with their codes:

**Table 4.3** Description of the variables and their codes

| Variables | Variables with binary codes |
|---|---|
| Child's age | Children of age 12–35 months (1), Others (0) |
| Hygiene | Children from kutcha households with no toilet facility and with inadequate drainage (1), Others (0) |
| Disease | Children suffering from any of the diseases: diarrhea, measles and ARI (1), Others (0) |
| Care | Children whose mothers took better diet, more rest and did less heavy work during the last three months of pregnancy (1), Others (0) |
| Literacy | Children of illiterate mothers (1), Others (0) |
| BMI | Children of mothers with BMI,18.5 (1), Others (0) |
| Complementary feeding | Children who were given complementary feeding at 4-6 months (1), Others (0) |
| Immunization | Children who were immunized (1), Others (0) |

Tables 4.4 and 4.5 give the results of undernourished vs. normal children and severely undernourished vs. normal children, respectively. Only those risk factors which have loading factor exceeding 1 have been reported.

**Table 4.4** Risk factors and their loadings (Undernourished children)

| Underweight | | Stunting | | Wasting | |
|---|---|---|---|---|---|
| Risk factor | Factor loading | Risk factor | Factor loading | Risk factor | Factor loading |
| BMI | 1.63 | BMI | 1.30 | Disease | 1.64 |
| Disease | 1.58 | Literacy | 1.27 | BMI | 1.29 |
| Child's age | 1.41 | Child's age | 1.26 | Child's age | 1.19 |
| Literacy | 1.28 | Hygiene | 1.19 | Literacy | 1.17 |

It is observed that BMI, disease, child's age and literacy are important risk factors for underweight, while BMI, literacy, child's age and hygiene are associated with stunting. For wasting, important risk factors are disease, BMI, child's age and literacy.

**Table 4.5** Risk factors and their loadings (Severely undernourished children)

| Underweight | | Stunting | | Wasting | |
|---|---|---|---|---|---|
| Risk factor | Factor loading | Risk factor | Factor loading | Risk factor | Factor loading |
| Literacy | 2.04 | Literacy | 1.84 | Care | 1.83 |
| Child's age | 1.79 | Child's age | 1.61 | Disease | 1.57 |
| Disease | 1.75 | Hygiene | 1.28 | BMI | 1.55 |
| BMI | 1.74 | BMI | 1.26 | Literacy | 1.39 |
| Care | 1.50 | | | Child's age | 1.31 |

For severe undernutrition, literacy, child's age, disease, BMI and care are important risk factors for underweight and wasting; while literacy, child's age, hygiene and BMI are associated risk factors for stunting.

Mishra et al. (2015) also fitted logistic regression using NFHS-3 data and carried out the analyses for each of the three indicators, namely, underweight, stunting and wasting. They took child's age in months, mother's literacy or educational status, birthweight or size, standard of living or wealth index, type of caste or tribe, birth order and mother's nutritional status, hygiene, diseases in the univariate analyses. In the multivariate logistic analyses, for underweight, wealth index is the dominant factor followed by mother's nutritional status, mother's educational status, child's age, size of child at birth, type of caste/tribe and birth order. For stunting, the child's age is the most dominant factor followed by mother's educational status, wealth index, and mother's nutritional status, size of child at birth, type of caste/tribe and birth order. For wasting, mother's nutritional status was the most dominant factor followed by child's age, mother's education, and wealth index, type of caste/tribe and size of child at birth.

Adhikari et al. (2015) also studied the association of various risk factors with the under-nutrition in under-2-year age children. The risk factors associated with high prevalence of underweight are found to be pertaining to the status of mothers viz. height of mother less than 145 cm had around double the risk of under-nutrition than the mothers with height more than 145cm, mothers with no education had 1.8 time more risk of having underweight-U2 children than the literate mothers, mothers who did not go for institutional delivery had 1.4 time more risk than the mothers otherwise, mothers who did not have the exposure of watching TV at least once a week had 1.4 time risk than the mothers who watch TV at least once a week, mothers who experienced emotional violence also were at higher risk of having underweight children, mothers who did not consume IFA tablets for at least 90 days, mothers experiencing emotional violence and mothers living in households with no toilet facility were also at higher risk of having underweight children.

Regarding prevalence of stunting, mothers with no formal education or mothers who had height < 145 cm have 1.6 times more risk than the other mothers. Similarly mothers who did not go for institutional delivery were at 1.4 times higher risk of having stunted children. Mothers who were living in household with no toilet facility or with low standard of living had higher risk of having stunted children.

The study findings supported the view that nutritional status of children was influenced not only by consumption of nutrients or food but also by a number of other development factors, i.e. infection/diseases in children, literacy of mothers, water and sanitation, etc. The need to address the problem of undernutrition in children through convergence of multi-sectoral development inputs is therefore of utmost importance. Nutritional status of children in fact needs to be viewed possibly as an important indicator of development along with infant mortality rate (IMR) and under-5 child mortality rate.

## 4.3 Nutritional status of adolescents

The use of anthropometry may be more difficult in adolescents than in other age groups because anthropometric indices in normally nourished adolescents change with age and sexual development. Moreover, survey and reference populations may differ in the age at which certain pubertal landmarks are attained, requiring adjustment for differences between survey and reference populations. Adolescent populations may also differ by ethnicity in various body proportions that affect anthropometric indices. Although no definitive recommendation can be made regarding which anthropometric indices are the most appropriate for adolescents, some revisions may improve current practices. Weight-for-height could be used for pre-pubertal adolescents and body mass index could be used for post-pubertal adolescents. Because cut-off points are age-specific, age should be collected as accurately as possible for all adolescents measured during screening or survey activities.

WHO (2007) has recommended BMI-for-age cut-offs for adolescents. This will go a long way in improving the methodology for assessing undernutrition in adolescents. An additional macro is now available to facilitate analysis of nutritional status in children and adolescents 5–19 years using R software. To develop this reference, the same statistical methodology was used as in the construction of the WHO standards. This reference complements the 2006 WHO child growth standards for 0–60 months. The Tables for BMI-for-age cut-offs for adolescents are available at http://www.who.int/entity/growthref/who2007_ bmi_for_age/en/-. Based upon these Tables, the BMI-for-age z-scores for boys and girls aged 5–19 years for meaningful combinations are given at the end of the book. Also given are height-for-age z-scores for 5–19 years and weight-for-age z-scores for 5–10 years. Weight-for-age Tables are restricted to only 5–10 years because as stated in the WHO document: *weight-for-age reference data are not available beyond age 10 because this indicator does not distinguish between height and body mass in an age period where many children are experiencing the pubertal growth spurt and may appear as having excess weight (by weight-for-age) when in fact they are just tall.*

## 4.4 Nutritional status of adults

### 4.4.1 Chronic energy deficiency

Chronic energy deficiency (CED) is a nutritional deficiency which refers to an intake of energy less than the requirement, for a period of several months or years. It is measured by BMI. It is given by [weight in kg/ (height in metres)$^2$] and is used to determine the nutritional status of the adults. The adults are grouped into different nutritional grades using the following BMI classification suggested by James, Ferro-Luzi and Waterlow (1988): BMI $<$ 18.5 as CED, $18.5 \leq$ BMI $<$ 25.0 normal, $25.0 \leq$ BMI $<$ 30.0 overweight, and BMI $\geq$ 30.0 obese. Those with BMI $<$ 16 are taken to be suffering from severe undernutrition.

## 4.4.2 Nutritional status of women

The health and nutritional status of the women of childbearing age has a direct bearing on the nutritional status of their children. Since mothers are the main providers of care and support for infants and children, their good health is imperative for the health and nutrition of children. Most of the women in developing countries are vulnerable to undernutrition throughout their life cycle for reasons, which are both social and biological in nature. Girls, particularly adolescents, are usually discriminated against in access to health care, education and diet. An undernourished mother is more likely to produce a child with low birthweight and hence an undernourished child. This completes the cycle of mal-nourishment:

Undernourished mother → undernourished children, and an undernourished girl child → undernourished mother.

According to Vir (2015), women's nutrition is a major contributor to stunting in South Asia. Poor women's nutritional status (poor height, thinness, BMI, anaemia) impacts not only maternal mortality but also childhood stunting. Poor women nutrition impairs foetal development, contributes to LBW and increases the risk of stunting (2.1 to 4.3 times). The assessment of the status of undernutrition and their causal factors among women is therefore quite important.

The levels and trends in women's nutritional status can be assessed through anthropometry, incidences of low birthweight and maternal mortality. The women with BMI less than has been static around 33–34 percent for the last several decades. In NFHS-3 it was 34.1 percent. However, there has been steady rise in obesity prevalence, being 11.1 percent in NFHS-3.

According to IASDS, 1995 study in Uttar Pradesh, 30 percent of women suffered from undernutrition (BMI < 18.5) out of which 5 percent were severely undernourished (BMI < 16). The prevalence of undernutrition increased to about 35 percent in subsequent studies (NFHS-2 and NIN-IASDS, 2002).

IASDS, 1995 study, also assessed prevalence of undernutrition among women in seventeen selected districts. Out of these, 5 districts from Eastern region, on an average had higher undernutrition among women as compared to other districts. Bahraich district had a very dismal picture as 53 percent women had BMI < 18.5. Interestingly, in Lucknow also, which is the state capital, undernutrition among women was higher than the state average (35 per cent).

It may be interesting to identify the factors, which are closely associated with undernutrition among women. According to studies by IASDS, 1995, and Department of Women and Child Development, 1999, some of the major factors which may have direct impact on women's undernutrition are: level of education, age at first marriage, number of abortions and live births, antenatal and post natal checkups, administration of TT injections, intake of IFA tablets, type of work load and diet during the last three months of last pregnancy and use of iodized salt. These findings reveal that the impact of pre-delivery maternal care services, particularly, the antenatal services have not been very effective.

## 4.5 Dietary surveys

### 4.5.1 Food and nutrient intake

Type, quantity and frequency of food and nutrient intakes are major factors affecting nutritional status of any individual. Dietary surveys are carried out with the purpose of evaluating the type and quantity of food and nutrient intakes at different household and individual levels. While household level consumption of foodstuffs gives the status of consumption of the whole family, the individual level exercise gives the variations among members within the family. It also gives vital information according to age groups and by gender. Most dietary surveys are based upon 24-hour recalls for dietary intake assessments giving details of food consumption during the past 24 hours. Further discussion on these surveys is based upon those conducted by NNMB.

In the dietary survey, consumptions of different category of foodstuffs are ascertained. The broad categories of foodstuffs are cereals and millets, pulses and legumes, green leafy vegetables, roots and tubers, other vegetables, nuts and oil seeds, condiments and spices, fruits, fishes and other sea foods, meat and poultry, milk and milk products, fats and edible oils, and sugar and jaggery. These foodstuffs when converted into nutrients provide information on nutrient intakes like protein, fat, energy, calcium, iron, retinol, thiamin, riboflavin, niacin, vitamin C, and folic free.

In addition to the above information, distribution of households according to consumption of foodstuffs as percentage of recommended dietary intakes (RDI) is also given. These percentages are according to the classes: < 50, 50–60, 60–70, 70–80, 80–90, 90–100, ≥ RDI.

### 4.5.2 Households

The daily intake of different foods and nutrients are computed per consumption unit (CU). The calorie requirements of a reference man aged 20–39 years, weighing 60 kg, doing sedentary work is taken as one CU and the calorie coefficients for all the other individuals in the households are calculated proportionately on the basis of energy requirements according to age, sex, physiological status and activity pattern. Average daily intake of various foods per CU is calculated. From this, the average daily intake of various nutrients is computed using Food Composition Tables. The average intakes of nutrients are compared with the levels suggested in nutrient requirements and RDA for Indians (1981, 1990) as suggested by the ICMR Expert Committee.

### 4.5.3 Individuals

The average daily food and nutrient intakes of individuals in the households surveyed are computed according to different age/sex groups. These are compared with RDA suggested by the ICMR Expert Committee.

### 4.5.4 Food frequency

In addition to the survey on dietary intake at household and individual levels, food frequency of food consumption is also assessed. Information of frequency of consumption of various food items by the households is collected from all the households covered for dietary assessment, using a separate pretested and pre-coded questionnaire. The food frequency enquiry gives an overall assessment of frequency patterns of different foodstuffs. It gives frequency of consumption food groups in terms of different patterns like daily, weekly, fortnightly, monthly, seasonal, and occasional.

## 4.6 KAP survey

Knowledge, attitude and practice (KAP) component of the surveys ascertain information on breast feeding, child rearing and socio-cultural aspects of food consumption carried out in all the households having at least one child of less than 5 years of age. In the households where there is more than one child below 5 years, the youngest child is considered as the index child. The respondent is the mother of the index child. In addition, it also ascertains information on foods that should be avoided during pregnancy.

In many surveys, in addition to KAP one more component – behavior – is added. Further, the information is sometimes also sought on a variety of issues like pre- and postnatal care, care during delivery, new born and infant care.

## 4.7 Discussion on dietary surveys

Use of 1-, 2- and 3-days, 24-hour recalls for dietary intake assessments is common, though 7-days recall also finds place in literature. Each of these methods has its own advantages and limitations. Food habits and dietary patterns are captured through food-frequency questionnaire using the columns like daily, once/twice a week, once in two weeks, monthly, seasonally, occasionally and never. Though the method is characterized by ease of administration and low costs of data analysis, it is highly subjective because of variations in perceptions regarding meaning of terms like occasionally and seasonally, and memory lag for information sought under once/twice a week, weekly, once in two weeks, monthly and seasonally.

The above variants of 1-, 2- and 3-days, 24 hour recalls and of food frequency were tried in an ICMR funded IASDS project in 2006 to assess intra-household gender disparity in dietary intakes and patterns in two districts in Uttar Pradesh. Some of its findings are reported by Nigam et al. (2010). ANOVA was applied to test for day-to-day differences in actual intakes of three days. The analysis revealed that a single-day dietary intake assessment may not be an efficient method. Instead, data based upon 3 days may provide more valid estimates of dietary intakes. Food frequency in its present form may also be an inefficient method for capturing dietary frequency patterns for reasons of ambiguity and memory lag. Food frequency patterns must be viewed with caution and their roles should be to complement 24-hour recall data repeated over 3 days. Reader may refer to Section 8.4 for more details.

A major limitation of most dietary surveys is that these are over ambitious and too many things are sought from a single survey. For instance, as pointed out by Nigam (2008), in NNMB and related surveys, while collecting information on anthropometry, dietary intakes and food frequency is directly linked with its objectives, collection of data on KAP is somewhat not justified in the time frame and mind set provided to the investigating teams. The investigators try hard to concentrate on quality in respect of height–weight measurements and on weighing of food items. This affects quality of data, particularly on KAP and food frequency. While we can dispense with the questionnaire dealing with KAP, there is a need to make the questionnaire more focused. Similarly, in NFHS-2, besides collecting information on health and anthropometric indicators, investigator is also asked to canvass food frequency, which is complete digression from the main focus of the survey.

Again, in NNMB and related surveys, the questionnaire on dietary intakes, both at the household as well as individual levels, needs revision for improvement. While information on major consumption of foodstuffs is readily recorded at each of the major meals-breakfast, lunch, tea & snacks and dinner, anything eaten in between is likely to be missed. As a result, the consumption figures are underestimated. It is desirable to re-devise the questionnaire where in addition to the major meals, more probing may be required on in-between eaten foodstuffs (including those eaten outside). This can be done by adding a row in the end with the caption "Foodstuffs eaten in addition to the above".

It may not be out of place to point out here that the *Handbook on Nutritive Values of Indian Foods* (1999) of NIN has South India bias, possibly because till recently only states from this part were being covered by NNMB. This Handbook needs to be revised, as some of the foodstuffs consumed in the north, particularly in hill states, are not included in the Handbook.

# 5

# Nutritional deficiency disorders and immunization

## 5.1 Vitamin A deficiency disorders

Vitamin A deficiency (VAD) is a major public health problem in 96 countries including India (WHO, 1994). Most vulnerable are preschool children and pregnant mothers. An estimated 5.7 percent children in India suffer from eye signs of VAD. Even mild VAD increases the morbidity and mortality in children. Further, episodes of illnesses such as ARI, diarrhea and measles deplete vitamin A reserves from the body of children. Bitot's Spots, night blindness and corneal xerosis are the most specific and recognizable clinical manifestations of VAD disorders in children. Among other manifestations are keratomalacia and corneal opacity. Vitamin A levels in children are assessed through serum retinol levels. Cut-off for vitamin A deficiency is serum retinol < 19.0. Very few studies have been carried out in India using serum retinol assessment method. As stated earlier, NIMS and IASDS have carried out some studies for WFP.

Night blindness and corneal xerosis have served as definite criteria for assessing vitamin A status of the community. Several small studies undertaken in various parts of the country have demonstrated that severe ocular manifestations caused by vitamin A deficiency have decreased with vitamin A supplementation. However, a large number of children and mothers may continue to have deficient serum retinol levels. The Ministry of Health and Family Welfare, Government of India, reported 68 percent coverage of vitamin A supplementation for children aged 6–11 months and 25 percent coverage of 1–5 years children in 1996. However, field reports suggest that coverage is considerably lower. According to NFHS-2 at the national level, wide interstate variations ranging between 4 percent (Nagaland) to 52 percent (Goa) in children who had received at least one dose within the past 6 months were reported. This data indicated that a large majority of children in India did not receive vitamin A supplementation at all and fewer children received it regularly. Almost similar scenario prevailed in NFHS-3.

Ordinarily, VAD contributes to decreased resistance to infections. VAD is often precipitated by a range of illnesses and infections like ARI, diarrhea, measles, which are also leading causes of child mortality and morbidity. The availability of vitamin A supplements, along with other vaccinations, therefore, now forms part of newly strengthened universal immunization program. Giving vitamin A supplements orally prevents eye damage, helps replace depleted body reserves and increases the chance of survival. However, some recent studies question the claims of the extent of protection provided by vitamin A supplementation.

The Indian Government launched the first vitamin A supplementation program in the world in 1970 to combat nutritionally caused blindness from VAD. The program was called National Program for the Prevention of Nutritional Blindness. In addition to the use of pharmaceutical supplements, the program also included promotion of dietary diversification as one of the key program strategies. As part of the program, massive dose of vitamin A (2 lakhs I.U.) is administered once in 6 months to children between 1 and 5 years of age. The children below 3 years are categorized as 'at risk' population and are covered on priority basis.

Under the RCH program, Ministry of Health and Family Welfare, Government of India, women and children are provided iron, folate and vitamin A supplementation. These micronutrients are also distributed through ICDS. In an effort to enhance the impact of food supplementation in the ICDS in general, CARE India had designed and initiated a program entitled Integrated Nutrition and Health Program (INHP) in 1996 with the ultimate objective to improve the health and nutrition status of women and children, especially that of girls.

Despite decades of operation of the above programs, the problems of vitamin A, iron and folic acid deficiency persist in the community. A few studies undertaken so far indicate that there may be difficulties and limitations in the process of implementing these two programs effectively. This includes problems of management of logistics and distribution of supplies at various levels. There might be other issues regarding the strategies of program implementation, social mobilization and people's response to national programs on prevention of nutritional blindness and anemia.

While discussing inadequacy of sample sizes with regard to district nutrition profile surveys by NNMB and others, Nigam (2004, 2008) and Vijayraghavan (2008) pointed out that though the sample size is adequate to assess dietary and nutritional status of communities and clinical deficiencies like Bitot's Spots at the state level; it is not amenable to dis-aggregated analysis or to represent district nutrition profile. As an example consider the case of assessment of Bitot's Spots. As its prevalence is expected to be around 4 percent, the required sample size at 10 percent relative margin of error is around 9600 which when multiplied with design effect say 1.5, comes to 14400. But district nutrition profile surveys take less than 400 children in each district. Because of grossly inadequate sample size, district nutrition profiles report the prevalence close to zero in most districts. Further, most previous studies by different workers/agencies also had very low sample sizes and their results lacked consistency and differed widely. After the inadequacy of sample size issue was raised in different forums reporting of deficiency disorders at district level was discontinued by NNMB.

Following these arguments, UNICEF supported a large-scale study to assess prevalence of Bitot's Spots with a sample size of over 14000 children of 6 months to 6 years age in rural areas of 4 districts in Uttar Pradesh (Srivastava and Nigam, 2004). Quite expectedly, the findings were much different from those reported earlier. The results showed a much higher prevalence of Bitot's Spots varying from 1.9 to 10.5 in the four districts.

## 5.2 Iodine deficiency disorders

Iodine is an important micronutrient for health, and lack of iodine can lead to disorders like miscarriage, cretinism, retarded psychomotor development and goiter. Iodine deficiency is the single most important cause of mental retardation worldwide. In India nearly 70 million people suffer from goiter. About one-fifth of pregnant women are at the risk of giving birth to children who will not reach their optimum physical and mental potential because of maternal iodine deficiency (Vir, 1995).

Iodine deficiency disorders (IDD) constitute the single largest cause of preventable brain damage worldwide. Majority of consequences of IDD are invisible and irreversible but at the same time these are preventable. Fortunately, iodine deficiency can easily be avoided by using iodized salt.

In India, the entire population is prone to IDD due to deficiency of iodine in the soil of the subcontinent and consequently the food derived from it. To combat the risk of IDD, salt is fortified with iodine. However, an estimated 350 million people do not consume adequately iodized salt and, therefore, are at risk for IDD. According to Pandav et al. (2013) of the 325 districts surveyed in India so far, 263 are IDD-endemic. The current household level iodized salt coverage in India as indicated by several studies is around 91 per cent with 71 per cent households consuming adequately iodized salt. The IDD control goal in India was to reduce the prevalence of IDD below 10 per cent in the entire country by 2012. Mainstreaming of IDD control in policy making, devising state-specific action plans to control IDD, strict implementation of Food Safety and Standards FSS Act, 2006, addressing inequities in iodized salt coverage (rural-urban, socio-economic), providing iodized salt in PDS, strengthening monitoring and evaluation of IDD programme and ensuring sustainability of IDD control activities are essential to achieve sustainable elimination of IDD in India.

IDD have been recognized as a major public health problem in India. Unlike other micronutrient deficiencies, IDD is due to deficiency of iodine in water, soil and foodstuffs and affects all socioeconomic groups living in specific geographic areas. ACC/SCN (2004) estimated that a third of India's population which is a sixth of the total global population was at risk of IDD. The number of children born mentally impaired due to IDD was highest in India and a third of all children born with IDD-related mental damage lived in India.

WHO/UNICEF/ICCIDD has given cut-offs of prevalence and criteria for classifying IDD as a significant public health problem. Goiters of different grades are classified as mild: 5.0–19.9 percent, moderate: 20–29.9 percent and severe: ≥30 percent. According to the WHO report (1994), the estimated prevalence of IDD in children in some countries in South Asia showed a gloomy picture. Total goiter rates and goiter rates in schoolchildren in India was high. UNICEF State of the World Children Report (2004) gave prevalence and number of IDD cases in the general population by region and country. Number of children born mentally impaired in the whole world was 19 million and 10 million of these were located in South Asia. Further, among countries in South Asia, highest number was in India (6.6 million), followed by Pakistan (2.1 million), Bangladesh (7.5 lakh), Afghanistan (5.35 lakh) and Nepal (2 lakh). Total goiter rate percentages in these countries were 26, 38, 18, 48 and 24, respectively. While Afghanistan and Pakistan were worst affected, India ranked third. India is also not badly placed in terms of total goiter rate percentage in schoolchildren (19) in comparison to Bangladesh (50) and Nepal (40).

Surveys carried out by Central and State Health Directorates, ICMR and various Medical Colleges have shown that no State or Union Territory of India is free from the problem of IDD. Out of 586 districts in the country, 281 districts have been surveyed for IDD and 41 districts have been found to be endemic. Universal use of iodized salt is a simple, inexpensive method of preventing IDD.

### 5.2.1 IDD in newborn and children

A study conducted in 22,000 newborns from different parts of India to determine the incidence of neonatal chemical hypothyroidism (NCH) as diagnosed by cord blood thyroxine level of less than 3 microgram percent and TSH of more than 50 MU/Ml showed that the incidence of NCH was a hundred-fold more in iodine deficient endemic districts of Terai regions of UP as compared to non-endemic areas like Delhi and Kerala. Subsequent studies in an endemic village of the region to determine the prevalence of known thyroxine deficiency related neurological deficits showed that a significant proportion of the village population had objective evidence of compromised brain development in the form of shift to left in IQ score distribution among school children from iodine deficient areas when compared to non-iodine deficient areas, 20 percent prevalence of nerve deafness and 3–5 percent prevalence of cretinism. Worst affected districts in U.P. have been Deoria, Gorakhpur and Gonda. For more details reader may refer to NNMB/ICMR surveys and the paper by Kochupillai (1986).

## 5.3 Zinc deficiencies

Zinc governs cell division in growth and stabilization of bio-membranes. It protects against free radicals and helps in production of sex hormones and brain development. The clinical manifestation of zinc deficiency is in the form of skin lesions, alopecia, failure to thrive and diarrhea. The daily requirement of zinc is around 1 mg/hg body weight per day. This is usually met from food and drinking water. There is not much work done on zinc deficiency. This is also limited to hospital based and that too on pediatric age.

Zinc deficiency is a link between these risk factors and the duration of diarrhea. Diarrhea is consistently found in children with severe zinc deficiency, as well as in animals with zinc depletion; it responds quickly to zinc supplementation. Zinc deficiency can result in growth retardation, especially stunting, and impairment of immune function. Finally, diarrhea leads to excess zinc losses and could contribute to zinc deficiency, especially if the zinc content of the diet is limited. The information on serum zinc levels of women and children in India is limited. Almost all studies carried out are hospital based and limited to pediatric age group.

The combined effects of inadequate sanitation, unsafe water supply and poor personal hygiene are responsible for 88 percent of childhood deaths from diarrhea. Poor sanitation and unsafe drinking water cause intestinal worm infections, which lead to undernutrition, anemia and retarded growth among children. Sanitation is one of the biggest challenges in India as in 2008, only 31 percent (UNICEF and WHO, 2010) of the population in the country benefitted from improved sanitation.

Uttar Pradesh Rural Water Supply and Environmental Sanitation Project was commonly called "Swajal" which signifies "one's own water" in Hindi and had two main objectives: (i) deliver sustainable health and hygiene benefits to the rural population through improvements in water supply and environmental sanitation services, which will increase rural incomes through time savings and income opportunities for women, test an alternative to the current supply driven service delivery mechanism and promote sanitation and gender awareness; and (ii) promote the long-term sustainability of the rural water supply and sanitation sector by providing assistance to Government of Uttar Pradesh to identify and implement an appropriate policy framework and strategic plan (World Bank, 2003).

The objective of the study was to evaluate the health benefits of Swajal project by comparing a set of indicators with baseline and first repeat study in the state of Uttar Pradesh, India. Part of the results is available in the paper by Srivastava et al. (2015).

The study was conducted in the two districts Banda and Jhansi of Uttar Pradesh. The 5 Swajal villages and 5 non-Swajal villages were selected. Non-Swajal villages were at 5 km distant from Swajal villages. The baseline study was conducted in 2000 and first repeat study was conducted 2002 in the same villages. In the baseline study, a total of 186 households and 3307 children under-5 years of age were interviewed and assessed for diarrhea in Swajal villages whereas 173 households and 302 children under 5 were covered in the Non-Swajal villages. A repeat study in both Swajal villages was conducted in 2002 in which 189 households and 323 children were covered in Swajal villages as against 165 households and 302 children in non-Swajal villages.

The incidence of diarrhea was lower among those who had proper hand washing practices. In a systematic review of number of studies (Matthew et al, 2014), 40 percent reduction in the risk of diarrhea from the promotion of hand washing with soap (RR 0.60, 95% CI 0.53–0.68) and a 24 percent reduction in the risk of diarrhea for general hygiene education alone (RR 0.76, 95% CI 0.67–0.86) was reported. The promotion of hand washing (with provision of soap or where soap was used) was thus associated with greater reduction of diarrhea than broader hygiene education ($p < 0.01$).

Good hygiene practices reduce diarrhea rates by 30–40 percent (Curtis and Cairncross, 2003; Fewtrell et al., 2005). This level of reduction can be achieved through a comprehensive approach: promoting improvements in key hygiene practices (hand washing, treatment and safe storage of drinking water, safe disposal of feces, and food hygiene); improving access to safe water and sanitation technologies and products; and facilitating or supporting an enabling environment (improved policies, community organization, institutional strengthening, and public–private partnerships).

Hand washing prevents diarrhea effectively when done properly and at critical times. A meta-analysis of hand washing studies conducted in developing countries concluded that hand washing can reduce the risk of diarrhea in the general population by 42–44 percent (Luby et al., 2011). A recent observational study in Bangladesh found that diarrhea occurred less often in households where residents washed at least one hand after defecation and before preparing food. The study suggested that washing hands before preparing food is particularly important to prevent diarrhea in children (Luby et al., 2011). The result of the present study is similar to the above-mentioned study.

In the present study, the safe storage of drinking water was also found to be significantly associated with the incidence of diarrhea. Similar finding had been shown in a meta-analysis in which the safe storage of drinking water in the household has been shown to reduce the risk of diarrheal disease by 30–40 percent (Clasen et al., 2006).

## 5.4 Immunization

Immunization can prevent various types of childhood diseases. The National Immunization Program is being implemented in our country by making free vaccination services easily available to all eligible children. The vaccination of child against serious but preventable diseases like tuberculosis, diphtheria, tetanus, poliomyelitis and measles is very important in order to reduce morbidity, mortality and disabilities from these diseases. Immunization, oral rehydration, and control of acute respiratory infections have reduced the post-neonatal component of the infant mortality rate.

Vaccination coverage information focuses on the age group 12–23 months, the age by which children should have received all basic vaccinations. According to the guidelines developed by the World Health Organization, children are considered fully vaccinated when they have received a vaccination against tuberculosis (BCG), three doses of the diphtheria, whooping cough (pertussis), and tetanus (DPT) vaccine; three doses of the poliomyelitis (polio) vaccine; and one dose of the measles vaccine by the age of 12 months. BCG should be given at birth or at first clinical contact, DPT and polio require three vaccinations at approximately 4, 8, and 12 weeks of age, and measles should be given at or soon after reaching 9 months of age.

Coverage of each individual vaccination is much higher than the percentage fully vaccinated. At the time of NFHS-2, 72 percent of children were vaccinated against tuberculosis (BCG), 55 percent had received all three doses of the DPT vaccine, 63 percent had received all three doses of the polio vaccine, and 51 percent had been vaccinated against measles. Sixty-one percent of urban children age 12–23 months were fully vaccinated compared with only 37 percent of rural children.

However, among children of age 12–35 months, 30 percent had received only one dose of vitamin A and fewer still (17%) had received a dose within the past 6 months.

According to NFHS-3, all India coverage percentages are: full – 43.5, BCG – 78, Polio – 78, DPT – 55 and measles – 59. These coverage levels differ widely among states. Though wide differences also exist in vaccination coverage among sub-groups of the population these are useful for program planning and targeting resources to areas most in need.

## 5.5 Coverage evaluation and validation

Realizing the importance of vitamin A supplementation for child's health, Government of India has recommended administration of 9 doses of vitamin A to children aged 6–59 months at every 6 months interval to reduce under-5 mortality. State Government of Uttar Pradesh has adopted a biannual strategy for vitamin A supplementation (VAS) through Bal Swasthya Poshan Mah (BSPM). The BSPM is implemented during fix months (June and December) in the entire state with the joint efforts of Departments of Health and ICDS.

Micronutrient Initiative (MI), India, started its operations in May 2010 in U.P. by providing technical and managerial assistance to the Government of U.P. in delivering vitamin A through BSPM and VHND (Village Health and Nutrition Day; usually Wednesday) months in 30 districts through implementation partner agency – Gorakhpur Environmental Action Group.

BSPM coverage of vitamin A is estimated by rolling up the reports received from the session sites, wards, health units and district in urban cities. The ANM administers doses of vitamin A to children and records the details in tally sheets and compiles the report of her ward after completing administration of vitamin A for all the session sites. These reports are further compiled at health unit level which is further aggregated at district level.

Errors take place during the process of roll up of these numbers which start at the health worker level as children are administered vitamin A without referring to a due list of target children to be administered vitamin A in the health worker's catchment. It is a pure numerator based reporting (i.e., based on number of children who were administered vitamin A).

In order to estimate the magnitude of difference between the VAS coverage reported by surveys and the health system and identify the errors occurring at the different stages of rolling up of health systems reports, a data validation exercise was undertaken in 2014–2015 by IASDS in MI-supported two urban cities Agra and Meerut of Uttar Pradesh. The scope and extent of the exercise was to validate and assess vitamin A supplementation coverage for June 2014 BSPM round in these urban intervention areas.

In both the cities, level of awareness about VAS/BSPM programme was found to be very low. Awareness about the next BSPM was also on lower side. Proportion of population having immunization cards was quite low. VAS coverage was quite low in both the cities; being 24 percent in Agra and 41.4 percent in Meerut.

### 5.5.1 First level of validation

In Agra the coverage of VAS as confirmed by mothers/caretakers was only 33.9 percent against 43.3 percent as per the tally sheets entries of ANMs. In Meerut corresponding figures were 39.4 and 47.1 percent, respectively.

### 5.5.2 Second level of validation

Significant discrepancies were noticed between health post and ANM data in both the cities. In fact ANMs were supposed to fill Form 3, which was not done and the records were completed as per information given by ANMs to health posts. In Agra, coverage as per health post data was 50 percent while the coverage reported by ANM/Vaccinator was 44.9 percent, leading to a discrepancy of 5.1 percent. In Meerut, coverage as per health post records was 57.3 percent, while that by ANM/Vaccinator was 48.8 percent, leading to a discrepancy of 8.5 percent.

### 5.5.3 Third level of validation

In Agra, coverage as reported at district level was 44.6 percent while that by all health posts together was 43.6 percent. In Meerut, coverage as reported at district level was 50.9 percent while that by health posts was 52.5 percent.

### 5.5.4 Fourth level of validation

The information for vitamin A supplementation is sent separately for rural and urban areas by district to state headquarter. For rural areas the data is of PHC level but for urban areas, the data of all health units is aggregated and then sent to state. Thus, calculated coverage percentage is same for both cities, and no variation is observed.

In general there appears to be no consistency at any level of data reporting except level 4. Steps are required to improve the reporting and recording of data.

## 5.6 Thirty cluster design

As stated in Chapter 1, cluster sampling gives more accurate results when most of the variation in the population is within the groups, not between them. However, in practice it may not be possible to ensure this as many times cluster sampling is also used for the sake of convenience and also to reduce cost.

A commonly used two-stage cluster sampling scheme, the 30×7 design was developed by WHO in 1978. This 30-cluster design has been adopted for other purposes such as rapid needs assessments with no or little modification. This sampling scheme is thought to be sufficient for most sampling of community health factors. In the 30×7 design, one can randomly select 30 first stage units, census blocks or villages from a list from all the census blocks/villages and then randomly select 7 target group members from each of these blocks/villages. This gives a total sample size of 210. The target group members could be selection sites or children of 12–23 months age or even pregnant women.

For an immunization coverage survey, the 30×7 design gives a total sample size of 210 children. This sample size may be adequate for higher coverage components, say, BCG and Polio each with 78 percent coverage. But it may be inadequate for other coverage components. It may be particularly inadequate for full immunization which is only 43.5 percent.

Complex surveys use a sampling technique other than simple random sampling. These surveys need an inflated sample size, the inflation factor being the design effect introduced by Leslie Kish in 1965. The design effect is the ratio of the theoretical variance for an estimator for a given sampling design to the theoretical variance for the same estimator under simple random sampling without replacement. As it is dependent on two theoretical variances, the computation of design effect is approximate being based upon sampling variances.

It is argued by Seshadri (2008) that use of complex designs like 30 clusters is more confusing as it is virtually impossible to correctly estimate the associated design effects. It is interesting to read her comments: It is important to keep in mind that these design effects are estimated from the data available and are therefore subject to their own sampling error. In circumstances such as this, it is possible that an imprecise correction adds more noise than clarity to the process. It is therefore felt that a simpler multi-stage stratified design with deep stratification even in the absence of complete frame may be more useful.

# 6
# Anemia

## 6.1 Introduction

Anemia usually results from nutritional deficiency of iron, folate, vitamin B12 and other micronutrients. Iron-deficiency anemia (IDA) is the most common and widespread form of micronutrient undernutrition. Iron deficiency anemia has been ranked as the third leading cause of disability for females aged 15–44 across the globe. According to NFHS-2 and -3, anemia prevalence in India is recognized to be high amongst pregnant women and young children. Studies by Tuteja et al. (2006) revealed that over 50 percent to as high as over 90 percent adolescent girls in India were anemic. Anemia has particularly high adverse impact on pregnant women and their fetuses. Anemia results in an increased risk of premature delivery, low birthweight babies and maternal mortality.

The National Nutritional Anemia Prophylaxis Program was launched in the year 1970. The program envisaged the use of iron and folic acid (IFA) supplementation for pregnant and lactating women, and children. The beneficiaries under the program were to receive iron-folic acid tablets for consumption at the rate of one tablet daily for a minimum of 100 continuous days in a year. For children, who are unable to swallow tablets, iron folic acid syrup is administered. It was realized at later stages, that anemia in adolescent girls was relatively a more serious problem. Early marriage, early conception and anemia during adolescence not only intercepts growth velocity but contributes to increased risk of maternal mortality, pregnancy complications, obstructed labor and low birthweights (see also, Section 6.3). Therefore, adolescent girls were also targeted for IFA supplementation.

According to NFHS-3, only 22.3 percent of women were consuming IFA for 90 days or more when they were pregnant with their last child. According to Sen and Kanani (2006) anemia is likely to adversely affect physical work capacity and cognition in young adolescent girls undergoing pubertal development.

As stated earlier in Chapter 1, evidence reviews were conducted by Vistaar of IntraHealth-USAID in 2007 with the help of expert groups on research studies carried out in India under different themes. One such review was on community-level interventions to prevent and treat anemia. The objective was to analyze the available evidence to make recommendations to the government about achieving impact in the area of anemia prevention and treatment.

The expert group identified 23 interventions and then short listed 9 of these based on the main selection criteria that the intervention should have a sound evaluation that documented results at the outcome or impact level (e.g., IFA consumption). Of the nine community level anemia interventions selected for the review, six focused on anemia among adolescent girls, two on maternal anemia and two on fortification. All of the interventions were community based with most in rural areas and only two were in the urban areas.

It is apparent that maximum focus of the interventions has been among adolescent girls. Seshadri and Gopaldas (1989) conducted a set of four studies to examine impacts of iron supplementation on cognitive functions in preschool and school-aged children of various ages and both sexes. The first study investigated impact of iron-folic acid supplements for 60 days on cognition in 94 boys and girls aged 5–8 years. Improvement in total scores of the anemics was significantly higher than the nonanemics in 7–8 years old children only. The second study assessed impacts of supplementation on cognition in 14 pairs of 5–6 years old anemic boys, with clear beneficial effects on cognitive function. The third study investigated effects of varying dosages of elemental iron on cognitive function in 48 boys aged 8–15 years, with different levels of improvement. The fourth study investigated impacts of iron supplementation on 163 anemic girls aged 8–15 years with treatment and evaluations at 4 and 8 months, with significantly improved scores in cognitive function after the 8th month.

IFA supplements have been shown to enhance adolescent growth. Spaced IFA supplementation is recognized as an effective public health strategy and effective preventive approach in combating anemia in adolescent girls. Spaced supplementation is also cost effective and results in fewer side effects. There are some studies to study the effect of bi-weekly supplementation of IFA with and without Albendazole administration on the status of hemoglobin level in school/college going adolescent girls. We discuss these studies later in Section 6.3.

## 6.2 Assessing anemia

Besides the studies focusing on undernutrition and nutritional deficiency disorders, another related area is the estimation of prevalence of anemia measured through surveys. The prevalence is measured on the basis of cut-off points on hemoglobin (Hb) levels, which are estimated through blood examination of surveyed individuals. Commonly used cut-offs for anemia are: Hb < 11 gm/dl for pregnant women and pre-school children below 5 years; Hb < 12 gm/dl for school children, adult women including lactating women and Hb < 13 gm/dl for adult men. Some other cut-offs are severe anemia (Hb% < 7 gm/dL), moderate anemia (Hb% 7–10 gm/dL) and mild anemia (Hb% 10–11.9 gm/dL).

The method usually adopted in India is either hemocue or cyanmethemoglobin. However, studies in India have found differences in the hemoglobin results estimated by the two methods. Some of these studies compared the hemocue estimates to estimates based on the indirect cyanmethemoglobin method (using filter paper cards), which was found to overestimate anemia (Sari et al., 2001). A discussion on different methods can also be found in Seshadri (2008). Very few large-scale surveys have been conducted on assessing anemia using hemoglobin estimation. NFHS-2 and NFHS-3 provide state level and region-wise estimates of anemia using hemocue method.

An excellent source of studies on anemia in India appears in Singh and Tuteja (2003). This publication also gives micronutrient profile of women and children in India. A similar profile for the state of Uttar Pradesh is by Srivastava and Nigam (2004) which also reports a state-level survey jointly by IASDS and King George Medical University (KGMU) on anemia in Uttar Pradesh (2002) using cyanmethemoglobin method for hemoglobin estimation. There are several other WFP-sponsored impact assessment studies involving hemoglobin and serum retinol estimation of ICDS and primary school children by National Institute of Medical Statistics and IASDS. These are baseline surveys of ICDS food fortification in districts – Kanpur Dehat (2002, 2003), Dehradun (2003) and Nahan (2004) and impact assessment studies for ICDS food fortification in district Nainital (2004) and in Madhya Pradesh, Uttar Pradesh and Uttarakhand (2005). In addition, there are baseline and impact assessments of nutrition interventions through food for Education by IASDS in Madhya Pradesh, Uttarakhand and Chhattisgarh (2004, 2005) and status of mid-day meal in Madhya Pradesh (2005). While some surveys are for one-time estimation of prevalence of anemia, undernutrition and nutrition deficiency disorders, others are for studying trends in prevalence.

There are also surveys for studying changes in prevalence levels after interventions like administration of IFA tablets (weekly or daily), vitamin A syrup, and food fortified with iron and vitamin A. There could be another interesting dimension added to it like assessing the sustainability of the intervention. For instance, it may be of interest to find out the impact of administration of IFA tablets even after a specified period of its withdrawal.

A major concern relates to wide variations between estimates derived from different studies. This is best understood through revisiting some estimates reported by Srivastava and Nigam (2004) from studies in Uttar Pradesh on anemia among pregnant women. The reported prevalence ranged from 14 percent (270 rural women) in one study, to 46 percent in NFHS-2, 48 percent in 8 districts in IASDS and KGMU (2002), and about 96 percent in 3 districts in ICMR (2001). Although standardized hemoglobin estimation techniques were used in these studies, the difference in estimates could possibly be due to varying sample sizes and also due to heterogeneity present in the targeted pregnant women. For instance, these women could be at different stages of pregnancy and even might have consumed IFA tablets, varying not only in quantity but also in duration.

## 6.3 Anemia in adolescent girls

Adolescent pregnancy and anemia are known to be primary factors responsible for high prevalence of low birthweight and subsequent undernutrition in children in the country. Moreover, iron deficiency with or without anemia during adolescence are documented to result not only in poor physical work capacity but poor concentration and lower school achievement. Prevention and control of IDA and iron deficiencies during adolescence is therefore critical for the development of the nation. Targeting adolescent girls will contribute to prevent iron deficiency during pregnancy and its serious consequences. A joint workshop of UNICEF, WHO and other agencies in 1998 recommended that in countries where anemia prevalence exceeds 40 percent, universal supplements to adolescent girls are warranted.

IFA supplementation during adolescence has been demonstrated to be effective in meeting the increase in requirements of iron and in building iron stores before the onset of pregnancy (Lynch, 2000). School-based programs, with strong assurance of supervision and compliance, have demonstrated that weekly IFA supplementation to adolescent girls is effective in addressing the problem of anemia (Beaton and McGabe, 1999; Tee et al., 1999). A study by Angeles et al. (1997) showed that weekly iron supplementation to adolescent girls has been effective for prevention of anemia. It also has fewer side effects (Schutlink, 1996) and lower costs (Gross et al., 1997).

IFA supplementation is also recommended for growth promotion by Kanani and Poojara (2000) for adolescents who are underweight. A study was conducted by them in urban areas of Vadodora district of Gujarat state to investigate the effect of IFA supplements on hemoglobin, hunger and growth in adolescent girls 10–18 years of age. Results showed that there was a high demand for IFA supplements and 90 percent of the girls consumed 85 out of 90 tablets provided. There was significant improvement in hemoglobin in the group of girls receiving IFA supplements, whereas hemoglobin decreased slightly in girls in the control group. Girls and parents reported that girls increased their food intake. A significant weight gain of 0.83 kg was seen in the intervention group, whereas girls in the control group showed little weight gain. The growth increment was greater in the 10–14 years age group than in the 15–18 years group, as expected, due to rapid growth during the adolescent spurt.

Sen and Kanani (2012) studied the impact of daily vs. intermittent (once and twice weekly) IFA supplementation on hemoglobin levels and pubertal growth among primary school girls in early adolescence (9–13 years) of Vadodara district. In three experimental schools (ES), IFA tablets were given daily, once weekly or twice weekly for one year. The fourth school (control: CS) did not receive any intervention. Hb levels significantly improved in all ES compared to CS. BMI increment in ES vs. CS was significant in twice weekly IFA and daily IFA. Within ES groups, mean Hb and BMI increments were comparable between twice weekly IFA and daily IFA. Anemic ES girls showed higher Hb and BMI increments vs. non-anemic girls. Better the Hb response, greater was the benefit on BMI. Thus, twice-weekly IFA supplementation was comparable to daily IFA as regards impact on Hb and growth; at less cost and greater feasibility. Once-weekly dose was inadequate to significantly improve growth.

An interventional study was conducted among 300 college going randomly selected girls in Agra by Lamba et al. (2014) in the age group of 16–19 years. Their hemoglobin levels were estimated before and after intervention by the cyanmethemoglobin method using Drabkin's solution. Three groups – two study groups A and B, and one control, of 100 girls each were randomly constituted. The study groups were administered supervised bi-weekly IFA with and without Albendazole for 3 months. The initial prevalence in study group A reduced significantly from 80.7 percent to 35.5 percent whereas in study group B it reduced from 73.5 percent to 58.8 percent and in control it remained almost same 84.3 percent and 81.2 percent pre- and post-intervention, respectively.

Recently, a large-scale study was reported by Vir et al. (2008). A comprehensive program entitled UMANG (Uplifting Marriage Age, Nutrition and Growth) for adolescent girls in school as well as those out of school was carried out in Lucknow district of Uttar Pradesh. The objective of the project was to develop an implementation strategy, integrated with the ongoing development programs, to reduce anemia in adolescent girls 10–18 years. The project focused on a set of interventions comprising weekly IFA supplements, six monthly deworming, and family life education. The efficiency of weekly IFA supplementation was assessed in terms of changes in anemia prevalence.

Hemoglobin levels were estimated using cyanmethemoglobin method at baseline and after 6 of intervention. Mean Hb levels improved from 10.8 to 11.8 mg/dL from baseline to endline stages (see example in Section 1.8.2). Impact of weekly iron folic acid supplementation on prevalence of anemia was noted to be significant within a short period of 6 months, the prevalence coming down from 73.3 percent to 46.3 percent.

During the project period, hemoglobin levels were assessed on a random sample of unsupervised non-school going (NSG) adolescent girls at an interval of 6 and 12 months and for the school going (SG) supervised adolescent girls after a period of 6 months of intervention. A comparison was made between mean Hb values of pre- and post-stages with mean Hb values of another two sets of adolescent girls. The comparative analysis is presented in the following figure. While the first set of adolescent girls were given weekly IFA tablets along with supplementary food, the mean hemoglobin level of girls of post-post category was measured after 12 months of their enrolment with the ICDS and these girls were continued to be given only weekly IFA tablets. Under the non-ICDS category of girls, while they were given IFA tablets for 6 months, at no time they were given any supplementary food from ICDS.

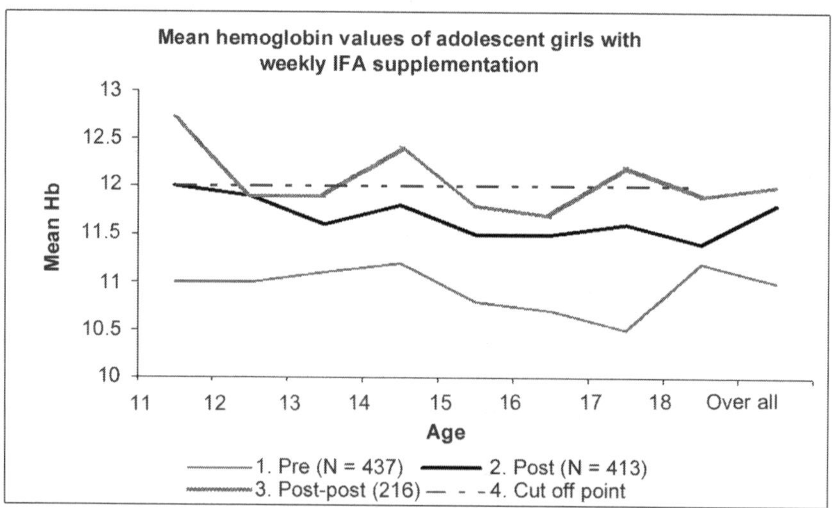


**Figure 6.1** Impact on hemoglobin levels following 6 and 12 months of weekly IFA consumption by non-school going (NSG) adolescent girls.

(non-ICDS girls taking iron for 6 months) once a week

- post once a week iron for 6 months
- post-post–once a week iron for 1 year

The findings confirmed that on a large-scale program, weekly iron folic acid supplementation is feasible and is effective in reducing anemia in both unsupervised non-school going as well as supervised school going adolescent girls.

The effects of supplementation on the prevalence of anemia and compliance rate were assessed over a 4-year period. In 4 years, prevalence of anemia reduced from 73.3 percent to 25.4 percent. The compliance rate was also very high, being around 85 percent.

# 7

# Adolescent reproductive sexual health

## 7.1 Introduction

Adolescent Reproductive and Sexual Health (ARSH) is recognized as a key development concern. Adolescence is both a transient stage, between childhood and adulthood, and a formative period during which many life patterns are learned and established. In India, the adolescents are generally identified in the age group of 10–19 years. Until recently, this age group as a distinct category with special needs barely got any attention by the policy makers. They were targeted within the larger interventions aimed at population stabilization. In India, there are over 240 million adolescents, which is roughly one-fifth of the total population of the country. This group constitutes the largest group among the victims of HIV infection – millions of new infections of STDs and of the reproductive tract occur every year.

Reproductive and sexual health is a major area of concern, as the adolescents do not have adequate awareness and knowledge about these. The chances of having sexually transmitted diseases (STD), teenage pregnancy and unsafe abortions are much higher among adolescents. In India, although traditional norms oppose premarital sex, some studies indicate a growing trend towards premarital sexual activities among adolescents (Nair, 2004). According to Futures group (2012), most sexual activities begin in adolescence; for example 3 percent of adolescent males and 8 percent of adolescent females had sex before age 15, 1 percent female and 63 percent males aged 15–19 had high risk sex with a non-marital, non-cohabitating partner and 31 percent adolescent males and 20 percent adolescent females used a condom during their last high risk sex. However, most of these estimates could be underestimates as these being sensitive questions. According to a UNICEF report (2012), there are 49,000 adolescent males and 46,000 adolescent females with human immune deficiency virus (HIV) positive in India. According to NFHS-3, almost 11 percent of females and 7 percent of males in age 15–24 had a history of sexually transmitted infections (STI) in the preceding 1 year of the survey. Among men, self-reported prevalence of the two STI symptoms – abnormal bad smelling genital discharge and genital sore or ulcer – is higher among adolescents than among men aged 20–24.

The adolescents should know how to protect themselves from HIV/STI/ reproductive tract infections (RTI) and should have easy access to adolescent friendly health services. Around 35 percent adolescent males and 19 percent adolescent females had comprehensive knowledge of HIV. DLHS–3 (2007–08) reported that only 30 percent of unmarried women aged 15–24 had heard about RTI/STI.

HIV prevalence is lower among young persons (age 15–24) than among persons in any other age group. Very few women or men of age 15–17 years are HIV positive. HIV prevalence remains low even at age 18–19. Even among women and men who never had sex, there are a few HIV positive cases. This is because there could be reasons other than sexual contact for getting infected with HIV.

The fertility pattern and contraceptive use among adolescents are crucial to the future fertility situation in the country. Knowledge of contraception among adolescents was more than 90 percent (NFHS-3). But, only a little more than 10 percent of adolescent girls were using any form of contraceptive (Nair, 2004). Many of these married women may not use contraceptives because they wish to bear a child.

An important aspect of neglect of adolescent girls is that they are married early and have their first child in their early teens. Although the legal age for marriage is 18, the majority of Indian women marry as adolescents. According to NFHS-3, 47.4 percent of women of age 20–24 married by the age 18, and 16 percent of women aged 15–19 were already mothers or pregnant at the time of the survey. NFHS-3 showed that 12 percent of all women aged 15–19 years and 44 percent of currently married women in the same age group had begun childbearing. Further, 30 percent of girls aged 15–19 were currently married or were in union, compared to only 5 percent of boys of the same age.

There are considerable disparities among girls according to their residence. According to UNICEF (2011) while the prevalence of child marriage among urban girls was around 29 percent, it was 56 percent for their rural counterparts. Further, young women in the poorest households were seven times more likely to give birth before age 18 than young women from the rich households in India. Along with prevailing illiteracy, ignorance and poverty, these adolescent mothers were not capable to take care of themselves and their children. This results in high maternal and infant mortality, chronic ill health and increased burden of disease for the nation. All this can be overcome with comprehensive care during adolescence including nutrition counseling, health education, delaying age of marriage and family planning.

Menstrual irregularities and ovarian disease among females and diabetes among both sexes, especially in urban affluent families, are emerging as major problems. More than half of females experience painful periods and around 40 percent reported passing of clots during menstruation. But, of the adolescent girls who experienced menstrual problems, only 26 percent had any consultation (Sachan et al., 2012).

Around 26 percent adolescents are less likely to visit public health facility or camps as compared to women of older age groups (Jejeebhoy and Santhya, 2011). As expected, private sector utilization was more prevalent in urban areas. The barriers in accessing health services by the adolescents and the young people are manifold – lack of confidentiality, privacy, odd hours of the clinics, feeling isolated among adults while waiting, stigma attached to visiting a clinic, etc. Around 50 percent women face many socio-economic challenges in accessing health services. The most common of these were distance to a health facility, transport, and concern over non-availability of female health provider, and/or drugs at the health facility (Jejeebhoy and Santhya, 2011).

## 7.2 How to address adolescents

In our country, there are very few services that respond to adolescents' needs. As interventions for children focus on the younger ages, adolescents are left out. They are also unreached by programs for adults. Adolescents' health problems must be addressed through a multidimensional holistic approach. For any effective program, role of different stakeholders like the schools, the parents, the community, and the politicians, the key persons of the community and most importantly the health care providers in providing health care services has to be ensured.

There is excessive pressure of expectations of parents, friends and teachers on adolescents. Parents are unaware about their role in improving adolescent health and addressing their reproductive sexual health concerns. There is no guidance available to them by elderly including parents and the only sources are friends, media and the literature creating more confusion. It is not surprising that some adolescents fall prey to premarital sex, risk-taking behavior and other self-destructive tendencies. It is, therefore, essential that parents and other elderly persons of the family devise ways to impart adequate knowledge on reproductive sexual health issues to this virgin section of the society.

As adolescents spend a major proportion of their time in their schools, teachers can play an effective role in screening adolescents for common disorders, providing nutritional counseling, reproductive and sex education, life-skill education, etc. School-level effective and focused health and counseling programs on reproductive sexual health can be one of the best ways to address the concerns of the adolescents.

Community and government can also play an important role in this direction. Awareness about harmful effects of early marriage and childbearing in community and knowledge of family planning can help a lot in not only reducing maternal and infant mortality rates but also preventing risk-taking behavior, unsafe sex and spread of STI and HIV. Adolescent friendly health and counseling centres should be established to provide services to the adolescents. The centres should ensure confidentiality and provide counseling not only regarding diet and lifestyle including hygiene but also on all aspects of sound health behavior including reproductive sexual health. These centres should also assist the adolescents on sexual violence and exploitation.

India's National Population Policy 2000 aims at ensuring that adolescents' need for information, counseling, population education, and contraceptive services are accessible and affordable; food supplements and nutrition services are available; and the legislation on restraint of child marriage is enforced (Gupta, 2003). The Pan American Health Organization and a WHO consultation held in October 2000 recommended provision of a package of services at an Adolescent Friendly Health Services Centre that includes monitoring of growth and development; management of behavioral problems, offering information and counseling on developmental changes, personal care and ways of seeking help; reproductive health including contraceptives, STI treatment, pregnancy care and postabortion management; voluntary counseling and testing for HIV; management of sexual violence and mental health services including management of substance abuse (McIntyre, 2003).

The National Rural Health Mission (NRHM) gives Adolescent Reproductive and Sexual Health (ARSH) top priority in its RCH-II program. The national strategy of the Indian government takes a three-pronged approach in improving the health of young people by building awareness among communities, creating conducive environment for service delivery and providing a comprehensive package of services to young people. This strategy focuses on reorganizing the existing public health system to enable it to meet the service needs of adolescents. The Medical Officers (MOs), ANMs and LHVs are required to ensure service delivery at sub-centres and PHCs at fixed day and timings. The services include preventive, promotive, curative and counseling aspects (Government of India, 2006). Safdarjung Hospital in Delhi set up the first Adolescent Friendly Health Services Centre. It provides a wide range of services which include clinical and mental health services, nutritional and reproductive counseling, growth monitoring and development, and immunization (Safdarjung Hospital Adolescent Healthcare Network, 2005). Haryana was one of the first states in the country to launch a distinct ARSH program providing 'Adolescent Friendly Health Services' at government health facilities.

## 7.3 Sex education

Sex education is the instruction on issues relating to *human sexuality*, including *human sexual anatomy, sexual reproduction, sexual activity, reproductive health,* emotional relations, *reproductive rights* and responsibilities, *sexual abstinence,* and birth control. Common avenues for sex education are parents or caregivers, formal school programs, media and public health campaigns.

Traditionally, adolescents are not given any information on sexual matters as discussion of these issues is considered *taboo*. Most of the efforts on providing sex education to adolescents originated from Western countries. The *progressive education* movement of the late 19th century, however, led to the introduction of *'social hygiene'* in North American school curricula and the advent of school-based sex education (Tupper, 2013). Despite these initiatives, most of the information on sexual matters in the mid-20th century was obtained informally from friends and the media, and much of this information was deficient and of doubtful value, especially during the period following puberty when curiosity of sexual matters was the most acute. This deficiency became increasingly evident by the increasing incidence of teenage pregnancies, especially in Western countries after the 1960s. To reduce such pregnancies, programs of sex education were instituted amidst strong opposition from parent and religious groups.

The outbreak of *AIDS* provided a sense of urgency to sex education. However, sex education is seen by most stakeholders as a vital *public health* strategy. Some international organizations such as *Planned Parenthood* consider that broad sex education programs have global benefits, such as controlling the risk of *overpopulation* and the advancement of *women's rights*. The use of mass media campaigns has sometimes resulted in high levels of awareness coupled with essentially superficial knowledge of HIV transmission (Piya Sorcar, 2010).

About 92 percent of adolescents reported that they wanted both to talk to their parents about sex and to have comprehensive in-school sex education (Sari Locker, 2001). Sex education can be informal, like someone receiving information from a conversation with a parent, friend, religious leader, or through the *media*. It may also be through sex *self-help* authors, magazine *advice columnists, sex columnists,* or sex education web sites. Formal sex education is usually provided by schools or health care providers. According to various experts, sex education is necessary to prepare the young for the future family and community life. It teaches the adolescents what they should know for their personal conduct and relationship with others. Officials generally agree that some kind of planned sex education is necessary.

It is debated whether formal sex education should be imparted as a full course in primary level or *junior high school* or high school. It is also debated whether it should be only one module within a wider *zoology, health, home economics, or physical education* curricula. Even today, some schools do not offer any sex education because of it being a *controversial* issue. In particular, there is no conscientiousness on many details like age at which children should start receiving such education, the amount of detail that can be revealed, including the topics dealing with *human sexual behavior*, e.g. *safe sex* practices, *masturbation, premarital sex,* and *sexual ethics*.

When sex education is a matter for debate, the main concern is whether covering *child sexuality* is valuable or detrimental. Whether the use of *birth control* such as *condoms* and *hormonal contraception;* and their impact on pregnancy outside marriage, *teenage pregnancy,* and the transmission of STIs should all form the curricula. Increasing support for *abstinence-only sex education* by conservative groups has been one of the primary causes of this controversy. Ironically, countries with conservative attitudes towards sex education have a higher incidence of STIs and teenage pregnancy.

In India, there are many programs promoting sex education including information on AIDS in schools as well public education and advertising. AIDS clinics providing information and assistance can be found in most cities and many small villages. India has a strong prevention program which goes hand in hand with care, support and treatment. We have been able to contain the epidemic with a prevalence of just 0.31 percent. We have also brought about a decline of 50 percent in new infections annually.

## 7.4 ARSH project in Bihar and Jharkhand

### 7.4.1 Introduction

National Foundation of India (NFI) launched a program in 2006 on Communication Initiative on Adolescent Reproductive and Sexual Health (ARSH) in the states of Bihar and Jharkhand with support from Packard Foundation. Working with adolescents has been challenging not only because it is new but also because the issues and actions involve matters of great cultural sensitivity. Indian society with its socio-cultural diversity has had a long tradition of what is accepted or what can be allowed regarding sexual information and values.

To start with, NFI sensitized a diverse group of stakeholders to design a culturally sensitive program for the adolescents. It tried to involve the NGOs as partners through distributing brochures, organizing meetings and inviting concept notes from those who were interested and had sensitivity to work on this. Such a process helped in identification of different resource organizations involved in ARSH related issues and more importantly, enabled them to explore strategic interventions and networking possibilities with support organizations and donors for complementing existing work on ARSH in these two states.

At the level of voluntary sector, it was evident that only a very few NGOs were working on ARSH related issues and most of them were working within a framework of mother and child program. Therefore, it was critical for NFI to strengthen the NGOs institutional capacity so as to enable them to contribute towards the goal of social transformation and well-being on a sustained basis.

### 7.4.2 Evaluation

Two types of evaluations were carried out by IASDS, viz. process evaluation and quantitative assessment. The evaluation studies concentrated on sensitizing civil society, knowledge building and environment building. These studies were expected to assess if the programme had created an environment on ARSH issues and had influenced any attitudinal change among the larger and direct community groups during the implementation.

The assessment covered different aspects of ARSH related knowledge, attitude but with limited practices with a focus on the following aspects: information and education on basic health, adolescents and youth reproductive and sexual health, gender and communication. The objective of the quantitative assessment was to assess the current status on the outcome indicators at the level of knowledge, group formation, skills of specific community on ARSH.

At the start of the project a total of ten NGOs were working on ARSH in 6 districts of Bihar and 4 districts of Jharkhand. Out of these two NGOs were to discontinue. Therefore, the target groups covered by remaining all the 8 NGOs were canvassed in the quantitative assessment.

### 7.4.3 Target groups

Different target groups were 10–14 and 15–19 years girls, and 15–19 years boys. These were in and out of school, in and out of Kishori-Samooh (a special group of adolescent girls). In addition, unmarried youth and newly married/ couples of 15–24 years with 0/1 child and community – key person in family, service providers and social/religious leaders. Some frontline workers were also included.

There was however a limitation in the assessment. The area selected for the intervention had more than one project in operation run by the same NGO.

In such a case, there was the likelihood of confounding (mixing up) of impacts on crucial indicators, and it was virtually impossible to accurately segregate and assign the exact quantum under any single project. This is a wider problem encountered in most intervention projects.

The analysis of data revealed some interesting features. One of these was on the issue of trafficking. On being asked about reasons for trafficking of young girls, most of the respondent boys cited lack of *money and education* as the major reasons for the evil. *Drug/alcohol addiction and irresponsibility of parents* were other significant reasons according to some. Educating girls and family to a large extent and de-addiction drive can prevent this evil. More than half to three-fourth of the responding girls knew about trafficking of young girls, and surprisingly, less number among boys put the reason lack of education as the reason for trafficking. But girls thought it to be lack of money as the foremost reason and irresponsibility of parents following by *lack of awareness*. However, prevention of trafficking among girls will be possible through *educating the family* and promoting education for *girls*.

There were many other interesting aspects of the study. Personal hygiene among girls, education, importance of girl child, improving negotiation skills and ANC/PNC remained the most commonly discussed issues among the 15–19 years adolescents covered by different NGOs. Awareness on nutrition deficiency disorders like anaemia and night blindness and their causes and prevention was good among the adolescents. The analysis reflects a large percentage of the target groups being unaware of the basic dietary source, where the programme needs to focus to overcome the concern. The awareness about HIV/AIDS was considerably lower among girls than the boys.

The target group having access to media raises the question whether the programme had a limited reach to the marginalized section. The social pressure on women regarding family, particularly ARSH issues, can be effectively addressed if the appropriate communication within the family and the spouse is created. It appears that the next generation feels the importance of their views in selecting the partners for better understanding. A strong life skill approach for the target groups can have a better impact in taking this decision.

Dowry as a social evil and often a form of violence against women is important to be addressed. May be, limited livelihood option leads to such a social evil. However, focused formative research needs to be done to address the issue which is a critical concern for all. Most of the respondents preferred to discuss with friends ARSH related issues. So, knowledge building of peer can influence in information dissemination.

For the unmarried youth, 20–24 years age, creating awareness on ARSH issues remained a major activity of the NGOs. Among females only few issues were discussed. Majority of the youth showed interest in gaining information on topics related to ARSH, gender, livelihood, life skill and MCH care. Hence, it is apparent that there is an urgent need to create space for dialogue with the concerned group to enable them for taking decisions on such critical issues and make a difference in their lives.

Among couples with 0–1 child, women showed a better understanding of reproductive and sexual health issues particularly related to women, though they were relatively less aware about male issues.

An impact of the intervention can be visualized by a sizeable number of respondents both male and female admitting the need to talk about choice of contraception, sex of the child, and delay in pregnancy or spacing with their spouse. A detailed analysis of the multiple responses data collected on functioning of NGOs addressing IEC issues relating to ARSH is presented in Chapter 11. It provides some interesting features which would not have been possible through the conventional analysis of overlapping responses.

The social pressure on women regarding family, particularly ARSH issues can be effectively addressed if the appropriate communication within the family and the spouse is created. Hence, behavioral change can be aimed in future from the programme intervention.

An impression which clearly emerges out of the NFI study is that it had a good wholesome strategy on ARSH, and environment building was the key achievement of the project. However, its implementation by most NGOs needs strengthening. These NGOs addressed only few of the ARSH issues, and that too in a superficial way. A key to further strengthening of the NFI project would be to focus only on issues having direct bearing on ARSH. It should have a uniform strategy and uniform indicators for effective monitoring/ evaluation.

# 8
# Gender disparity

## 8.1 Gender disparity

Gender inequality is an integral part of our social system. Women in rural areas live in serious deprivation while urban women comparatively have better access and opportunities to housing, schooling, safe water, sanitation, fuel, electricity, etc. Women have the primary responsibility for household works – cooking, dishwashing, shopping, cleaning, and caring not only for children but also for other family members. In contrast, men generally do fewer household chores. These aspects do have an effect on the social and economic status of women and the extent of disparity within the household.

Gender discrimination is widely prevalent with regard to literacy in most states in India. Dropout rates are much higher among girls, and are particularly more visible in the age group 11–14 years. Besides literacy, there are many other inequalities, which prevail in most parts of our country. Amartya Sen (2001) has discussed seven types of inequalities. These are mortality, natality, basic facility, special opportunity, professional, ownership and household.

Mortality inequality is the higher rates of death among women and girls compared to men and boys. Higher rates of disease and mortality among women and girls are manifestation of a failure to give them medical care, food and social services, compared to that given to their male counterparts. Given a preference for boys over girls that many male-dominated societies have, gender inequality can manifest itself in the form of the parents wanting the newborn to be a boy rather than a girl. With the availability of modern techniques to determine the gender of the fetus, sex-selective abortion has become common in many countries. This gives rise to natality inequality. Basic facility and inequalities of opportunity refer to fewer opportunities for girls in respect of schooling, higher education and professional training. The professional inequality refers to far greater handicap women have in terms of employment and promotion in their career. Ownership inequality refers to imbalances in men's favour with regard to ownership of property and assets, while household inequality is characterized by the division of work among men and women: household chores by women and outside work by men. Although this categorization of inequalities is very informative, there is paucity of data on these at district levels. There is also a need to develop suitable methodology for evaluation of some of these inequalities.

The preference for sons is deep rooted in India for cultural and economic reasons. A major reason why a son is preferred over a daughter among Hindus is the widespread belief that only a son can perform rituals at his parent's cremation and at every death anniversary. Further, the daughter is perceived to be of little economic benefit to her parents as she leaves the parental home to live with her in-laws. A daughter's wedding can be a cause of stress and a grave financial burden for parents because of the widely prevalent dowry system despite laws against dowry in 1961.

Throughout their lifecycle, from pre-birth till death, females are subjected to gender discrimination. Starting from feticide (female), there is widespread prevalence of discrimination in dietary intake (both in quality and content), schooling, clothing and even decision making during adulthood towards health, care and utilization of health services and goods. Sex ratios at different stages of age are main indicators of sex discrimination. This is discussed in Section 8.2. Another component of gender inequality is the imbalance in intra household consumption expenditure and dietary intakes and patterns. Both these types of disparities are discussed later in Sections 8.3 and 8.4.

## 8.2 Sex ratios

Sex ratio is an indicator to find the inequality of males and females in a society at a given period of time. Three important stages for sex ratios are: at birth, at child attaining age 5 and at adulthood. Sex ratio is expressed as the number of women per thousand men in a given population at a given time. It is used to assess relative excess or deficit of men or women in a population at a given point of time. Sex differentials can be due to difference in mortality rate, migration, sex ratio at birth and even due to the undercounting of women at the time of population enumeration. Indian Census provides dis-aggregated information by sex on various aspects of population. According to Census 2001, there were 532 million (52%) males and 497 million (48%) females in the population. This shows significant imbalance in favor of males. In 2011 Census, this composition was 624 million males and 586 million females. Percentage-wise this was approximately 51.6 males and 48.4 females showing some improvement in favor of females.

Sex ratios in most of Indian states are in favor of males. North Indian states have persistent high sex inequalities. As stated earlier, mortality inequality between women and men is characterized by unusually high mortality rates of women. Inequality in newborn is directly linked with female feticide arising out of son preference by parents. Majority of parents desire to have at least one male child and availability of modern medical techniques to determine the gender of the fetus contribute to sex-selective abortions. As a result, there is a sharp decline in the child sex ratio (CSR) in most of the northern states of India. Such a decline is observed in 48 out of 70 districts of Uttar Pradesh. Ironically most of these districts are located in the western UP which is a developed region of the state.

### 8.2.1 Overall sex ratio

According to United Nations estimates, the world had 986 females against 1000 males in 2000. Except Indonesia and Japan, all other Asian countries had low sex ratios. Though most of the developed European countries have high sex ratio, highly populated China (944) and India (933) with low sex ratio create the imbalance in favor of males in the world.

There is a list of ranks according to 2011 census of the states and union territories of India ranked in order of sex ratio for the years 2001 and 2011. Data are as per the Census of India 2001 and provisional census totals for 2011 results. According to Census of 2011, Kerala has the highest sex ratio while Haryana has the lowest sex ratio among states and Daman & Diu has the lowest among all states and territories (Table 8.1).

Though Census has shown an increase in the sex ratio of total population from 927 in 1991 to 940 in 2011, it still needs further improvement. In 2001, eighteen states/union territories recorded sex ratio above the national average of 933, while remaining seventeen were below this. Chandigarh and Daman & Diu occupied the bottom positions with less than 800 females per 1000 males. Only Kerala and Pondicherry had sex ratio in favor of females having registered more than 1000 females. The sex ratio has gone up from 933 in 2001 to 940 in 2011 Census. In rural areas this was higher, 947, compared to 926 in urban areas. Migration of males to urban areas could be one of the reasons for lower sex ratios in urban areas.

Table 8.1 gives sex ratio changes from 2001 to 2011. There has been some improvement in the sex ratio of India but it has gone down badly in some states like Haryana. The state of Kerala which has the best sex ratio in India has also shown a tremendous improvement in these 10 years. On the other hand, Daman & Diu has shown the steepest decline during this period.

Sex ratio varies from region to region in the country. Kerala and Puducherry are the only two places in India where total female population continues to be more than the male population. As a matter of fact, Puducherry has the highest female sex ratio among union territories. The states of South India have the best sex ratio of females per 1000 males. States like Andhra Pradesh, Maharashtra and Karnataka also show increase in their sex ratios.

**Table 8.1** Sex ratios of states and union territories in 2001 and 2011

| Rank | State | Sex Ratio 2011 | Sex Ratio 2001 | Sex Ratio Change 2001 to 2011 |
|---|---|---|---|---|
| 1 | Kerala | 1,084 | 1,058 | +26 |
| 2 | Puducherry (2011)<br>Pondicherry (2001) | 1,038 | 1,001 | (not meaningful) |
| 3 | Tamil Nadu | 995 | 986 | +9 |
| 4 | Andhra Pradesh | 992 | 978 | +14 |
| 5 | Chhattisgarh | 991 | 990 | +1 |
| 6 | Manipur | 987 | 978 | +9 |
| 7 | Meghalaya | 986 | 975 | +11 |
| 8 | Odisha (2011)<br>Orissa (2001) | 978 | 972 | +6 |
| 9 | Mizoram | 975 | 938 | +37 |
| 10 | Himachal Pradesh | 974 | 970 | +4 |
| 11 | Karnataka | 968 | 964 | +4 |
| 12 | Goa | 968 | 960 | +8 |
| 13 | Uttarakhand (2011)<br>Uttaranchal (2001) | 963 | 964 | -1 |
| 14 | Tripura | 961 | 950 | +11 |
| 15 | Assam | 954 | 932 | +22 |
| 16 | Lakshadweep | 946 | 947 | −1 |
| 17 | Jharkhand | 947 | 941 | +6 |
| 18 | West Bengal | 947 | 934 | +13 |
| 19 | Nagaland | 931 | 909 | +22 |
| 20 | Madhya Pradesh | 930 | 920 | +10 |
| 21 | Rajasthan | 926 | 922 | +4 |
| 22 | Maharashtra | 925 | 922 | +3 |
| 23 | Arunachal Pradesh | 920 | 901 | +19 |
| 24 | Gujarat | 918 | 921 | −3 |
| 25 | Bihar | 916 | 921 | −5 |
| 26 | Uttar Pradesh | 908 | 898 | +10 |
| 27 | Punjab | 893 | 874 | +19 |
| 28 | Sikkim | 889 | 875 | +14 |
| 29 | Jammu & Kashmir | 883 | 900 | −17 |
| 30 | Andaman & Nicobar Islands | 878 | 846 | +32 |

*Contd...*

*Contd...*

| Rank | State | Sex Ratio 2011 | Sex Ratio 2001 | Sex Ratio Change 2001 to 2011 |
|---|---|---|---|---|
| 31 | Haryana | 877 | 861 | +16 |
| 32 | Delhi | 866 | 821 | +45 |
| 33 | Chandigarh | 818 | 773 | +45 |
| 34 | Dadra & Nagar Haveli | 775 | 811 | −36 |
| 35 | Daman & Diu | 618 | 709 | −91 |
| | Total average | 940 | 933 | +10 |

The sex ratio of population in villages and towns helps to know the composition of population distribution at lower levels and is also useful in micro-level planning. Table 8.2 gives the distribution of sex ratios in 2001 Census by districts, villages and towns. It is observed that out of 593 districts, 164 (close to 26%) had sex ratio below 900, 48 had sex ratio below 850 and 9 had it below 800. The distribution is also different in rural and urban areas, the latter having relatively poorer sex ratios. Out of 582699 villages 163871 (28.1%) had ratio below 900; and out of 4378 urban areas 1611 (36.8%) had sex ratio below 900.

**Table 8.2** Number of districts villages and urban agglomerations (UA)/towns by sex ratio of total population: India

| Sex ratio | No. of districts | No. of villages | No. UAs/towns |
|---|---|---|---|
| Less than 800 | 9 | 33,876 | 201 |
| 800–849 | 39 | 44,636 | 270 |
| 850–899 | 116 | 86,359 | 1,140 |
| 900–949 | 193 | 125,542 | 1,261 |
| 950–999 | 162 | 117,935 | 948 |
| 1000 and above | 74 | 174,351 | 558 |
| Total | 593 | 582,699 | 4,378 |

### 8.2.2 Sex ratio at birth

The sex ratio at birth (SRB) is the ratio of the number of girls born per 1000 boys born. It is one of the major social indicators. A low sex ratio is an indicator of biased attitude of society against the females. It is an indicator of the extent of prenatal sex selection. Internationally accepted norm for SRB is 952 or more. In India, a normal SRB is taken as 950 female births per 1,000 male births. Accurate information regarding SRB is not available, though in the recent past some data on this are available through AHS.

Data on sex ratio at birth is periodically collected at the national level by the Civil Registration System and the Sample Registration System (SRS), both under the Office of the Registrar General of India. A detailed discussion of these is given in Kulkarni (2007) and the major reporting here is based upon this article. The Civil Registration System data is not reliable due to gross under registration of births in some states. This makes SRS estimates as the most frequently used source of sex ratio at birth data. However, these estimates are only at state and national levels. SRS utilizes data from a sample and, therefore, has the problem of large sampling errors for annual estimates, and to overcome this, it gives 3-year moving averages of the sex ratio at birth.

Another limitation with SRS estimates is that it does not provide data at district and lower levels. Such data can become available only if coverage of birth registration under the Civil Registration System improves. A few states, such as Kerala, Himachal Pradesh, Punjab and Tamil Nadu have achieved cent percent birth registration while states like Bihar, Uttar Pradesh and Madhya Pradesh have reported coverage only in the range of 17–53 percent.

### 8.2.3 Child sex ratio

Like the sex composition of the total population, the sex composition by age groups is vital for studying the demographic trends of young population, its future patterns and particularly, the status of the girl child. As per the 2001 Census, sex ratio of the population in the age group 0–6 years was 927, declining from 945 in 1991 and 962 in 1981. The decreasing sex ratio in this age group adversely affects the population over a period of time leading to diminishing sex ratio. Imbalance at the early age group is difficult to be removed and would continue its negative impact on the population for a long time to come.

Child sex ratio is mainly influenced by sex ratio at birth and mortality in the early childhood. The natural sex ratio at birth usually has higher male births. It ranges between 943 and 954. But the advantage of higher sex ratio at birth (SRB) is neutralized due to higher male infant mortality in the normal population. Prior to 2001, the child sex ratio was close to sex ratio at birth but it fell even below the natural SRB in Census 2001. This reflects the poor status of the girl child in the country and majority of its states.

According to provisional estimates of Census (2011), CSR in India declined from 927 to 914; maximum decline from 2001 to 2011 was recorded in J&K (−82, from 941 to 859), though Punjab had a rise of 48, up from

798 to 846. Other major declines of more than 20 points were noted from Maharashtra (−30), Rajasthan (−26), Jharkhand and Uttarakhand (−22 each), and Madhya Pradesh (−20).

Table 8.3 gives CSR in rural and urban areas at three time points: 1991, 2011 and 2011. It is observed that CSR has declined in both rural and urban areas. The decline is, however, much higher in rural areas in 2011.

**Table 8.3** CSR in rural and urban areas (1991–2011)

| Census | Total | Rural | Urban |
|---|---|---|---|
| 1991 | 945 | 948 | 935 |
| 2001 | 927 | 933 | 906 |
| 2011* | 914 | 919 | 902 |

*Provisional totals

As per Census 2001, the CSR (in UP was 916 girls per 1000 boys, a drop of 11 points from 927 in 1991. Alarmingly, the CSR was below 900 in 23 districts of western UP. The worst-hit 20 districts of the state are given in the following table:

**Table 8.4** Districts with adverse child sex ratio in UP

| S. no. | Name of district | 0–6 Sex ratio |
|---|---|---|
| 1 | Baghpat | 850 |
| 2 | Ghaziabad | 854 |
| 3 | Gautam Budh Nagar | 854 |
| 4 | Meerut | 857 |
| 5 | Muzaffarnagar | 859 |
| 6 | Agra | 866 |
| 7 | Bulandshahr | 867 |
| 8 | Kanpur Nagar | 869 |
| 9 | Saharanpur | 872 |
| 10 | Mathura | 872 |
| 11 | Aligarh | 885 |
| 12 | Hathras | 886 |
| 13 | Jhansi | 886 |
| 14 | Jalaun | 889 |
| 15 | Etah | 891 |
| 16 | Kanpur Dehat | 892 |

*Contd...*

*Contd...*

| S. no. | Name of district | 0–6 Sex ratio |
|---|---|---|
| 17 | Auraiya | 894 |
| 18 | Etawah | 895 |
| 19 | Shahjahanpur | 897 |
| 20 | Farrukhabad | 897 |

Interestingly, the CSR was above 950 in backward districts such as Sonbhadra, Maharajganj, Kushinagar, Gonda, Balrampur, Bahraich and Siddharthnagar.

## 8.2.4 Trends in sex ratio at birth

It has been discussed earlier that there is a need to improve the Civil Registration System. Sincere efforts need to be undertaken by central and state governments. It is also important to assess whether improvements in sex ratio at birth have been due to better reporting of girls, or due to increase in the actual number of girls born.

There have been considerable concerns regarding distortions in reporting sex ratios in India. An excellent discussion on these aspects appears in Kulkarni (2007). Present Section derives heavily from his write-up. Distorted sex ratios in early ages have taken place mainly due to age misreporting giving a wrong impression of changes during 1901 to 1981. In the early censuses the ratio seemed to be very low in the 0–4 age group and high in the 10–14 age group mainly on account of sex-selective age misreporting the tendency of which had declined over the period yielding a near constancy in the ratios. However, a notable rise in the ratio in the 0–4 age group was seen after 1981. While in earlier census results, adult women constituted the bulk of 'missing women'; it were young ages who contributed the most in the recent census enumerations. This phenomenon provided evidence that the sex ratio at birth had altered perhaps due to the practice of sex-selective abortions. This was further corroborated by the regional variations in sex ratios at birth.

As discussed in Kulkarni (2007), in the 2001 census, a small improvement was observed in the overall sex ratio, to 107.2 from 107.9, but a greater imbalance noted in the young ages, 0–6 years, from 105.8 to 107.9. By then, the sex ratio at birth had emerged as a factor in the sex ratio imbalance in India. Independent investigations showed the existence of the practice of sex-selective abortions on a non-negligible scale.

Imbalances in sex ratios as discussed in the preceding sections are indicative of sex selective births caused by prenatal sex selection. Intensive efforts are called for to control this problem. The strong preference for sons is evident in some Indian states. The practice of sex-selective abortion to ensure a male child has been documented in many parts of India and even among Indians living abroad. The increasing availability of ultrasound has been linked to the sharp rise in the ratio of male births to female births in some parts of India in recent decades. Female infanticide continues to be practiced in the poorest areas, although its extent is unknown. The situation is likely to change in near future due to the concerted efforts by the central and state governments to discourage the abortion of female fetuses, by way of enacting a law in 1994 against the misuse of Pre-Natal Diagnostic Techniques.

The issue of sex-selective abortion was indicated in 2001 census showing the sex ratio of the total population ages 0–6 as 927 girls per 1,000 boys, down from 945 in 1991. The situation had deteriorated to the point where one district, Fatehgarh Sahib in Punjab state, had a ratio of only 754 girls for every 1,000 boys under age 7. But as stated earlier, the situation has changed since 2001.

Skewness towards male child has been a major concern over the decades. Many reasons like preference for son, neglect of girl child, social structure, etc., can be attributed to low sex ratio in India. There are region specific reasons like in J&K – social security of girls, and in Punjab – land reforms. Other reasons are like poor economic condition, dowry, earning, old age security, etc.

Annual statistics on births and deaths are regularly published in our country. The SRS is the most regular source of demographic statistics in India. The sample size of SRS in 2006 was about 5.1 million rural and 1.8 million urban households. Following the 2001 census, the SRS began publishing sex ratios for births in the more populous states. The SRS data show that the sex ratio crisis has shown improvement in most of these states. The lowest SRBs are in two of India's wealthiest states, Punjab and Haryana (which itself was once part of Punjab) in northwest India. Many of the earliest efforts to combat the crisis were focused on this area. In Punjab, the SRB has improved from 775 in 1999–2001 to 808 in 2004–2006; while in Haryana, it rose from 803 to 837 over this period. These data indicate that a slow reversal has indeed begun.

Couples who want to limit their family to two children, at least one of them a boy, they are more likely to abort a female fetus. The pressure to have a son is often felt most intensively by young wives, who want to please their husband's family. Punjab which has India's most unbalanced ratio of boys to girls has a total fertility rate (TFR) as 2.1. TFR of a population is the average number of children that would be born to a woman over her lifetime if she was subject to prevailing fertility rates at all ages from a single given year, and survives throughout all her childbearing years. The southern state of Kerala had a sex ratio at birth below 900, suggesting a strong son preference. That state's TFR is only 1.7. However, Tamil Nadu, with the same TFR, had normal SRB for some time. This state has excelled in promoting health and combating sex-selective abortion. Its example shows that the practice can be controlled.

The somewhat higher sex ratios in relatively poor and higher TFR states such as Uttar Pradesh and Bihar may largely reflect the fact that the average of over four children per woman in those states makes the birth of a son much more likely.

As discussed above, low SRB is major concern at national level. Lower SRB is an indication of female feticide. In the absence of reliable data on SRB no valid inferences can be drawn. It is therefore necessary to arrive at valid estimates of SRB. In recent past some attempts have been made to estimate SRB. Data for the sex ratio at birth for different countries of the world are generally not available on a continuous time series basis. Indian Census child sex ratio (0–6 years) data were used to adjust the SRS sex ratio at birth for India and Indian states. As expected, there is no agreement between the SRS estimates and the census and the NFHS estimates; the SRS estimates being higher than others. Hence, while in the recent years India's SRB has undoubtedly risen above 105, one cannot be so sure about its being as high as 111. Therefore, we use both the given SRB values from the SRS as well as the implied SRB obtained from the census sex distribution.

For better understanding of the complexities involved in sex selective abortions, it may be desirable to assess the reasons for feticide. Reasons behind sex selective abortions should cover different socio-economic characteristics of social groups preferring/performing sex selective abortions. There can be many reasons for opting for illegal medical termination of pregnancy. To ascertain reasons for termination of pregnancy or going for ultrasound for sex determination is rather tricky, as respondents find it difficult to answer the related questions or they may provide wrong answers as the questions are embarrassing for them. In order to arrive at correct answers, one may adopt randomized response technique which is specially developed for ascertaining information on sensitive characteristics. It is discussed in details later in Chapter 12. Such an approach would enable us to develop an estimate of proportion of population resorting to feticide.

Proper monitoring of social indicators and precise estimates of female feticides will help planners and administrators to devise appropriate strategies to eliminate the existing bias towards girl child. It will also help to stop misuse of technologies for unlawful activities like pre-natal determination of sex, which in turn will lower the chances of female feticide. Proper and justified intervention will reduce the level of atrocities towards girl child.

The comparison of observed sex ratio at birth with normal sex ratio at birth gives an idea of girls missing at birth. Sex ratio at birth in India for the period (2007–09) was 906, while the internationally observed normal sex ratio at birth is 952 or more girls born per 1000 boys. The number of missing girls was computed by Kulkarni (2007) from the difference between observed numbers of girls born during the period 2001–07, and the numbers of girls that would have been born if the sex ratio at birth was normal, i.e. 952. Accordingly, it is estimated that the practice of prenatal sex selection has resulted in approximately 5.7 lakh girls being missed annually in India during the period 2001–08.

## 8.3 Intra household gender inequality in consumption expenditure

The best way of investigating the concept of intra household gender inequality is to compare the extent of inequality in household consumption. It would be of significant interest to compare gender differences in the distribution of consumption expenditure. Even though the surveys of National Sample Surveys Office (NSSO) provide time series data on household consumer expenditure, the surveys do not have the desired focus to provide aggregated or dis-aggregated data needed for studying the gender bias. As a result, no standardized methodology is available for adoption in a large-scale survey.

IASDS in 2003 conducted a research study for Central Statistical Office (CSO), Ministry of Planning and Program Implementation, Government of India, to develop a methodology for evaluating gender inequality in intra-household consumption expenditure. The study was conducted in three districts of Eastern Region of UP.

Gender inequality is a very sensitive issue and quantifying it even in the restricted area of household consumption expenditure is a difficult task. Development of a viable methodology for measuring the intra household inequality in household consumer expenditure is rather an intricate task necessitating field research and investigation in many phases and stages. The structure of NSSO household consumption expenditure surveys was taken as the nucleus.

The field investigation comprised of a *bench line* survey, followed by two *repeat* enquiries with a gap of at least two months to capture seasonal variations. These periods were also likely to facilitate study of any possible variations in consumption pattern during major festival times. The study focused on four broad age groups, 6–10, 11–17, 18–39 and 40–59. This was done with the assumption of homogeneity of consumption requirements in the two sexes under each age group.

The study was confined to three districts of Eastern Region of Uttar Pradesh. These districts were so selected that one each was from three distinct agro-climatic as well as socio-cultural belts. Three districts – Bahraich from Terai belt, Varanasi from Gangetic plains and Mirzapur from dry Vindhyachal region – were selected. Two panchayat wards were selected from each of these districts and from each panchayat ward; four villages were selected through stratified sampling. The stratification variable for village selection was the population $\leq 750$, $750 \leq 1500$, $1500 \leq 2500$ and $\geq 2500$.

In each of the panchayat wards, 200 households were selected across different socio-economic groups on proportional basis. Not only was socio-economic categorization a criteria for selection of households but also special care was taken to capture those households which specifically contain the broad age groups required for studying gender inequality.

Each of the sampled households was contacted thrice during the course of investigation, the first contact for collecting information was the bench line survey and the subsequent two contacts, and each spaced out in an interval of at least 2 months, for canvassing the specially structured schedule of enquiry focused on inequality in household consumption expenditure.

There were three different aspects of the analyses considered in this investigation:

- *To estimate average household monthly consumption expenditure.*

  For estimating this, three reference periods, namely 7, 30 and 365 days were considered. Based upon the relative consistency and other analytical arguments, feasibility of using one reference period was probed. Both mean and median were computed as average with a view to investigate which of these two would be more meaningful. This is important in view of the skewed distribution of consumption expenditure.

- *To evaluate gender-wise intra-household disparities in expenditure under different major household items.*

  This has been done under four age groups, namely, 6–10, 11–17, 18–39 and 40–59 age groups. The particular choice of these age groups assumes homogeneity within each age group, the first one being childhood, second as adolescent, third as young and the last as the middle-aged groups. This analysis was attempted in two ways. First, the gender bias was evaluated against gender-wise expenditure on each consumption item within each age group; and second, against the proportion of males and females consuming the particular item. The basic assumption was that disparity is of two types: first, females are denied access to many of the consumer items; and second, in the event of their taking some consumer items the expenditure incurred by them is lower in comparison to their male counterparts.

- *To evaluate intra-household, gender-wise disparities according to homogeneous broad age groups as above in the consumption of food items during the past 24 hours.*

### 8.3.1 Limitations of the study

As in NSSO consumption surveys, the list of household consumption items are too varied and diversified, necessitating enquiry through different recall periods. In spite of the best tools, efforts and care, the bias due to memory lag cannot be ruled out. However, since the objective is to investigate the gender bias necessitating the study of differentials, and not to develop the consumption estimates as such, these biases are not likely to affect the findings.

Another limitation of the study is inadequate sample sizes. The information was collected for four broad age groups, 6–10, 11–17, 18–39 and 40–59. Thus a restriction was that within the family, for a given age group, there should be at least one member form the two sexes. This resulted in reduction of sample sizes which were already small due to budget and time constraints. The sample sizes get further reduced, even drastically, when we make dis-aggregated comparisons by religion and castes.

### 8.3.2 Findings

The findings revealed similarity in the expenditure patterns among males and females in the 6–10 years age group both in terms of percentages and amount.

Slightly different trends were visible for the adolescent age group. Higher percentage of males had spending on education possibly because of relatively higher dropout rates among adolescent girls. Small differentials were also observed in expenditures on clothing and footwear in terms of amount spent on these items. Males were allocated higher amounts in comparison to female counterparts. Some degree of differentials was also noticed on consumption patterns relating to education. Higher percentage of males had higher spending on education possibly because of preference and higher dropout rates among adolescent girls which is a well-known phenomenon across the entire state of Uttar Pradesh. There was also higher spending in favor of boys towards wristwatch. This was in addition to the fact that boys were also shown favor in terms of providing them with a wristwatch. It is therefore noticed that some element of gender bias gets in to our system at the adolescent age, the age when the roles of boys and girls are conceived to be different by the elders of the family. The element of gender inequality continued in higher age groups also, though with reduced pace in the 40–59 years age group.

Although there seemed to be evidence of gender inequality in respect of consumption expenditures of different household items, the inequality in terms of dietary intakes was not that evident.

The results though do not markedly highlight the existing disparity but are encouraging enough to provide momentum for further probing with larger sample size. Further probing is also required as many times the disparity is not due to gender bias but may arise due to self-requirement and likings. For example, for wristwatch, a housewife might not need it as much as a working man. Hence here instead of simply asking whether *received a watch*, it would be more appropriate to probe and ask if the respondent had asked for a watch and then denied which might indicate gender bias. Similarly for dietary pattern, likes and dislikes for particular food item may hinder the result.

## 8.4 Gender inequality in dietary intakes

The household consumption expenditure survey did not reveal significant differences in dietary intakes by gender. This was mainly because of small sample sizes for different age groups. Further, the study did not include children below 6 years. A comprehensive study on gender inequality exclusively on dietary intakes and patterns was conducted by IASDS in an ICMR funded project in 2006.

For food intakes, the 24-hour recall was done over a period of three consecutive days. Food frequency questionnaire (FFQ) was also canvassed over each of these days and on every individual of same households. The information was sought in a format under the columns daily, once/twice a week, weekly, monthly, seasonally, and never. Standard bowls of different sizes were used for weighing food intakes.

Actual quantities of food servings (cooked instead of raw) were recorded. This may appear inadequate for deriving the estimate of food quantity consumed, but it may be reasonable in the present setting as the objective was not to derive estimates of intakes of food items or the nutrients but to perform a comparative analysis by days (and gender).

The study was confined to two blocks each of districts Kanpur Dehat and Mathura in Uttar Pradesh. Twenty villages were selected in each block and as the final stage units, 24 households per village were selected. Thus the total targeted sample size was 1920 households which were selected so as to represent different socio-economic groups on proportional basis and each household had at least one male and one female child of the same (defined) age group from same mother. The individual in a household was canvassed in two rounds, once in summer and the other in winter to capture seasonal variations if any. The households were visited on three consecutive days in both rounds in order to capture day-to-day variability.

The targeted population (children below 18 years) was divided into three broadly homogeneous age groups, viz. (i) below 72 months, (ii) 6 years to below 11 years, and (iii) 11 years to below 18 years. The first age group was further split into two sub-groups, viz. 'below 36 months' and '36 months and above', and in respect of former, the information about breastfeeding and complementary feeding practices was collected from the mothers on the basis of current practices for the younger child and allowing up to 3 year recall for the older child. The findings of the project also appeared in a paper by Nigam et al. (2010).

## 8.4.1 Analytical framework

ANOVA was applied to test for day-to-day differences in actual intakes of 3 days. This was done for data sets of each of the two rounds. Gender disparity was assessed by comparing how the food was distributed to the two sexes – (i) whether the food was served first to males, (ii) whether more food was served to males and (iii) whether leftover food was first given to males. Disparity was also assessed by comparing food intakes on gm/cu/day basis for individuals over 3 years of age, while for children below 3 years, breastfeeding and complementary feeding practices formed the basis for comparison. For these comparisons, t-tests were applied. This analysis was done on the data set pooled over two rounds as there was no significant difference between the rounds.

## 8.4.2 Results and discussion

### *8.4.2.1 Breast feeding practices*

It was observed that almost all the children below 36 months age, irrespective of the sex were breast fed except when the mother had insufficient milk. There was virtually no difference between the boys and girls regarding colostrums feeding and the frequency of breast-feeding. No significant difference between the sexes was also noted in 'average number of times breast fed'.

There was no difference in initiation of water before 4 months between the two sexes. The difference in initiation of top milk (any milk other than breast milk) among children of different sexes within the same households was significant (t = 2.5 with a probability level <0.05) in Kanpur Dehat (25.8% boys than 38.5% girls) but it was not significant in Mathura (39.5% boys than 42.0% girls). The mothers also reported higher percentages for not giving top milk to boys (43.2% in Kanpur Dehat and 32.8% in Mathura) which indicated that the male child was breastfed for a longer period of time compared to female in the family. The results in both districts in respect of reasons for weaning away a child from breast feed do indicate that this may be possibly because of their desire of getting pregnant again to have a male child (both t-values were highly significant: t = 3.50 at Kanpur Dehat and t = 6.68 at Mathura).

Timely initiation of complementary food was significantly different by gender in both the districts. In Kanpur Dehat, the difference in initiation percentages before 6 months had a t-value of 2.57, while it was 7.77 in Mathura. However, none of the other variables, like differences between *breast milk and semisolid food was given together, ghee was added, green leafy vegetables were added, initiative was taken by the mother to feed the child, breast feeding was stopped at <1 year* were statistically significant.

#### 8.4.2.2 Food distribution at home

In order to investigate the presence of gender disparity among children aged 6 months and above, responses from mothers of targeted children by age groups (both sexes) were analyzed. There was significant evidence of gender disparity (almost all t-tests were highly significant) in terms of all the three distribution characteristics, though it was in favor of males on whether the food was served first to males and whether more food was served to males. It was exactly opposite in case of whether leftover food was first given to males. A possible reason for this could be the fact that more boys than girls were going to school early in the morning, and were being given the leftover food of the previous day.

#### 8.4.2.3 Average food intake

An analysis of differences in average food intakes averaged over two rounds was also carried out by gender of different age groups in the two districts. It was revealed that for the age group 36 ≤ 72 months, none of the differences in food intakes by gender were significant. However, differences in the intakes of milk & milk products in 6 ≤ 11 years were significant in Mathura

($t = 2.09$), as males had received higher amount of milk and milk products. For the age group $11 \leq 18$ years, pulses & legumes, fats & oils and sugar & jaggery in Mathura, and roots & tubers and other vegetables in both the districts had significant t-values, but contrary to popular belief all these were in favor of females. It may be observed that with growing ages, children have more pronounced likes and dislikes about food items and they are likely to eat accordingly. Disparity is likely to be confounded with likes and dislikes of adolescents.

#### *8.4.2.4 Consistency of 3 days food intakes*

The consistency of intakes of 17 food items comprising Indian rural diets was probed. Respondents were asked on consecutive 3 days whether they had consumed these items on the previous day. The ANOVA on the food intakes over 3 days revealed that intakes of most of food items were statistically not different over days for younger children. However, with increase in age, there was higher evidence of difference in intakes over days. Further, the variations were seen mostly for important foodstuffs like cereals, pulses and vegetables. This indicates the superiority of 3-day recalls over single day (last 24 hour) recall.

The ANOVA on the food intakes over 3 days revealed that intakes of important food stuffs like cereals, pulses and vegetables were significantly different over days for children aged 6 years and above. This indicates that a single-day dietary intake assessment may not be an efficient method.

## 8.5 Consistency of food frequencies

It was stated earlier that FFQ formats currently in use often lead to highly subjective information because of variations in perceptions regarding meaning of terms like occasionally and seasonally, and memory lag. Memory lag is likely to be more serious for information sought under once/twice a week, weekly, once in two weeks, monthly and seasonally. This aspect was not difficult to probe as there was sufficient data available in both formats (actual intakes and food frequency) for the same three consecutive days. For analytical purpose, a common indicator for both data sets (as in NFHS-2) – *'at least once a week'*, i.e., percent of respondents who consumed a food item at least once a week was used.

In the 24-hour recall repeated for three consecutive days, the frequencies for 'at least once a week' were derived by counting such days when the food item was consumed on any of the 3 days, whether on a single day, or any of the two days, or on all the 3 days. As it captures food intakes up to 3 days out of total 7 days, it has the potential to provide a reasonably good estimate of *'at least once a week'*. For food frequency, an exact estimate is provided by combining entries from columns daily, once/twice a week and weekly.

The differences between two estimates were tested for significance using independent two sample t-tests. The results reveal that across all age groups, estimates by conventional food frequency were significantly higher than those of frequency by 24-hour recall for almost all the food items in both the districts. Possible reasons for this could be variations in perceptions regarding meaning of terms like occasionally and seasonally, and memory lag, particularly for information sought under once/twice a week, weekly, once in two weeks, monthly and seasonally. Another interesting feature is that of highest t-values for green leafy vegetables, indicating the memory lag and the possible confusion among the respondents in differentiating between green leafy and other non-leafy vegetables.

# 9

# Food insecurity and hunger

## 9.1 Introduction

Poverty, high levels of illiteracy, social discrimination and neglect besides other factors like poor health facilities, inadequate availability of nutritious food and poor hygiene are some of the major factors leading to food insecurity of the states. Failed governance has also a fair share in food insecurity. There is a cycle: poverty → poor purchasing power and lower literacy levels → poor awareness → social discrimination and denial of opportunities. All these factors combined with many other factors lead to poor levels of food security. Food insecurity leads to the feeling of hunger. It is therefore necessary to identify food insecure areas based on various indicators. It may be also be necessary to develop a suitable methodology for identifying types of hunger.

## 9.2 Food insecurity

Food insecurity has basically three components, viz. *food availability, food access* and *food absorption*. All of these components have their own importance concerning the food insecurity. M. S. Swaminathan Research Foundation (MSSRF) in 2001 in its document *'Food Insecurity Atlas of Rural India'* used nineteen indicators to capture the three components of food insecurity encompassing wide ranging factors besides many others like agriculture, sustainability, environment and ecology, health and nutrition, hygiene, living style and poverty, dietary intakes, demographic structure, etc. This was followed by two more publications, viz. *'Food Insecurity Atlas of Urban India'* in 2002, and *'Atlas of the Sustainability of Food Security' in 2004*. These documents present state-wise scenario on food insecurity/ sustainability with the help of chosen indicators, indices and maps. Such mappings are directly useful to planners and policy makers to readily visualize state-level disparities and identify problem states for remedial measures. IASDS conducted a district-level study for CSO on food insecurity atlas in rural Uttar Pradesh in 2010 and identified food insecure districts on the basis of these components, using 21 indicators. The present write up on food insecurity atlas is based upon this study. Part of this work also appeared in Nigam et al. (2014).

### 9.2.1 Food availability, access and absorption

Availability of food is a pre-requisite for food security and economic development. Domestic production and imports together play a significant role in food availability. For food availability, agriculture plays a very significant role. In this era of globalization, there is the possibility of food imports and industrial exports. Import of food items can be utilized to stabilize the prices of food items if the production of food falls short. In Indian context, however, the industrial exports are very much limited, to permit any dependence on food import. One thus finds that enhancing domestic production of food is the best option.

With rapid changes taking place with advancement of technology and globalization, importance of contribution of agriculture to national economy is coming down. Further, dependence of population on agriculture is decreasing. Even though there appears to be a shift from dependence on agriculture to industry, India has yet to go a long way to complete the process. The change has to be accompanied by improved productivity per worker both in industry and agriculture. Till higher paid jobs are not available in non-agricultural sector, agriculture will continue to provide livelihood. Thus, the role of agriculture in food production and employment will continue to be crucial for India.

Food access essentially consists of a package of entitlements. By entitlements is meant the acquirement of different things including food items. Apart from food items, it includes endowments like land, assets, physical ability and the things that can be obtained through exchange. Non-availability of enough food items in entitlements leads to hunger. This situation can arise due to certain changes like loss of assets or crops or/and change in exchange such as fall in prices of produce or wages. Physical disability also many a times leads to loss in endowments.

The problem of food access in the case of disadvantaged sections of the society is more acute and depends on food affordability. Shortage of food affordability leads to discrimination against women, children, old people and scheduled castes and scheduled tribes. Enhancement of food affordability through access to livelihood helps disadvantaged groups to escape from starvation and the related problems like undernutrition and premature mortality, etc.

Food absorption or ability to assimilate the food consumed is the final step towards healthy life, besides availability and accessibility of food. Food absorption essentially depends upon (i) food containing all nutrients and micronutrients and consumed in such a manner that it is absorbed well in the body, (ii) state of health of individual, and (ii) pure water supply, environment and hygiene.

Food absorption related problems lead to unhealthy under-nourished adult population having low BMI. Undernutrition leads to stunted growth of children. They are generally found to be underweight for their age. Further, food absorption problems are the root cause of many diseases.

### 9.2.2 Limitation of state level estimates

A major limitation of the state-level mapping as done by MSSRF is that the state-level aggregation may not capture inter- and intra-regional variations for large states with lot of heterogeneity in the underlying indicators and sub-indicators. This may happen because of masking effects. This issue was also highlighted by MSSRF. Quite rightly, it was pointed out that village-level and block-level mapping would be most useful, as it would enable to take up speedy and location-specific action. But, they ruled out attempting this exercise thinking that it would be formidable in view of the enormity of the work involved and the non-availability of data on virtually all sub-indicators particularly at the village/block level. The problem however is not that complicated at the district level and only some of the sub-indicators may not be available at this level.

The argument that the state-level aggregation may not capture inter- and intra-regional variations for large states with lot of heterogeneity is also valid for Uttar Pradesh which has not only large variations between its four regions: terribly backward Eastern and Bundelkhand, moderately backward Central and rather developed Western regions, but also between districts within the same region. For instance, some of the districts in the neighborhood of Bijnor of Western region are backward.

In view of the discussions as above, a district-wise atlas of rural UP using small area estimates was prepared. It is expected that this would be much more useful to the policy planners and implementers. Small area estimates have been derived wherever necessary to obtain district-level estimates of the crucial indicator namely percentage of population with chronic energy deficiency.

The study was carried out in 70 districts of Uttar Pradesh that existed at the time of the study. Data pertaining to these districts were collected from secondary sources. As stated earlier, the study uses 21 indicators as against 19 in MSSRF food insecurity atlas in rural India (2001). The district-level study of IASDS used a slightly modified version of MSSRF methodology.

Details of the indicators and modified methodology are:

(i) Deficit in production represented by the ratio of consumption to production of cereals,

(ii) Instability in cereal production in percent,

(iii) Sustainability index in percent,

(iv) Population affected by flood /heavy rain (in lakhs),

(v) Percentage of total crop loss by drought,

(vi) Calorie intake of the lowest decile (Kcal) per cu per day,

(vii) Percentage of population consuming less than 1890 Kcal,

(viii) Percentage of households dependent on labour income,

(ix) Rural Infrastructure index in percent,

(x) Juvenile sex ratio female per 1000 male,

(xi) Percentage of female literacy,

(xii) Percentage of SC & ST population,

(xiii) Percentage of households below poverty line,

(xiv) Maternal health index,

(xv) Percentage of population with chronic energy deficiency,

(xvi) Percentage of severely stunted children (under 5),

(xvii) Percentage of severely wasted children (under 5),

(xviii) Infant Mortality Rate (IMR),

(xix) Health infrastructure index,

(xx) Percentage distribution of households according to consumption of iron below 90 percent RDA,

(xxi) Percentage distribution of households according to consumption of Vitamin-A below 90 percent RDA.

First 5 of these indicators relate to food availability and next 8 each relate to food access and food absorption, respectively. The indicator, 'life expectancy at age one', used in MSSRF study was dropped as its reliable district-level estimates were not available and it is also not considered crucial for food insecurity. Two new indicators namely 'percentage distribution of households having consumption of iron below 90 percent RDA' and 'percentage distribution of households having consumption of vitamin A below 90 percent RDA' were used to capture iron and vitamin A deficiency. These indicators helped in capturing the status of undernutrition on account of iron and vitamin A deficiency. A third indicator 'maternal health index' was also included as it is considered crucial towards health of mother and child by health experts and nutritionists.

MSSRF used 19 indicators for food availability, access and absorption. These were combined into a single composite development indicator of food insecurity at a sectoral and/or aggregate level. The most commonly used methods for preparing a composite index are the ranking method, indexing method and multivariate data analysis techniques like principal component analysis and cluster analysis.

MSSRF used ranking method which is the simplest and the most commonly used method for preparing composite index of food insecurity. This method consists of assigning ranks for each indicator separately and simply totaling the ranks for each state/region/district to arrive at the aggregate rank. In this method all indicators are implicitly assigned equal weights, which may not always be appropriate. This method also fails to take into account the extent of variations in the magnitude of differences between units. MSSRF has discussed the problem of aggregation of indicators in the section on methodology. It is stated that the simple adding up of the ranks of indicators in skewed distribution influences the interpretation of the relative position of the various states.

The methodology used by MSSRF was modified by IASDS. The modified approach used geometric mean (GM) instead of arithmetic mean (AM) used by the MSSRF. Geometric mean was preferred over arithmetic mean as AM is greatly influenced by large values in the data. In fact a single large value can influence the AM and thus may lead to erroneous conclusion; on the other hand GM is preferred when data is not homogeneous. Principal Component Analysis (PCA) technique was also tried in the IASDS study. The principal component method is statistically a more sophisticated method of analysis than the ranking of the index method. Under this method, weights are assigned to each variable on the basis of the correlation matrix. The PCA analysis was not fruitful as seen from the following Section.

## 9.2.3 Principal component analysis

Principal component analysis (PCA) is a statistical procedure that uses an orthogonal transformation to convert a set of observations of possibly correlated variables into a set of values of linearly uncorrelated variables called principal components. The number of principal components is less than or equal to the number of original variables. This transformation is defined in such a way that the first principal component has the largest possible variance (that is, accounts for as much of the variability in the data as possible), and each succeeding component in turn has the highest variance possible under the constraint that it is orthogonal to (i.e., uncorrelated with) the preceding components. The technique is computer intensive and needs the application of software like SAS, SPSS, R, etc., with the association of a statistician.

In PCA, the eigenvectors correspond to principal components and the Eigen values to the variance explained by the principal components. Generally, all Eigen values greater than 1 and explained total variations exceeding 50 percent for all such Eigen values indicate the corresponding vectors (components) being significant contributors. For details please see Jollife (2002). A limitation of PCA is that it is useful only under certain underlying assumptions. These are non-normality, non-linearity and inadequacy of sample size. This is best explained through the use of PCA to identify important factors leading to food insecurity.

Principal component analysis using extraction method (Jollife, 2010) was done on all the 21 variables. In PCA, the eigenvectors correspond to principal components and the Eigen values to the variance explained by the principal components. Generally, all Eigen values greater than 1 and explained total variations exceeding 50 percent for all such Eigen values indicate the corresponding vectors (components) being significant contributors. The variables were standardized for PCA. This was done by dividing the deviation of the value of a variable from the mean by standard deviation. Eight Eigen values were greater than 1, explaining over 74 percent of total variation. However, the first two components explained only 31.3 (18.9 and 12.4 respectively) percent of this variation. The third component was also close enough with a value of 10.2. Possible reasons for low levels of explained variation by first two components may be the non-normality, inadequate sample size, inappropriate and/or improper choice of indicators, as also revealed by low values in correlation matrix; or else, non-linear relationship among variables. There are 70 districts against 21 indicators. Thus, we have sample size of 70 districts which is over 3 times the number of indicators (21), whereas the recommended sample size is 5 times the number of variables (here indicators). The non-normality test based upon Shapiro-Wilk's test (1965) which is a test of normality revealed that all group 1 (availability) variables are non-normal, in group 2, out of 8 variables 3 are non-normal and in group 3 (absorption) out of 7, 3 are non-normal.

It may, therefore, not be a sound idea to pursue further analysis with PCA. Yet, we proceeded with PCA to gain insight. A further effort was made for carrying out PCA separately for each of different groups – indicators of each of food availability, food access, and food absorption. Quite surprisingly, the results showed marked improvements.

Out of 5 indicators of food availability, all related to agriculture, three Eigen values were greater than 1, and first two principal components accounted for 54 percent, while the third contributed another 20 percent. The fourth one with an Eigen value of 0.88 also contributed 18 percent of total variation. Out of 8 indicators of food access, four Eigen values were either greater than 1 or close to 1; first two principal components accounted for 53 percent, while the third and fourth one, together, also contributed over 25 percent of total variation. Out of 8 indicators of food absorption, infant mortality was dropped as it contained several missing values. Out of remaining 7, three Eigen values were greater than 1, the fourth one had the value 0.95; first two principal components accounted for 41 percent, while the next two contributed another 31 percent.

It was observed from the analyses of separate groups that PCA performed reasonably well. However, this was not the case when all groups were combined to perform an overall PCA. A possible reason for this could be the non-linearity among variables of different groups. The PCA results, besides non-normality, also suggest presence of non-linearity among variables of three different groups indicating inappropriateness of PCA.

The above discussion clearly cautions against using PCA without validating underlying assumptions. PCA is likely to be useful for within group analysis and may be inappropriate for between group analyses.

### 9.2.4 Food insecurity map of rural Uttar Pradesh

All the 70 districts were classified according to 'extremely insecure', 'severely insecure', 'moderately insecure', moderately secure' and 'secure' based upon composite mapping index. Class intervals of each typology were determined by GIS software Arc View, following natural breaks in the series. Two types of mapping indices and typologies of food insecurity situation based upon arithmetic and geometric means were computed. On comparing the two approaches, it was found that the insecurity ranks matched for 50 out of 70 districts. For the remaining 20 districts, in all but one case the two results differed by one level on either side depending upon the type of skewness in mapping indices.

In the map abbreviations used for districts are as under:

AG – Agra, AL – Aligarh, AH – Allahabad, AN – Ambedkar Nagar, AU – Auraiya, AZ – Azamgarh, BG – Baghpat, BH – Bahraich, BL – Ballia, BP – Balrampur, BN – Banda, BB – Barabanki, BR – Bareilly, BS – Basti, BI – Bijnor, BD – Budaun, BU – Bulandshahar, CD – Chandauli, CT – Chitrakoot, DE – Deoria, ET – Etah, EW – Etawah, FZ – Faizabad, FR – Farukkhabad, FT – Fatehpur, FI – Firozabad, GB – Ghaziabad, GZ – Gautam Buddha Nagar, GP – Ghazipur, GN – Gonda, GR – Gorakhpur, HM – Hamirpur, HR

– Hardoi, HT – Hathras (Mahamaya Nagar), JL – Jalaun, JP – J.P. Nagar (Jyotiba Phoole Nagar), KJ – Kannauj, KD – Kanpur Dehat, KN – Kanpur Nagar, KS – Kaushambi, KU – Kushi Nagar, LK – Lakhimpur Kheri, LA – Lalitpur, LU – Lucknow, MG – Maharajganj, MH – Mahoba, MP – Mainpuri, MT – Mathura, MB – Mau (Maunathbhanjan), ME – Meerut, MI – Mirzapur, MO – Moradabad, MU – Muzaffar Nagar, PI – Pilibhit, PR – Pratapgarh, RB – Raebareli, RA – Rampur, SA – Saharanpur, SK – Sant Kabir Nagar, SR – Sant Ravidas Nagar, SJ – Shahjahanpur, SV – Shravasti, SN – Siddharth Nagar, SI – Sitapur, SO – Sonbhadra, SU – Sultanpur, UN – Unnao, VA – Varanasi.

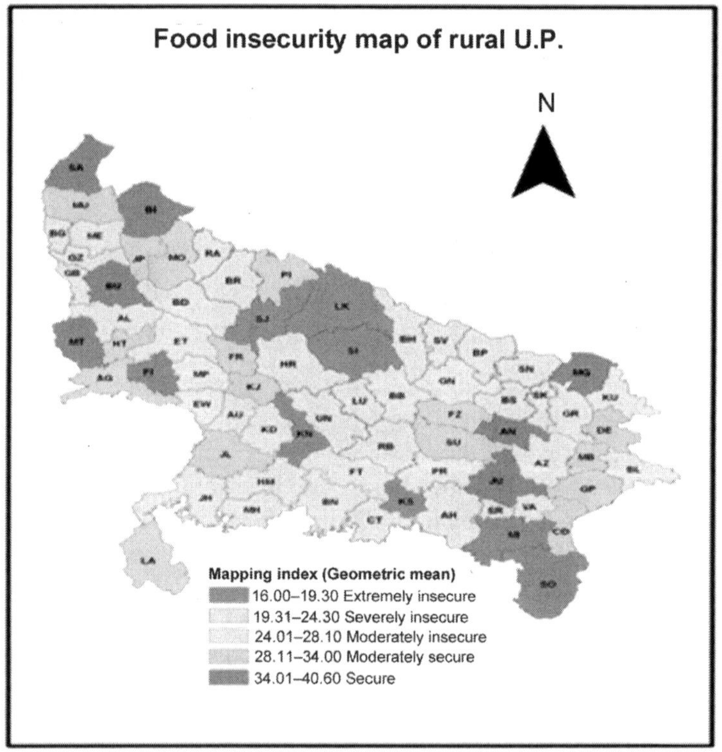


**Figure 9.1** Food insecurity map based upon GM

## 9.2.5 Food insecurity pattern

There are three important categories of food insecurity. These are extremely insecure, severely insecure and moderately insecure.

i. *Extremely insecure districts:* There are 7 districts in this category. Kanpur Nagar, Kaushambi, Lakhimpur Kheri, Mirzapur, Shahjahanpur, Sitapur and Sonbhadra are extremely food insecure districts of Uttar Pradesh. These are shown in red colour in the map. These are the districts with lowest mapping indices. These districts form small clusters, showing that the problems are common inside the clusters. Lakhimpur Kheri, Shahjahanpur and Sitapur constitute one cluster, followed by another cluster of Mirzapur and Sonbhadra. In these districts major factors responsible for poor food availability are floods and instability in cereal production. For poor food access factors like poor rural infrastructure, low female literacy, and large population of SC/ST are responsible. As for poor food absorption poor maternal health, low CED, wasted children and high rate of infant mortality are some of the responsible factors.
ii. *Severely insecure districts:* There are 18 districts in this category. Allahabad, Baghpat, Bahraich, Balrampur, Bareilly, Basti, Budaun, Chitrakoot, Ghaziabad, Hardoi, Lucknow, Raebareli, Rampur, Sant Kabir Nagar, Sant Ravidas Nagar, Shravasti, Siddharth Nagar and Unnao are severely food insecure districts of Uttar Pradesh. These are depicted in mustard colour in the map. In this typology also one can observe 'neighbor affinity' in the form of clusters. The factors responsible are more or less the same as for 'extremely insecure' category.
iii. *Moderately food insecure districts:* Twenty one districts shown in light green colour fall in this category. Aligarh, Auraiya, Azamgarh, Ballia, Banda, Barabanki, Etah, Etawah, Fatehpur, Gautam Buddha Nagar, Gonda, Gorakhpur, Hamirpur, Jhansi, Kanpur Dehat, Kushi Nagar, Mahoba, Mainpuri, Meerut, Pratapgarh and Varanasi are moderately food insecure districts. Here also formation of clusters can be seen.

Sitapur with lowest mapping index has emerged as the most food insecure district. The indicators contributing significantly to food insecurity are instability in cereal production, floods, and rural infrastructure. In Sitapur, about 35 percent of the population belongs to SC/ST segment and more than 60 percent population suffers from CED. The district with highest mapping index is Mathura and is therefore most secure district. Even this district suffers from problems. Total crop loss due to drought is more than 73 percent and juvenile sex ratio is only 867 per thousand in Mathura district. Thus, each district has its own problems and should be addressed very carefully.

## 9.2.6 Recommendations

The recommendations reported here are taken from Nigam et al. (2014). First reported are the recommendations of general type and then follow some specific recommendations for each category of districts.

### *9.2.6.1 General*

It is observed that major contributors to inadequate food availability are instability in food production, deficit in cereal production, poor sustainability and loss of crops due to natural calamities like floods, etc. Food instability and deficit crop production needs to be tackled vigorously. Rural infrastructure needs immediate push up. Cropping and irrigation intensities play significant roles in food availability. In Uttar Pradesh irrigation intensity is much higher than cropping intensity warranting efforts to enhance the cropping intensity. Better supply and efficient use of seeds, fertilizers and pesticides are also required for a push to agricultural growth.

This can be achieved by bringing new technologies in agriculture through proper and effective coordination between agricultural universities and extension agencies. Agencies like Krishi Vigyan Kendras need strengthening. The promotion of Village Food Banks, Seed Banks and Forage and Feed Banks is highly desirable for food and feed security during distress times. Farmers should be provided with a single card which should fetch them different facilities like credits/loans/ seeds/fertilizers, etc. Panchayats can play effective roles in this direction. It is also necessary to invent special packages for marginal and landless farmers. This group must be given extra fillip to make them competitive with medium and large farmers. Marginal farmers must be given credit at reduced interest rates and flexible repayment schedule.

Banking and credit facilities is another area of concern. Banking facilities are available to only 21.3 percent villages at state level. At district level availability of banking facility is highly skewed. This varies from zero to 90 percent. As for loaning facilities for agriculture, at state level this is 46.6 percent of the total loan provided. At district level this varies from one percent to 92 percent, and is highly skewed.

In India, agriculture that comprises of crops, animal husbandry, fisheries and agro-forestry, etc., form the backbone of rural economy. In India farming is still farmers' oriented and not industry oriented. As most of the rural employment is dependent on agriculture, it is desirable to create better opportunities in agriculture by converting unskilled labors to skilled labors.

Besides improved performance in agriculture and related sectors, efficient public distribution of food grains is the key to food availability and access.

The welfare schemes like MGNREGA and PDS are intended to ensure access. However, the functioning of both these is far from satisfactory.

Maternal health, CED, consumption of less than 1890 cals/day, consumption of less quantity of iron and vitamin A lead to poor food absorption. In Uttar Pradesh 35 districts have lower calories consumption than the state average. Similarly, iron and vitamin A consumption is at very low levels across all districts of the state. Very low calorie consumption among the poorest is a matter of concern. The situation pertaining to calorie intake by landless households and marginal cultivators is grim. All these issues and those related to caste, gender and female literacy need to be addressed. In addition to these, better disaster management is required to meet the challenges due to natural calamities like floods, etc.

### *9.2.6.2 Specific*

The implementations of suggestions as above are likely to make improvements in food and nutrition security across all districts. However, there has to be special focus on extremely and severely insecure districts. Out of 70 districts, 46 districts were found to be food insecure at different levels (7 extremely insecure, 18 severely insecure and 21 moderately insecure). Reasons for their being food insecure varies from district to district.

As noted above, 7 districts are extremely food insecure, and 18 are severely food insecure. All these districts lack in varying extent in each of food availability, access and absorption.

*Food availability:* Among the extremely insecure districts, Kanpur Nagar, Kaushambi, Mirzapur, Sitapur and Sonbhadra have deficit in production over cereal consumption, Sitapur has low sustainability, and Lakhimpur Kheri, Shahjahanpur, Sitapur, Mirzapur, Sonbhadra and Kaushambi suffer recurrent crop losses due to floods and draught.

Similarly, amongst severely insecure districts, Lucknow has very high level of deficit in production over cereal consumption. Other districts having deficit are Allahabad, Bahraich, Chitrakoot, Ghaziabad, Raebareli and Siddharth Nagar. Baghpat, Ghaziabad, Chitrakoot, Sant Ravidas Nagar, Budaun, Lucknow and Raebareli have either low sustainability or instability in crop production. Ghaziabad, Bareilly, Lucknow, Unnao, Basti, Sant Kabir Nagar, Siddharth Nagar Allahabad, Chitrakoot and Sant Ravidas Nagar have the recurrent problem of crop loss due to floods and drought.

In view of the above it is necessary to enhance the production in sustainable manner through innovative technologies and sustained efforts towards strengthening extension of lab to land. Further, it is essential to effectively manage natural disasters like floods and droughts.

*Food access:* Among the extremely insecure districts, Mirzapur and Sonbhadra have dependence on labour income for livelihood resulting in poor purchasing power, while Rampur, Hardoi, Bahraich, Shravasti and Siddharth Nagar of severely insecure category have this problem.

Mirzapur, Sonbhadra and Kanpur Nagar among the first category and Hardoi, Lucknow, Raebareli, Unnao, Bahraich, Basti, Shravasti and Chitrakoot of the second category have a sizable population in BPL/SC, ST category.

Shahjahanpur, Sitapur, Mirzapur and Sonbhadra among extremely insecure districts and Unnao, Balrampur, Basti, Sant Kabir Nagar, Shravasti, Siddharth Nagar and Sant Ravidas Nagar of the other category have very poor rural infrastructure.

Kaushambi, Budaun, Bareilly, Rampur, Bahraich, Balrampur, Shravasti and Siddharth Nagar have very low female literacy rate, while Kanpur Nagar, Baghpat, Ghaziabad, Budaun, Bareilly, Rampur, Unnao, Balrampur, Basti, Sant Kabir Nagar and Chitrakoot, have low calorie intake.

Poor purchasing power is the greatest roadblock towards food access. It is therefore necessary to enhance the employment opportunities for the population. The solution lies in creating jobs/livelihoods through agriculture and related sectors. Since the share of agricultural workers is declining in workforce, it is necessary to enhance the productivity. As most of families engaged in rural areas are unskilled, their income levels are low. Thus, there is a need to convert unskilled workers into skilled workers. This can be achieved by providing proper training facilities through agricultural universities, KVK's, etc. Besides this, rural infrastructure can be improved by providing seed centres and pesticides/insecticides stores and improved banking facilities, etc. Proper schooling facilities are also essential for development.

*Food absorption:* Poor health infrastructure and maternal health, high infant mortality, CED and low consumption of iron and vitamin A contribute to poor food absorption. Mirzapur and Sonbhadra among extremely insecure and Budaun, Bareilly, Rampur, Allahabad, Chitrakoot and Sant Ravidas Nagar among severely insecure districts have poor maternal health. Bareilly, Budaun, Raebareli, Unnao, Balrampur, Basti, Sant Kabir Nagar, Allahabad and Chitrakoot of the later category have high infant mortality rates, whereas Ghaziabad, Budaun, Bareilly, Rampur, Bahraich, Sant Kabir Nagar, Shravasti and Siddharth Nagar of the same category have high prevalence of CED. Among the extremely insecure category, Lakhimpur Kheri, Shahjahanpur, Sitapur and Kanpur Nagar have high prevalence of CED.

Majority of population in Mirzapur, Sonbhadra and Kanpur Nagar among extremely insecure districts and Baghpat, Ghaziabad, Bahraich, Balrampur and Siddharth Nagar among severely insecure districts have very low consumption of iron. Similarly, those with very low consumption of vitamin A are Lakhimpur Kheri and Kaushambi of the first category and Baghpat, Ghaziabad, Bahraich, Balrampur, Basti and Sant Ravidas Nagar of the second category. Bareilly, Lucknow and Basti among this category also have poor health infrastructure.

Health facilities need revamping with effective implementation of food, health and nutrition security schemes like ICDS, mid-day meals and PDS. Programs like food fortification need to be implemented rigorously. Health infrastructure needs to be improved.

## 9.3 Hunger

Even though we have achieved self-sufficiency in the production of food grains in our country, there still exist problems of poverty, undernutrition and hunger among large segment of the population across the states. A large population finds it hard to meet nutritional requirements and is still living below the poverty line. Nearly half of young children are undernourished. There is an urgent need to address the issues relating to undernutrition and food insecurity. Hunger is related both to undernutrition and food insecurity both of which have already been discussed.

It is a common knowledge that a very small percentage of the gains of development percolate down to the urban and rural poor. For inclusive growth, we must identify the poor and downtrodden and ensure through a series of welfare measures in public–private partnership mode that they remain no more deprived, and instead, feel empowered to join the mainstream. We must pay highest attention to livelihood and food insecurity.

There have been several social, health and nutrition protection and promotion programs run by the government like PDS for food at subsidized rates for the poor, ICDS for growth monitoring and supplementary nutrition, nutrition and health education, mid-day meal programs and food for work schemes. Though these schemes were started with novel intentions, they lack in their proper implementation. Many reasons like gender discrimination, failed governance and improper monitoring can be attributed to rather poor performance of these schemes.

Though MGNREGA has helped increasing the purchasing power of various poverty-ridden sections, these have not been uniform across all states. According to Panda (2015), NSSO survey of 2009–10 indicates that 35 percent of rural households had job cards, 24 percent got work and had worked on an average for 37 days during the year. There have been problems in distribution of quantity and quality of food grains under the PDS and the performance of the PDS as a delivery mechanism varies considerably across states.

Besides ICDS, mid-day meal program for schoolchildren also aims at food and nutrition security. The mid-day meal program intends to improve enrolment and retention. Reports suggest that while both the programs have problems like pilferage, there have been complaints of inadequate quantity and poor quality of meals for mid-day meal program. There have also been reports of lack of hygiene in preparation of food.

Studies by IASDS on baseline and impact assessments of nutrition interventions through food for education in Madhya Pradesh, Uttarakhand and Chhattisgarh (2004, 2005) and status of mid-day meal in Madhya Pradesh (2005) reveal that there is still huge nutrition gap as both iron and vitamin A intakes are far below recommended levels. This makes a strong case for fortified foods. In recent times there have been sincere efforts to fortify foods with micronutrients. Agricultural scientists are engaged in developing protein and vitamin rich varieties. It is hoped that in near future fortified version of cereals, pulses, oils, vegetables and fruits with enhanced nutrients will be made available to all sections of the population.

Many of the government projects encompass several ministries and departments and for their successful implementation inter-departmental coordination is necessary. It is common knowledge that most of the government-run projects excepting the Prime Minister's Jana Dhan Yojana have not achieved the desired results. Most of the schemes need careful evaluations by external agencies on identifying reasons for their dismal performance and whether the benefits are being availed by actual target groups. Immediate remedial measures are thus required at the government level for delivering these schemes to the intended people.

## 9.4 Food for security act

India has serious problems of population, pollution and poverty. The UNDP Human Development Index for India continues to be very disappointing. The Institution of Panchayati Raj which was supposed to take us to the path of balanced development is still in its infancy. Large section of the population still lives below the poverty line and nearly half of young children are undernourished. Defining poverty line is an important step for planning and evolving of appropriate policies and programs for the provision of assistance to the weaker sections of the society. The methodologies of identifying below poverty line (BPL) families are being evolved over the last few decades. Unfortunately, there are competing methodologies leading to widely different estimates of poverty line. The latest revisions by Tendulkar and Rangarajan Committees on poverty have already generated heat and need to be assessed thoroughly.

Indian government recently enacted the food security act that allows the right to avail specified amount of food by two-third of the population at a very low price. It seems to be an ambitious extension of PDS. Main challenge for its effective implementation would be proper identification of target groups, coordination between involved ministries, effective movement, storage and distribution of food grains, and effective monitoring and evaluation by external agencies of repute. While it is doubtable to include such huge population as target group, food and nutrition security demands inclusion of a whole range of foodstuffs like vegetables, milk, fruits, fats, etc., at highly subsided rates.

## 9.5 Hunger and food insecurity

Food security implies access by all people at all time to enough food for an active, healthy life. Food security includes at a minimum (i) the ready availability of nutritionally adequate and safe foods and (ii) an assured ability to acquire acceptable foods in socially acceptable ways (i.e. without resorting to emergency food supplies, scavenging, stealing or other coping strategies).

Hunger, when defined as the uneasy or painful sensation caused by lack of food, is a potential, although not necessary, consequence of food insecurity. Similarly, the cutoff point between food insecure without the experience of hunger and insecure with moderate hunger is identified by the inability of households to economize food budgets any further without adults reducing food intake or cutting meals. Hunger in this third category is characterized by reduced food intakes with the physical sensation caused by lack of food. The category, food insecure with severe hunger, is characterized by reduced food intake and hunger in children and more severe hunger in adults.

The questions in the food security module should measure four underlying conditions or behaviors in the households: (i) anxiety about the food budget or food supply, (ii) perceptions that food is inadequate in quantity or quality, (iii) reduced food intake in adults, and (iv) reduced food intake in children.

## 9.6 Assessing hunger

NSSO has been collecting information on ‘hunger’ as part of regular countrywide surveys on “household consumption expenditure”. The specific questions asked on hunger/food adequacy in these surveys are: whether all members of households get two square meals (enough food every day) and if yes, whether it is throughout the year (termed as seasonal hunger) or during some months in the year (chronic hunger).

## 9.7 FANTA project

FANTA (Food and Nutrition Technical Assistance) is the project supported by USAID (2002–2017) and has focus on maternal and child health and nutrition, nutrition in emergencies and management of acute malnutrition, nutrition and infectious diseases, food security, and agriculture and nutrition linkages. It has effectively demonstrated that the approach to constructing measures of hunger and food security (as previously validated for use in the United States) can also be used in developing countries. For more than 15 years, FANTA has been working to improve the health and well-being of vulnerable individuals, families, and communities in developing countries by strengthening food security and nutrition policies, programs, and systems. FANTA assists USAID's efforts to collect and analyze the best available data to rigorously and credibly support programmatic decision making, systematic learning, and documentation of program effectiveness. FANTA has developed and tested several food security and nutrition indicators, many of which are now used globally, and has created guidance documents to support data collection for these indicators.

### 9.7.1 FAST module

Using the United States 'food security core module' as a model, extensive ethnographic research and concept testing was used to develop an experimental food security survey tool adapted to the Bangladesh context. The US 'food security core module' is a validated set of 18 questions that collectively distinguishes individuals and households experiencing food insecurity related to insufficient quantity and quality of food, food procured through personally and socially unacceptable means, and a feeling of vulnerability to downturns in supply.

A nine-question set of FAST (Food Access Survey Tools) questions was created and tested against indicators of household status relating to poverty, undernutrition and food consumption. The FAST module's stability against other indicators over time and its sensitivity to change were tested using a variety of rigorous statistical tools. The nine question FAST module had significant correlation with (a) indicators commonly used in the analysis of poverty and undernutrition, (b) the food security status rating of each household, and (c) indicators of food insecurity.

Thus, FANTA-supported research effectively demonstrated that the approach to constructing a measure of hunger and food security (as used in the United States), can also be applied in a very different, developing country context. The FAST module constructed for use in Bangladesh (2003) passed all the validation tests that were applied to the US module, and it is transparent in both the underlying concepts and the meaning of the questions used. Common measures of 'poverty' and 'food insecurity' also correlated well, some even better, with the FAST module as applied in 2003.

The FAST module does not substitute for more intensive food consumption and expenditure surveys or anthropometric surveys where those are required to answer specific questions relating either to poverty or nutrition. It cannot be used in place of surveys seeking information that guides an operational response, e.g., assessing hygiene in order to target a latrine-building intervention. This research demonstrates that the FAST module is a complement to more common measures either of nutritional status or of food production and marketing. In this sense, the FAST tool serves to address the multi-faceted 'access' dimension of food insecurity that until now was insufficiently measured using traditional indicators that typically captured only one particular aspect of the problem.

Through this module, it is possible to classify a household into one of the following categories: food secure, food insecure without hunger, and food insecure with hunger. However, the FAST module does not substitute for more intensive food consumption and expenditure survey or anthropometric survey. While the format of FAST module is a complement to more common measures either of nutritional status or of food production and the nutritional status of individuals is assessed through anthropometric measurements and the dietary intake could be measured through food consumption surveys.

There is therefore a need to recommend a standardized mechanism and instrument(s) for defining and obtaining data on the prevalence of 'food insecurity' or 'food insufficiency' and recommend methodologies that can be used across the nation and at state and local level.

## 9.8 Hunger mapping

The present section is based upon an ICMR-funded study on hunger mapping at Gram Panchayat level in Banda district of Bundelkhand region of Uttar Pradesh which is one of the most deprived and underdeveloped regions in terms of almost all human-developed indicators. In recent past, there had been media reports of deaths due to hunger in the district. For identifying hunger, the study used FAST (as used in Bangladesh) and other modified modules after adaptation to local (Bundelkhand region) conditions. The FAST was modified not only in content but was also tried sequentially. The modifications were decided after a preliminary probing on the food habits in the district. The study also used other instruments for measuring undernutrition and dietary intake and related these with hunger.

The study was at gram panchayat level, which is the core grass root unit for administrative action. Bundelkhand region is one of the most deprived and underdeveloped regions in terms of almost all human developed indicators. Banda district is not only among the worst in terms of underweight and stunting indicators of undernutrition in children, it also falls under border cluster districts. As per joint NIN-IASDS Nutrition Profile of Indian Studies (2002), the prevalence of severe stunting in Banda was 59.3 percent and of severe underweight was 40 percent.

The gram panchayats have been identified as food secure, food insecure without hunger and food insecure with hunger on the basis of MFAST which is a modified version of FAST and anthropometric measurements and related indicators. The hunger mapping actually would enable to zero down to areas of concentration of deprived hunger stricken families. The effort is first ever micro-level scientifically planned exercise (not just a data gathering exercise) in the area of hunger and undernutrition. Such an effort would ultimately lead to proper targeted distribution of aids/funds.

### 9.8.1 Adopted methodology

There are 436 gram panchayats and 592 villages in Banda. Gram panchayats were grouped in 44 strata of neighboring 10 gram panchayats. A household survey was carried out in each such group of gram panchayats. For this, a sample of 10 villages was selected by PPS and from each village, 20 households were selected for the detailed study. Thus, a total of 8,800 household (48,400 individuals assuming the household size 5.5) spread over 440 selected villages were covered.

Clearly, it is assumed that there is homogeneity in the 10 neighboring panchayats. This assumption does not seem to be unrealistic. The households within village were selected as per standard procedure ensuring due representation of different socio-economic groups. The modified version of the hunger tool – MFAST was canvassed in each of the selected households.

Information on anthropometric measurements to assess the nutritional status as per NFHS questionnaire and on dietary intake using 24-hour recall method of NIN (ICMR) was obtained on a sub-sample of 10 households per village. At the district level, information on various nutritional supplementation schemes in the area such as APL, BPL, Anthyodaya Aahaar Yojna (AAY), MDM, ICDS, Food for Work, Mahatma Gandhi National Rural Employment Guarantee Act (MGNREGA), etc., was also collected. At the household level also, this information was also collected to categorize them as beneficiary households or otherwise.

The data collected was analyzed both for estimation of hunger at the gram panchayat levels and also for identifying the target areas and groups which require intervention for hunger. The inter-relationship of hunger and undernutrition was also attempted. In order to carry out the study, 436 gram panchayats were grouped in 44 strata comprising of 10 neighboring panchayats each. A total of 592 villages were covered.

### 9.8.2 Modified FAST (MFAST)

For the present study FAST was modified as per the local requirements. At the time of pretesting it was noted that the FAST module had questions having ambiguity causing overlapping. In FAST module, housewife was not included, though it is the housewife which is the main victim of food insecurity and hence of hunger. Taking into consideration all these concerns, it was considered appropriate to modify it from 11 items to 9 as below:

1. The family ate few meals per day on a regular basis;
2. Obliged to eat non-preferred instead of preferred food;
3. Members of the household who had to skip the meal due to lack of food

   (i) working adult (ii) housewife (iii) working adult and housewife (iv) entire family;

5. There were times when food stored in the house ran out and no cash to buy more;
6. Worried frequently about where the next meal would come from;
7. Needed to purchase food frequently (because own production or purchased stores ran out);
8. Took food on credit from a local store;
9. Needed to borrow food from relatives or neighbors to make a meal (making ends meet on a day-to-day (hand-to-mouth) basis); and
10. Needed to borrow food in order to meet social obligations (to serve a meal to guests or relatives).

Based upon different classifications of hunger, it may be appropriate to classify different types of hunger: (1) anxiety about the food budget or food supply; (2) perceptions that food is inadequate in either quantity or quality;

(3) reduced food intake in men; (4) reduced food intake in women; and (5) reduced food intake in children. On the basis of responses on above groups, it may be possible to classify a household in to one of the following categories:

- Food secure,
- Food insecure without hunger, and
- Food insecure with hunger

The households were classified as food secure, food insecure without hunger, or food insecure with hunger on the basis of responses on 9 questions of MFAST module. The concern here was to restrict only to the category – food insecure with hunger. The mapping was done only for this indicator. As the unit of selection was a group of 10 neighbouring panchayats, the mapping of the panchayats (groups) was done on the basis of some cut-off points derived from the distribution of food insecure with hunger.

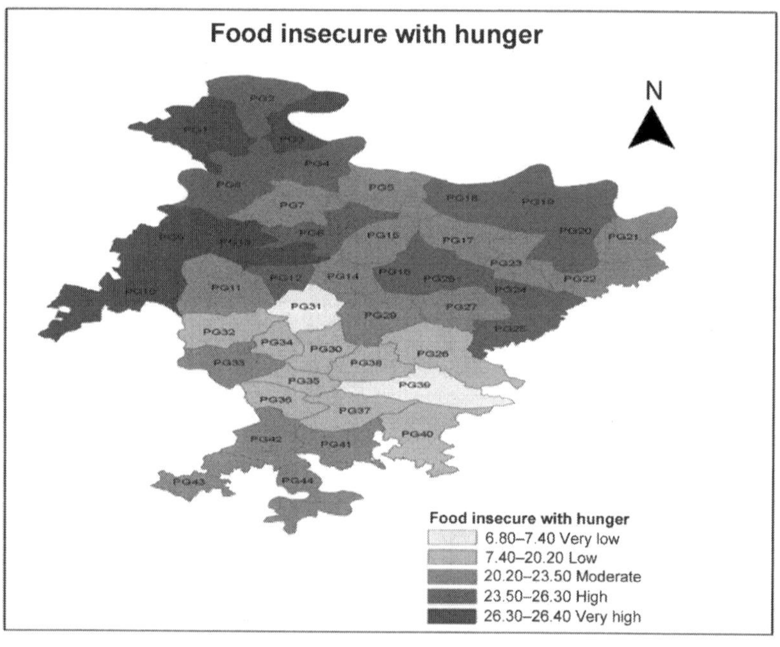


**Figure 9.2** Food insecure panchayats with hunger

The mapping index gives the combined intensity of 7 items (Q3-9) of MFAST. The panchayat group with severe problems in one aspect may be relatively problem-free in other aspects. Hence, the mapping index gives the relative position of a panchayat group vis-à-vis others as per the combined intensity of the problem of hunger. Unlike the human development index, where the position of a state is measured against the total distance between the best and the worst, or a price index that measures the price position vis-à-vis the base year's position, the mapping index indicates the average position of the panchayat group with respect to others.

'Arc-view' Geographical Information System software was used for mapping gram panchayats. The software detects the natural breaks in the series, so that the error in detecting natural breaks is minimized. Figure 9.1 gives hunger mapping of panchayats which are in different categories of food insecurity with hunger.

### 9.8.3 Salient findings

The study revealed that in general, the study area was vulnerable to hunger situations. Infrastructure relating to all the sectors like, agriculture, health education, etc., was poor across all panchayat groups. Socioeconomic indicators and household characteristics like type of houses, source of drinking water, economic status, land holdings and irrigation facilities; PDS and MNREGA also presented a poor scenario. Salient findings of the study were as under.

Seventeen panchayat groups were found to be food insecure with hunger. Of these 6 were in the category very high hunger. In general, panchayat groups had very poor infrastructure. Out of 17 panchayat groups of the category food insecure with hunger, 6 had poor infrastructure, and 6 groups had poor dietary intakes and poor nutritional status.

Dietary intake was below RDA for all the food items across all the panchayat groups. Prevalence of CED among adults was found to vary from 36.9 to 60.1 percent as against 33 at national level. Similarly, prevalence of stunting, underweight and wasting was very high.

Based on 11 socioeconomic level indicators (SLI), scores of SLI were calculated for each panchayat group and the households were categorized in 3 categories: low, medium and high. As majority of the population belonged to low and medium categories, the panchayat groups were ranked on this basis. These were combined with the access to government programs and 5 typologies were obtained. Out of 17 panchayat groups, 8 groups were in the category of poor socioeconomic level indicators and access to government programs.

An attempt was made to identify the factors that related to hunger, using logistic regression analysis. Prevalence of underweight in children, poor irrigation facilities to farmers and poor performance of PDS emerged as major correlates of hunger.

### 9.8.4 Recommendations

One of the major problems of the district was the unavailability of seeds of improved variety and quality. Seed replacement ratio is also very low in the district. Concerted efforts are therefore required to correct these scenarios. Other concern is the lack of irrigation facilities. The area has large tracks of degraded lands which prohibit adaption of efficient cultivation practices. Conservation of water and micro irrigation is recommended. Agro forestry on ravine and degraded soil should be encouraged and given financial and technical support. Use of diversified techniques of agriculture and use organic farming is recommended.

Roads to villages, electricity and potable water are the basic facilities which need upgradation. The district requires more high schools. Banking system needs to be improved. Grain banks may be established at panchayat level. Marketing facilities for milk should be strengthened. Government schemes like PDS, MGNREGA, MDM, ICDS, etc., are in poor shape and need overhauling.

There is largescale migration of youth due to unemployment. This has to be checked though skilled job creation. There should be opportunities of training for skilled jobs in order to increase availability of manpower for agricultural and other purposes.

Health care system needs to be revamped. Awareness camps on health care, good hygiene practices, sanitation and intake of balanced diet should be organized.

# 10
# Diseases in community clusters

## 10.1 Diseases in community clusters

In this chapter we discuss about different methods of disease cluster detection and some diseases which have spatial and space-time disease clusters in the community, with special reference to India. The basic problems in geographical surveillance for a spatially distributed disease are the identification of areas of exceptionally high prevalence, to test their statistical significance and to identify the reasons behind the elevated prevalence of the disease. Various methods have been suggested by different authors to overcome these problems. Some of these methods are either able to detect clusters with no inference involved, or they do inference without the ability to detect the location of clusters. However, the spatial scan statistic developed by Martin Kulldorff (1997) can both detect and provide inference for spatial and space-time disease clusters. The spatial scan statistic implemented in SaTScan software Kulldorff (2006) offers several advantages over the existing techniques for detection of disease clusters. Temporal, spatial and space-time scan statistics are now commonly used for disease cluster detection and evaluation, for many diseases including cancer (Kulldorff et al., 1998; Viel et al., 2000; and Michelozzi et al., 2002), Creutzfeldt-Jakob disease (Cousens et al., 2001), granulocytic ehrlichiosis (Chaput et al., 2002), sclerosis (Sabel et al., 2003), diabetes (Green et al., 2003), and giardiasis (Odoi et al., 2004).

The use of geographic information system (GIS) with spatial statistics, including spatial filtering and cluster analysis has been applied to many diseases to analyze and more clearly display the spatial patterns of disease (Curtis, 1999). GIS is a computer system designed to capture, store, manipulate, analyze, manage, and present all types of spatial or geographical data. The acronym GIS is also used for geographical information science or geospatial information studies to refer to the academic discipline or career of working with geographic information systems and is a large domain within the broader academic discipline of Geoinformatics. What goes beyond a GIS is a spatial data infrastructure, a concept that has no such restrictive boundaries.

In a general sense, the term describes any information system that integrates stores, edits, analyzes, shares, and displays geographic information. GIS applications are tools that allow users to create interactive queries (user-created searches), analyze spatial information, edit data in maps, and present the results of all these operations. GIS is a broad term that can refer to a number of different technologies, processes, and methods. It is attached to many operations and has many applications related to engineering, planning, management, transport/logistics, insurance, telecommunications, and business. For that reason, GIS and location intelligence applications can be the foundation for many location-enabled services that rely on analysis and visualization. Spatial scan statistic implemented in SaTScan software was successfully used to detect the clusters of different diseases worldwide.

## 10.2 Geospatial hotspot

A hotspot is an area of high response or an elevated cluster for an event. Temporal, spatial and space-time scan statistics are now commonly used for disease cluster detection and evaluation, for many diseases including cancer, granulocytic ehrlichiosis, sclerosis, diabetes, and giardiasis.

A 30-month (January 1994 to June 1996), prospective, city-wide study of all cases of TB using traditional contact investigations, GIS data, and molecular epidemiological comparison of *Mycobacterium tuberculosis* was carried out at Baltimore, in which clusters of recently transmitted cases of TB were detected in geographically distinct areas of Baltimore (Bishai et al., 1998). A population-based cross-sectional study on all incident culture-positive TB cases reported in New Jersey from January 1996 to September 1998 using multiple molecular techniques in conjunction with surveillance data was used to identify a previously unidentified outbreak of *Mycobacterium tuberculosis* in a defined geographical setting (Bifani et al., 1999). Transmission of TB during a 9-year period (1988–1996) in a countrywide community-based cohort of HIV-infected persons in Switzerland was investigated and it was found that one-fourth of TB cases were grouped in clusters of 138 HIV-infected patients (Sudre et al., 1999). A study was conducted in the municipality of São Paulo, Brazil, from 1994 to 1998 to describe the distribution of TB mortality by area and to evaluate its statistical association with several population characteristics (Antunes and Waldman, 2003). Nunes (2007) used GIS and spatial scan statistic to study the tuberculosis incidence in Portugal.

The spatial scan statistic developed by Kulldorff is used to test the presence of statistically significant spatial clusters of TB and to identify their approximate locations. Purely spatial analysis, which does not take time into account, is performed to detect the TB clusters in the study region. The theory behind the spatial scan statistic is a generalization of a test proposed by Turnbull et al. (1990). The number of events may be assumed to be either Poisson or Bernoulli distributed, depending on the application of the data under study. The spatial scan statistic imposes a circular window on the map and lets the centre of the circle move over the area so that at different positions the window includes different sets of neighboring census areas. If the window contains the centroid of the census area, then that whole area is included in the window. For each circle centroid, the radius of the circular window is varied continuously from 0 up to a maximum radius so that the window never includes more than 50% of the total population at risk. The spatial scan statistic is based on the likelihood ratio test. As the likelihood ratio is maximized over all the circles, it identifies the circle that constitutes the most likely cluster. Its p-value is obtained through Monte Carlo hypothesis testing technique proposed by Dwass (1957). To find the distribution of the test statistic, 999 random Monte Carlo replicates (see, Chapter 1) of the data set under the null hypothesis of no significant clusters are generated, calculating the test statistic for each replica.

## 10.3 Tuberculosis geo hotspots in India

Tuberculosis has been known as a major public health problem in India since time immemorial. A nationwide disease survey conducted by the Indian Council of Medical Research (ICMR) in 1955–1958 provided for the first time an insight into the enormity of the problem. Most epidemiological studies on TB, subsequent to the ICMR disease survey have been conducted in smaller geographical areas mostly in southern part of the country. To assess the prevailing epidemiological situation of TB, a nationwide survey was conducted during 2000–2003. The objective of the survey was to establish the prevalence of TB infection among children 1–9 years of age and to compute annual risk of infection in each of the four defined zones (north, south, east and west) into which the country was stratified for the purpose of survey (Chadha et al., 2002, 2003; Kollappan et al., 2004; Chadha et al., 2004). Molecular and conventional epidemiological techniques were used to study the mechanism and risk factors for TB transmission in a small area with high prevalence of TB in South India (Narayanan et al., 2002).

Tiwari et al. (2006) used GIS and spatial scan statistic to detect the geo-spatial hotspots of tuberculosis in Almora district of India and found significant high rate spatial and space-time clusters in three areas of the district. The identification of spatial high/low clusters was done under Poisson probability model assumption. The maximum spatial cluster size was first set to include up to 50 percent of population for both excesses and deficits and then set at 10 percent and 5 percent, to test the excesses and deficits separately because testing at the 10 percent and 5 percent levels can identify smaller, more defined areas. For statistical inference, 999 Monte Carlo replications were performed. For purely spatial analysis, the null hypothesis of no significant clusters is to be rejected when the simulated p-value was less than or equal to 0.05 for the primary clusters and 0.1 for the secondary clusters since the later have conservative p-values. For geographical analysis, they had used the techniques available through the Geographical Information System (GIS). All the geographical and cartographic outputs have been presented using the ArcGIS 9 application software.

There are two other studies carried out by Tiwari et al. (2010, 2012) for identifying tuberculosis geo hotspots in Dehradun district and Almora, Nainital and Udham Singh Nagar districts of Uttarakhand, respectively. These studies provide an opportunity to clarify and quantify the health burden of TB in hilly region of Uttarakhand. We discuss some of the results and methodologies carried out in the first of these two studies. The details of the second study are omitted for brevity.

In what follows is a detailed discussion on identification of tuberculosis geo hotspots in Dehradun. The studies utilized secondary data for the tuberculosis patients treated in Dehradun Tuberculosis Unit of Dehradun district, situated at Doon hospital Dehradun. The data had information on age, sex, religion, address, etc., of the patient and also regarding his/her treatment details. On the basis of these details, patients were divided according to different wards of Dehradun municipal area.

(a) *Detection and identification of tuberculosis clusters*

The spatial scan statistic developed by Kulldorff (1997) implemented in SaTScan v6.1 (2006) was used to test the presence of statistically significant spatial clusters of TB and to identify their approximate locations. Spatial analysis, which does not take time into account, was performed to detect the TB clusters in the study region. The theory behind the spatial scan statistic is a generalization of a test proposed by Turnbull et al. (1990). The number of events may be assumed to be either Poisson or Bernoulli distributed, depending on the application of the data under study. The spatial scan statistic imposes a circular window on the map and lets the centre of the circle move over the area so that at different positions the window includes different sets of neighboring census areas. If the window contains the centroid of the census area, then that whole area is included in the window. For each circle centroid, the radius of the circular window is varied continuously from 0 up to a maximum radius so that the window never includes more than 50 percent of the total population at risk. The spatial scan statistic is based on the likelihood ratio test. As the likelihood ratio is maximized over all the circles, it identifies the circle that constitutes the most likely cluster. Its p-value is obtained through Monte Carlo hypothesis testing technique proposed by Dwass (1957). To find the distribution of the test statistic, 999 random Monte Carlo replicates of the data set under the null hypothesis of no significant clusters are generated, calculating the test statistic for each replica. The result is significant at 5 percent level if the value of the test statistic from the real data set is among the 5 percent highest of all 1000 values, including those calculated from the 999 replicas. In addition to the most likely clusters, the method also identifies secondary clusters in the data set and orders them according to their likelihood ratio.

(b) *Geographical analyses*

For geographical analysis, the techniques available through the GIS are used. All the geographical and cartographic outputs can be presented in Arc GIS 9 software having UTM co-ordinate system and information can be retrieved using any compatible software.

### 10.3.1 An example

Using the maximum spatial cluster size of ≤5 percent of the total population, the spatial cluster analysis identified the most likely significant cluster for high occurrence of TB in the Dharampur ward of Dehradun for 2008. The overall relative risk (RR) within the cluster was 2.806 with an observed number of 29 cases treated between January 1, 2008, and May 31, 2008, compared with 10.75 expected cases. Statistically significant secondary clusters for high occurrence of TB were also detected at Khudbura, Ajabpur, Adhoiwala and Patel Nagar wards with 25, 35, 33 and 18 cases and 10.19, 5.19, 4.85 and 4.54 relative risks, respectively.

A similar analysis of low rate clusters for 2008 revealed Mansinghwala, Arya Nagar, Maha ranibag and Salawala wards with 0, 1, 2 and 1 cases and all relative risks far below one, respectively.

Both the high and low rate analyses for 2008 were strengthened by utilizing the information of 2007. The combined analysis revealed that there were 19 high zone wards for 2008 with total number of 274 TB cases reported during January–May 2008. These ward numbers were 14, 38, 28, 37, 29, 30, 39, 13, 16, 12, 15, 27, 26, 32, 36, 17, 10, 31 and 33 with relative risk of 1.655.

## 10.4 Associated risk factors

The studies also suggest investigation of the effect of various socioeconomic and environmental factors on the occurrence of TB in the hilly region of the state. It is known that the incidence of TB increases with age (Comstock, Livesay and Woolpert, 1974). They also report several other risk factors associated with the disease like cigarette smoking, alcohol abuse, injection drug use and undernutrition. They adversely affect immune system, and so could influence the TB incidence. Several other medical conditions are commonly associated with TB such as silicosis, where the risk has been shown to be 26 times higher to develop TB (Paul, 1961). It has also been found to be three times more in diabetics than in the general population (Opsahl et al., 1961). The risk of TB is 10–15 times higher in patients with end stage renal failure and those on hemodialysis and five times higher in male gastrectomy patients (Andrew et al., 1980; Belcon et al., 1982; Thorn et al., 1956). The factors mainly responsible for high occurrence of TB in hills are the poor socio-economic conditions of the people, low nutrients in the diet, smoke due to timber used for cooking purposes, high level of smoking, and high intake of liquor due to extreme cold in the region. After detecting the statistically significant clusters of TB in the region, a survey-based study may be helpful to identify the role of these factors in the spread of TB. A critical evaluation of Revised National Tuberculosis Control Programme (RNTCP) can also be done to verify whether the benefits of the high profile program are actually reaching to the people for whom it has been implemented.

## 10.5 Japanese encephalitis

There are some other diseases like the prevalence of Japanese encephalitis Bitot's Spots and polio in children which are located in clusters. We discuss here some further details on Japanese encephalitis.

Japanese encephalitis is the leading viral cause of Acute Encephalitis Syndrome (AES). Seventy percent of those who develop illness either die or survive with a long-term neurological disability. Seasonal outbreaks of acute encephalitis syndrome (AES) occur with striking regularity in India and lead to substantial mortality. Data of National Vector Borne Disease Control Program Directorate reveals that Uttar Pradesh has the maximum disease load. Uttar Pradesh has 20 districts listed for the epidemic of JE/AES.

Human vaccination is the only effective long-term control measure against JE. All at-risk population should receive a safe and efficacious vaccine as part of their national immunization program for which it is essential to identify the hotspots of the disease. Temporal, spatial, and space-time scan statistics are commonly used for disease cluster detection and evaluation. The spatial scan statistic developed by Martin Kulldorff can both detect and provide inference for spatial and space-time disease clusters. It is felt that one can also identify statistically significant clusters of JE/AES which has seasonal outbreaks with striking regularity leading to substantial mortality. The detection of these clusters may be highly useful in surveillance of the disease, finding the factors behind the spread of the disease, and making suitable policies to control these factors. The effect of various socio-economical and environmental factors on the occurrence of JE in U.P. can also be studied. The geographical correlation analysis can be used to study the association between JE and its causative factors.

## 10.6 Detecting influenza epidemics using search engine query data

A very interesting study was reported by Ginsberg et al. (2009) at Google which allows detection of influenza epidemics. Epidemics of seasonal influenza cause tens of millions of respiratory illnesses and 250,000 to 500,000 deaths worldwide each year. Internet itself could be used as a source of identifying outbreak of diseases as shown by research paper from Google. It leverages online web search queries, which are submitted by millions of users around the world each day. The paper on Google Flu Trends analyzes submitted queries in the context of influenza-like illness. The basic premise of research is that relative frequency of certain queries should be highly correlated with the percentage of physician visits in influenza-like symptoms are reported. Using this correlation, the current level of weekly influenza activity is predicted accurately with a reporting lag of only one day. Utilizing an automated method of finding search queries related to influenza-like symptoms, the approach makes itself a viable tool to analyze and predict such outbreaks in areas where the concentration of web users is high.

Authors have suggested a simple model which estimates the probability that a random physician visit in a particular region is related to an influenza-like illness. This has the potential that once a best-fit model is chosen it can be exploited to predict the influenza outbreak.

The potential of this approach in Indian context may need to be checked. Most of the cities have good number of internet surfers and hence may be submitting queries which can be used to predict disease clusters. The approach should be useful because by 2016, India is forecasted to have the 2nd largest online user-base after China. As per forecasts, the online population of India will touch a whopping 283 million by that year leaving even the US behind.

However, in areas where online web search queries are not made or are not recorded, an alternative could be to monitor health-seeking behavior in the form of visits to the physicians, hospitals and clinics. This would require sending data over network from these channels to an aggregation point where models can be run and predictions made. Even medical stores can be a good source. However, its potential remains to be investigated.

# 11

# Analysis of multiple response data

## 11.1 Introduction

Multiple response categorical variables are common in surveys where respondents are instructed to 'mark all that apply' from a list of items. For example it may be of interest to analyze of reasons of failures of some intervention like administering IFA to pregnant women. As there could be several reasons of failures, the responses could be multiple in natures requiring careful diagnostics. Possible types of answers sought by any survey-based study could be related to interventions for the targeted population – whether all components of antenatal checkup are being provided, whether all aspects of IEC are being covered, and even, which out of several NGOs involved at the grass root level for a large-scale intervention are poor performers of implementation. The current practice to analyze such questions is counting of the frequencies for a single code and then reporting its percentage. But, it hardly reveals any useful information, since the total percentage of all options exceeds hundred which does not clearly depict the actual data characteristics. This type of analysis conceals more than it reveals and, as would be seen later, it does not fully exploit some of the peculiar data characteristics.

## 11.2 Alternative method of analysis

An alternative method of analyzing data with multiple responses was proposed by Nigam et al. (2013). It provides answers to both important queries as discussed in the previous paragraph, that is, whether all types of intended services are being provided and which out of several NGOs involved at the grass root level for a large-scale intervention are poor performers of implementation. The method is best described through examples.

**Example 1:** Under the ANC given to pregnant women, there is a check list of 16 or 17 services that should be included in the check up, like examination of eyes, tongue, stomach/abdomen, nails, palms, providing medicine, dietary suggestions, pulse checking, collection of urine sample, providing immunization card, blood test, BP testing, weighing, awareness regarding the precautions to be taken just before the delivery, injection, arrangement of the things required during the delivery. In addition to the ANC, paramedical service providers like Anganwadi Worker (AWW), Auxiliary Nurse Midwife (ANM) and other mobilization functionaries are also supposed to advise pregnant women, like take TT injections, IFA tablets, enough rest during the day, eat enough nutritious food at least 3–4 times in a day, do not eat sour food and carry heavy weights, go for health check-ups, consult doctor for complications and start breast-feeding on first day itself.

These services are provided to the pregnant women through a doctor at primary/community health centres/government hospital, private doctor, ANM or AWW. In a study on assessment of CARE, India project on maternal and infant survival in the state Madhya Pradesh, done by IASDS in 2005, lactating women of children below 1 year were asked that during the pregnancy which of the services were provided in ANC and what advice were given by AWW/ANM/Community Mobilizer. The responses were multiple and were analyzed in the traditional manner.

A ready inference drawn from this analysis was that almost every ANC service and advice was being provided at varying levels. An alternative analysis of the same data, however, reveals some more information. In the alternative approach, ANC data were again analyzed to ascertain percent of women who were provided only one, only two, only three, and so on…, of the 16–17 services under ANC.

While 55 percent women were given medicine, 44.4 percent had weight measurement, 32.7 percent blood test, and 28.9 percent had urine tests. All other components had extremely low coverage levels. One-fourth of women were provided only one, 12 percent only two, 17.1 percent only three, and 15.5 percent only four of these services. Thus nearly 70 percent of women were provided four services or less. Coverage above these had less than 10 percent rates, there were none receiving more than twelve services. These results provide striking value-added information.

Analysis of the services provided by ANM/AWW/ Community Mobilizers revealed similar findings. Out of 12 to 13 components of advice, 54.5 percent were given only one, 7.6 percent two, 9.7 percent three, and 13.9 percent four of these. Coverage above these was also very low.

**Example 2:** Project managers implementing large-scale targeted interventions through a consortium of NGOs at the grass root level usually want to ascertain whether all the intended interventions are being made and which of the NGOs are poor performers. In the National Foundation for India study on mid-term assessment of communication initiative for Adolescent Reproductive Sexual Health (ARSH) in the states Bihar and Jharkhand, evaluated by IASDS in 2007, it was intended to assess whether the NGOs were discussing as a part of IEC all the ARSH issues like empowerment, sexual and reproductive health, gender issues, delaying first child birth, life skill, safe MCH, HIV/AIDS, RTI/STI, contraception, and hygiene with the adolescents or not.

The analysis was done on the basis of number of topics addressed by the NGOs in the format only one, only two, and so on, and the issues addressed by them to at least 30 percent of the targeted adolescents. It was observed that not only most of the NGOs touched upon merely 2–3 topics; they concentrated upon only one of the covered topics. Hygiene and sexual and reproductive health issues were the topics addressed by most of the NGOs. Sexual and reproductive health issues were discussed with mostly boys, and girls were hardly covered. Only two NGOs number 1 (53.3%) and 6 (52.8%) covered girls under this crucial topic.

Two inferences are readily drawn from the above analysis: None of the NGOs implemented the targeted interventions satisfactorily as they covered far fewer topics than assigned; and among the NGOs, one easily notices that most of them are poor performers.

# 12

# Randomized response technique

## *(for sensitive characteristics)*

## 12.1 Sensitive characteristics

In the conduct of surveys related to socioeconomic and the related fields, researchers are often faced with the problem of ascertaining accurate information on sensitive issues like drug abuse, improper sexual behavior and tax evasion, etc. Respondents are generally reluctant to respond truthfully to 'sensitive questions'. This leads to erroneous conclusions.

Some examples of this are information on: abortions by unmarried girls, high risk sex behavior before and after marriage, child sexual abuse, domestic violence, and female feticide. A similar concern is the extent of child labor engaged in hazardous activities in industries like carpet, glass, etc.

The Indian experience shows that the information on such sensitive characters is still being ascertained through traditional methods based upon direct questioning. This has resulted in either complete refusal to respond or give an incorrect or misleading response. There are also some qualitative ways of extracting such information usually by social scientists, but all such responses cannot be assigned any standard errors and are, therefore, not useful.

NFHS-3 included questions on respondents' (male and female) sexual partners during the 12 months preceding the survey. Information on the use of condoms at the acts of sexual intercourse with each of these partners during the previous 12 months was collected from both women and men. Respondents were also asked to identify what their relationship was with each sexual partner and the duration of the sexual relationship. All women and men who ever had sex were asked how many sexual partners they had during their lifetime. Men were also asked whether they paid for sex at any time in the 12 months preceding the survey. NFHS-3 also put a note of caution that the results should be interpreted with caution. This is because due to the sensitivity of questions on sexual behavior, there is a potential for reporting bias of an unknown extent.

## 12.2 Randomized response technique

Randomized response technique (RRT) introduced by Warner (1965) allows estimation of the proportion of the population possessing a sensitive characteristic. It utilizes a randomized device on a probability basis, which ensures confidentiality of the respondent. As the status of the respondent (whether he belongs to a sensitive group) is not revealed to the interviewer, the technique is likely to provide a much more efficient estimate, than the one obtained through direct questioning. As randomized response methods work by adding extra noise, they suffer from large standard errors and for this reason these methods require larger sample size than the direct question methods. For details please see Gerty et al. (2005).

Warner's technique was modified by Greenberg et al. (1969). There are several other more efficient methods. A good source of literature on randomized response is the book by Chaudhari and Mukerjee (1988). In Warner's version, the sensitive question is worded in two dichotomous alternatives, and chance decides, unknown to the interviewer, which one is to be answered honestly. The interviewer gets a 'yes' or 'no' response without knowing to which of the two questions it belongs. The two alternatives can be related or unrelated. In case of unrelated alternatives A and B, the two proportions which need to be estimated are $\pi_A$ and $\pi_B$. The probability of a 'yes' answer $\lambda_1$ based upon a sample of size, say, $n_1$ is given by

$$\lambda_1 = p_1\pi_A + (1-p_1)\,\pi_B$$

where $p_1$ and $1-p_1$ are the probabilities with which the first and second options are answered. As there are two unknowns, $\pi_A$ and $\pi_B$, to be estimated, we need another independent sample of size, say $n_2$, with probabilities $p_2$ and $1-p_2$ with which the first and second options are answered. This gives another equation for estimating the two proportions. The second equation is then

$$\lambda_2 = p_2\pi_A + (1-p_2)\,\pi_B$$

If the two groups are related with each other, $\pi_B$ is the same as $1-\pi_A$, then $\pi_A$ can be estimated only from one sample. Let p be the probability to answer the sensitive question and $\pi$ the true proportion of those interviewed having the sensitive characteristic, then the proportion of 'yes' –answers $\lambda$ is given by:

$$\lambda = p\pi + (1-p)\,(1-\pi)$$

This gives $\pi = (\lambda + p - 1)/(2p - 1)$.

The variance of the estimate of $\pi$ is given by $[\pi\,(1-\pi)/n] + [p(1-p)/n(2p-1)^2]$.

Though the randomized response technique has been used extensively in other parts of the world, its use in India appears to be negligible. Two of its applications in India are illustrated through examples, one on estimating the proportions of truck drivers involved in high-risk sexual behavior and the other on child sexual abuse.

### 12.2.1 Examples

**Example 1:** First example is of a World Bank funded study by IASDS on HIV/AIDS (1997). It was an intervention project among national and state highway truck operators in Lucknow district of Uttar Pradesh. The objective of the project was to increase the levels of STD/HIV/AIDS information and awareness and distribution of condoms. Ascertaining high-risk sexual behavior among highway truck operators was an important component of the project. Randomized response technique was used to obtain the proportion of truckers engaged in unsafe sex.

Truckers showed keen interest in responding to the question on unsafe sex in spite of this being a sensitive question. To answer this question, the truckers were first asked to draw one of the slips at random, which were of two colors with unequal numbers – 7 blue and 3 red. They were then to answer in 'yes' or 'no' to one of the two options as below depending upon the color the slip drawn.

1. I did not have sex with other than wife/I had sex with other than wife but invariably used condoms
2. I had sex outside but did not always use condoms.

This procedure looked attractive to them because of the confidentiality of their response. However, it needed considerable explanation on how to respond in a randomized way as required under the procedure. It was observed that once the truckers were convinced that their confidentiality of belonging to high-risk behavior group was ensured, they responded in an overwhelming manner to this sensitive question. Whereas the first group indicates safe sex, the second group reflects high-risk behavior.

The randomized response estimate of the second group of truckers after adjusting it for a few direct responses was 52.8 percent. The percentages of truckers belonging to high-risk behavior group for the National and UP/local categories were respectively 57.9 and 45.0. Thus, a large proportion of truckers have the risk of contracting HIV infection because of unsafe sex. It is worth noticing that the percentage of truckers belonging to high-risk behavior category is lower for UP/local highway category. The reason for this is the fact that these truckers have to travel shorter distance destinations and the absence from home is of lesser durations. From the survey, it was found that the average durations of absence from home were around 15 days for the National and 3 days for the UP/local truckers.

**Example 2:** The second study was a state-level study from Plan India on status of assessment of child sexual abuse in Uttar Pradesh. The study was undertaken in 2011 by Vatsalya with IASDS as a partner. The survey was carried out in Mau and Maharajganj (Eastern UP), Lucknow and Ambedkar Nagar (Central UP), Baghpat and Etawah (Western UP) and Jhansi and Jalaun (Bundelkhand) districts.

Some of its results are also given in Srivastava, Nigam and Neelam Singh (2015). Focus of the study was to assess the status of sexual abuse in children in the age groups 5–10 years and 11–17 years. For children in the age group 5–10 years, information was gathered by direct questioning method. The children belonging to 11–17 years age group were classified into four categories viz.: (i) children in family environment, (ii) school going children, (iii) working children and (iv) children in institutional care. The coverage of these was 162, 167, 512 and 630, respectively. The category-wise breakup according to males was 72, 93, 223, 292 and that of females was 90, 74, 289 and 338, respectively.

Child abuse is not only violation of their rights but it can also make them psychologically depressed and even place them in long-term *psychological trauma.* It is really difficult to get accurate responses due to stigma attached to it. No reliable estimates are available in our country on child sexual abuse. Ministry of Women and Child Development, Government of India, in its report entitled 'Study on Child Abuse India 2007' has data on child sexual abuse obtained through direct questioning at National level in 5–18 year age group children. These data are, however, not reliable as direct questioning does not allow accurate responses due to the stigma attached to the topic.

According to Wikipedia, child sexual abuse is not only a violation of children's rights it can also place them in *post-traumatic stress disorder, anxiety,* propensity to further *victimization* in adulthood, and physical injury to the child. Sexual abuse by a family member can result in more serious and long-term *psychological trauma.* It is really difficult to get accurate direct responses due to stigma attached to it. We now demonstrate that RRT can be successfully used in the problem of child sexual abuse.

Following indicators of sexual abuse were used.

**Table 12.1** Indicators of child sexual abuse

| Sexual abuse (severe form) | Sexual abuse (mild form) |
|---|---|
| • Sexual assault<br>• Make the child fondle private parts<br>• Make the child exhibit private parts<br>• Exhibit private parts to the child<br>• Photograph the child in the nude | • Forcible kissing<br>• Forcible kissing during travel situations<br>• Kissing/molestation attempt during marriage<br>• Forced to view private body parts of others<br>• Forced to view pornographic video/ photographs |

The study was carried out in five zones of the state. Information regarding sexual abuse in the children in the age group 11–17 years belonging to family environment and school going children was gathered using direct questioning method while for working children and children in institutional care it was obtained by using randomized response technique. An overall sample of 512 (223 males, 289 females) for school going children and 630 (292 males, 338 females) for children in institutional care was used in the study.

Working children and the children in institutional care were divided into two groups. Two sets of different urns containing tokens of different colors as given in Table 12.2 were used for drawing the samples.

**Table 12.2** Details of colors in urns

| Color of the token | Urn 1 | Urn 2 |
|---|---|---|
| Red | 4 | 3 |
| Green | 3 | 4 |
| Yellow | 3 | 3 |
| Total | 10 | 10 |

Group 1 was asked to pick a token from Urn 1 and the following schedule was followed depending upon the color of the urn.

**Table 12.3** Action taken according to colors from Urn 1

| Color of the token | Action |
|---|---|
| Red | Ask the child to respond YES/NO whether anytime in the past there was a sexual assault, or the child was made to fondle or exhibit private parts, or he/she exhibited his/her private parts, or was photographed in the nude.<br>Put the answer sheet in box 1 |

*Contd...*

*Contd...*

| Color of the token | Action |
|---|---|
| Green | Ask the child to respond YES/NO whether he/she was kissed forcibly, or somebody tried to kiss/molest him/her during travel, or somebody tried to kiss/molest him/her during marriage, or he/she was forced to view private body parts of others, or he/she was forced to view pornographic video/photographs |
| | Put the answer sheet in box 1 |
| Yellow | Ask the child to respond YES/NO whether he/she was never sexually abused. |
| | Put the answer sheet in box 1 |

Similar procedure was carried out for Group 2 and answer sheets were collected in box 2. Mathematical details for obtaining randomized response estimates are given at the end of the Chapter.

Table 12.4 provides a comparative scenario of incidence of overall child sexual abuse across various categories of children. It may be observed that randomized response technique has been able to capture higher incidence of abuse among children of school going and institutional care categories with the latter category having higher percentages. A possible reason of this could be relatively higher exposure to outsiders for 'children in institutional care' category and children due to residential nature of the institution. However, one should also take note of the fact that children of family environment spend more time at home and are more protected.

**Table 12.4** Comparative view of incidence of sexual abuse in children (11–17 yrs) across the categories (percent)

| Zone | Category | | | |
|---|---|---|---|---|
| | Family environment | Working | School going* | In institutional care* |
| Eastern UP | 64.1 | 61.3 | 76.4 | 94.6 |
| Central UP | 45.5 | 53.8 | 75.0 | 90.4 |
| Western UP | 71.1 | 65.1 | 76.8 | 86.1 |
| Bundelkhand | 36.6 | 41.5 | 91.1 | 84.2 |
| UP overall | 53.7 | 55.1 | 80.2 | 88.7 |

*Estimated using Randomized Response Technique

Table 12.5 relates to severity of sexual abuse. Here the reporting gives higher percentages (over 20%) in all categories of children who were put to direct questioning. However, the children who were administered randomized response technique had lower percentages of severe abuse. It could be because of this technique capturing the two types of abuse more correctly and because of confounding (mix-up) between severe and mild abuses when the questions are put directly.

**Table 12.5** Age-wise child sexual abuse in UP

| Type of sexual abuse (%) | 5–10 years | 11–17 yrs | | | |
|---|---|---|---|---|---|
| | | Family environment | Working | School going* | In institutional care* |
| Sexual abuse | 41.1 | 53.7 | 55.1 | 80.2 | 88.7 |
| Severe sexual abuse | 22.7 | 24.1 | 27.6 | 16.6 | 18.4 |

*Estimated using Randomized Response Technique

Ministry of Women and Child Development, in its report on Child Abuse has provided information (Table 12.6) on child sexual abuse relating to above categories at national level.

**Table 12.6** Percentage of children reporting sexual abuse (5–18 years)

| Family environment | Working | School going | Institutional care |
|---|---|---|---|
| 53.18 | 61.61 | 49.92 | 47.08 |

This study has considered children in the age group 5–18 years, while present study has two classifications, viz. 5–10 years and 11–17 years. Thus a comparison between the two studies will be only indicative. It is seen that the estimates obtained using RRT for school going and in institutional care children are fairly high in Table 12.5 compared to direct estimates (Table 12.6) establishing the advantage of using RRT.

## Methodology for randomized response estimates

The problem now is to estimate $\pi_1, \pi_2, \pi_3$ the true proportions of each statement: $0 < \pi_j <$ and $\sum_{j=1}^{3} \pi_j = 1$. The randomized response formulation of Abul-Ela et al. (1967) was utilized for this. Under this formulation, two simple random samples of sizes $n_1$ and $n_2$ are drawn independently without replacement from the population. For I = 1, 2 and j = 1, 2, 3 $P_{ij}$ denotes the proportion of cards belonging to jth statement from i$^{th}$ sample. Then $\sum_{j=1}^{3} P_{ij}$ and the probability of 'yes' for any interviewee in i$^{th}$ sample is $\lambda_i = \sum_{j=1}^{3} P_{ij}\pi_j$ , i = 1, 21

In our case

$$\begin{aligned} \lambda_1 &= P_{11}\lambda_1 + P_{12}\pi_2 + P_{12}\pi_3 \\ \lambda_2 &= P_{21}\lambda_2 + P_{22}\pi_2 + P_{23}\pi_3 \end{aligned}$$

Remembering that $\sum_{j=1}^{3} P_{ij}\pi_j$ we have in matrix notation

$$P\pi = \xi$$

Where

$$P = \begin{pmatrix} P_{11} - P_{13} & P_{12} - P_{13} \\ P_{21} - P_{23} & P_{22} - P_{23} \end{pmatrix}$$

$$\pi = \begin{pmatrix} \pi_1 \\ \pi_1 \end{pmatrix} \text{ and } \xi = \begin{pmatrix} \lambda_1 - P_{13} \\ \lambda_1 - P_{13} \end{pmatrix}$$

If in the i$^{th}$ sample $n_{i1}$ persons report 'yes' then an unbiased estimate of $\lambda_i$ is $\hat{\lambda}_i = n_{i1}.n_i$. Therefore writing $c = \begin{pmatrix} \hat{\lambda}_1 - P_{13} \\ \lambda_2 - P_{23} \end{pmatrix}$ we have

$\hat{\pi} = P^{-1}c$ provided inverse exists: we may otherwise use Moore-Penrose inverse. Since $\pi_1$ and $\pi_2$ have been estimated, $\pi_3$ can easily be estimated. Dispersion matrix of c is given by disp (c) = diag ($V_{11}, V_{22}, V_{33}$) and dispersion matrix of $\pi$ is given by disp ($\pi$) = $P^{-1}$ diag ($V_{11}, V_{22}, V_{33}$) and $V_{ii} = \lambda_i (1 - \lambda_i)/n_i$

In our case

$$\begin{aligned} P_{11} &= P_{22} = 4/10 \\ P_{12} &= P_{13} = P_{21} = P_{23} = 3/10 \end{aligned}$$

The estimating equations are

$$\hat{\pi}_1 = 10\hat{\lambda}_1 - 3,$$
$$\hat{\pi}_2 = 10\hat{\lambda}_2 - 3,$$
$$\hat{\pi}_3 = 1 - (\hat{\lambda}_1 + \hat{\lambda}_2)$$

Where

$\pi_1$ = Proportion of severe sexual abuse

$\pi_2$ = Proportion of mild sexual abuse

$\pi_3$ = Proportion of no sexual abuse

$\lambda_1$ = Proportion of yes response in group 1

$\lambda_2$ = Proportion of yes response in group 2

It can be seen from estimating equations that following should hold under the above set up

$$0.3 < \lambda_1, \lambda_2 < 0.4$$

and $$0.6 < \lambda_1 + \lambda_2 < 0.7$$

This in simple term means that proportions of 'yes' responses in individual groups should be between 30 to 40 percents and when two groups are taken together the total of 'yes' responses should be between 60 to 70 percents.

# 13

# Small area estimation

*(for inadequate sample size)*

## 13.1 Introduction

We now discuss an aspect of improved estimation which has a direct bearing on development planning. Creation of a reliable and wide database is essential for effective planning. Although substantial efforts are being made towards data collection, gaps still occur in some sectors of development. One of the areas of data gaps is related to micro-level planning, which requires estimates of different activities for 'smaller' areas. For instance, though district-level estimates may be available for certain characteristics we may instead be interested in block-level estimates. The question now is whether block-level estimates can be obtained by using secondary data already collected at district level which were targeted to provide reliable estimates only at the district level. Traditional block-level estimates, if developed from these data, are not reliable. This happens because sample sizes for blocks may be very small.

There has been a growing demand for reliable small area estimates (SAE) both from the public and private sectors. The term 'small area' or small domain generally refers to a small geographical area such as a tehsil/block/gram panchayat or even a small demographic or socioeconomic sub-group. The term 'small area' is generally used to denote any domain for which direct estimates of adequate precision cannot be produced. In India, with such large variations, there is an increasing concern about issues of distribution, equity and disparity. For instance, some sub-groups may be far below the average in certain respects and may need upgrading. As a matter of fact these arguments extend to states and even regions also because of diversity.

The small area estimates can be obtained for a variety of domains or subpopulations. A domain is regarded as large if the domain-specific sample is large enough to yield estimates of adequate precision. A domain is regarded as 'small' if the domain-specific sample is not large enough to support direct estimates of adequate precision. It should be noted that while a smaller sample size leads to invalid estimates, with unduly large standard errors, a larger sample involves avoidable wasteful expenditure.

Small area estimation deals with the estimation of parameters for small sub-populations, when the sub-population of interest is included in a larger survey. If a survey has been carried out for the population as a whole (for example, a nation or state-wide survey), the sample size within any particular small area may be too small to generate accurate estimates from the data. It is practically not possible to have a large enough overall sample size to support reliable direct estimates for all domains. However, it may be possible to use additional data such as census records or past records or records of highly correlated variables that exist for these small areas in order to obtain efficient estimates. In making estimates for small areas with adequate level of precision, it is often necessary to use 'indirect' estimators that 'borrow strength' by using values of the variable of interest, y, from related areas and/or time periods and thus increase the 'effective' sample size. These values are brought into the estimation process through a model (either implicit or explicit) that provides a link to related areas and/or time periods through the use of auxiliary information related to y.

Section 1.14 describes many research studies in which though adequate sample size is taken for the whole population, there is an attempt to present analysis by sub-groups in terms of related socioeconomic, demographic, housing or household characteristics. Reporting of indicators in most of the large-scale surveys is usually done by sub-groups like caste, religion, gender, age group, grades of nutritional status, grades of anemia, etc. In most situations, sample size for these sub-groups is inadequate. Examples of this are found in reporting of NNMB, NFHS, RCH and DLHS, and many others. In all these studies the sample size was determined for all the groups together keeping in mind the precision, complexity of the design and expected non-response. But the reporting is also done by sub-groups. Several examples of these types of dis-aggregated reporting for undernutrition and anemia prevalence by region, caste and of self-employed parents are described in that Section. One easily notices that sample sizes are not adequate for any of these sub-group estimates.

It is discussed in Chapter 1 that sample sizes rapidly increase with the decline in expected prevalence rates. For determining sample sizes for infant mortality around 50 gives p as 0.05, and expected maternal mortality around 230 gives p as 0.0023. The sample sizes for 10 percent relative margin of error are 7600 and 199600, respectively. These are to be multiplied by the design effect which is usually taken as 1.5. This raises the sample sizes to 11400 and 299400. If infant mortality is taken as 40, giving $p = 0.04$, then the sample size required is 14400 live births, and for MMR as 200 ($p = 0.002$) then the sample size is approximately 3 lakhs live births. In the IRMS example of Section 3.5.3 with expected MMR around 400 per lakh births, 3.8 lakh births were required. For tracking such huge number of births, if we assume the birth rate of 28.5 per thousand population, a population of 1.30 crores (13 millions) needs to be tracked. Similarly, for IMR at 40, the population that needs to be tracked is over 5 lakhs.

For the estimation of MMR/IMR, information on all the characters which have close association with maternal/infant survival is to be ascertained. These as elaborated in Chapter 3 for maternal mortality are pre-intra-post natal practices, and availability, access and utilization of maternal health services. Also needed are the information on maternal and delivery complications, accurate classification of mother's death as the maternal death and data on factors associated with maternal mortality. All this information is required for the several past years to be able to get to such huge number of births. It was also discussed that we have virtually a failed health service system with unreliable and inconsistent record keeping. It is difficult, time-consuming and costly task to get quality data on so many births and health practices and services. In addition to tracking maternal deaths within the health system, there is also the problem of omission of deaths occurring outside the system (say, deaths occurring outside maternity wards).

Almost a similar scenario exists for IMR, though of smaller magnitude. The sample size requirement is lower in comparison to MMR, and so is the requirement of information on covariates – variables closely associated with IMR.

All this calls for resorting to small area estimation as this would enable seeking information on these characteristics at a much smaller scale.

## 13.2 Small area estimation

'Small area estimation' is a statistical technique which makes it possible to enhance the precision of sub-group estimates. The technique uses the idea of 'borrow strength' from similar other areas to develop more accurate estimates for a given area. Availability of good auxiliary data and determination of suitable linking models are crucial to the formation of indirect estimators. If the implicit linking model is approximately true, then the design bias will be small, leading to significantly smaller MSE compared to the MSE of a direct estimator. Reduction in MSE is the main reason for using indirect estimators. Inferences from model-based estimators refer to the distribution implied by the assumed model. Model selection and validation, therefore, play a vital role in model-based estimation. If the assumed models do not provide a good fit to the data, the model-based estimators will be model biased which, in turn, can lead to erroneous inferences.

The term best linear unbiased predictor (BLUP) is used in linear mixed models for the estimation of random effects. BLUPs of random effects are similar to BLUE (see Section 1.10) of fixed effects. In practice, it is often the case that the parameters associated with the random effect(s) term(s) are unknown; these parameters are the variances of the random effects and residuals. Typically the parameters are estimated and plugged into the predictor, leading to the Empirical Best Linear Unbiased Predictor (EBLUP). Notice that by simply plugging in the estimated parameter into the predictor, additional variability is unaccounted for, leading to overly optimistic prediction variances for the EBLUP.

The EBLUP method for general linear mixed models has been extensively used in animal breeding and other applications to estimate realized values of linear combinations of fixed and random effects. An EBLUP estimator is obtained in two steps: (i) the best linear unbiased predictor (BLUP), which minimizes the model MSE in the class of linear model unbiased estimators of the quantity of interest is first obtained. It depends on the variances (and covariances) of random effects in the model. (ii) An EBLUP estimator is obtained from the BLUP by substituting suitable estimators of variance parameters. This technique is also computer intensive and needs the application of software like SAS, SPSS, R, etc., with the help of a statistician. An excellent source of material on small area estimation is the book by Rao (2010).

### 13.2.1 An example of SAE

The technique of deriving small area estimates is best explained through an example. We continue with the research project carried out by IASDS on food insecurity (Chapter 9).

A major limitation of the state-level mapping as done by MSSRF is that the state-level aggregation may not capture inter- and intra-regional variations for large states with lot of heterogeneity in the underlying indicators and sub-indicators. This may happen because of masking effects. This issue was also highlighted by MSSRF. Quite rightly, they have pointed out that village-level and block-level mapping would be most useful, as it would enable us to take up speedy and location-specific action. But, attempting this exercise would be formidable in view of the enormity of the work involved and the non-availability of data on virtually all sub-indicators particularly at the village/block level. Further, in MSSRF study, whenever comparable data was not available for some states and some periods, data from another source for the same year or a year close to was taken. Sometimes even data for the same state for a previous period was used. To explain this further, at the time of MSSRF study Jharkhand state was already carved out of Bihar but the state-level data were available for Bihar only. The study used erstwhile Bihar figures for both the newly carved out Bihar and Jharkhand states. This was not a satisfactory situation. Indeed, in such cases, the technique of statistical imputation as discussed in Chapter 1 is extremely useful.

### 13.2.2 SAEs of CEDs

As already indicated, small area estimation methodology is useful for deriving efficient estimates for smaller domains. The technique is explained by applying it for a crucial indicator, namely, chronic energy deficiency (CED). The necessity arose because of a peculiar reason. District-wise CED estimates were already available in the NIN, IASDS study (Nutrition Profile of Community, Uttar Pradesh, 2002). However, the study whose data were collected in 1999–2000 was for 54 districts which were in existence at the time of survey. In subsequent years there was reorganization of districts and in 2008 there were 70 districts in the state. Many new districts were carved out of some of the older districts. Now the problem was to obtain reliable estimates of CED for these 70 reorganized districts by using already available CED estimates of 54 districts which were in existence in 1991. The reorganization occurred in 33 out of 54 districts leaving out 21 districts unaffected due to reorganization. Thus in all, there were 49 new affected districts. Each of these affected districts had much smaller sample size. This necessitated the use of small area estimation technique to estimate CED. The list of 33 districts is given at the end of the chapter.

An 'area level random effect model' by Fay and Herriot (1979) has been used for application of small area estimation technique as information on the covariates is available only at the area/district level. Specifically, EBLUP methodology has been utilized to arrive at the SAEs for CED. EBLUP methodology basically uses appropriate covariates related to direct estimate to arrive at SAE of CED. As a first step, therefore, direct estimates of proportion of population having BMI less than 18.5 were calculated. The methodology adopted for SAE is described at the end of the chapter.

### 13.2.3 Covariate selection

The first step is to choose certain covariates which may have significant correlation with CED. To start with, social variables available in census 2001 which were significantly correlated with direct estimates were used to arrive at SAE of CED for males, females and total population. The covariates used were as follows.

**Table 13.1** Selected covariates

| S. no. | Variable name |
|---|---|
| 1 | Main Cultivator Male Population |
| 2 | Scheduled Castes (SC) Percentage |
| 3 | Population Literacy Percentage |
| 4 | Male Literacy Percentage |
| 5 | Female Literacy Percentage |

The criterion used to compare direct estimates with SAE was coefficient of variation. This however did not show any improvement in the estimates. As an alternative, nutrition related dietary intake variables as given in Table 13.2 were used. Only those variables were used as covariates which were significantly correlated with direct estimate. In case of males, per unit consumption of vitamin A and vitamin C only were found to be significantly correlated to direct estimate. Unit for vitamin A, vitamin C, Fat, etc., was cu/day i.e., per unit consumption per day. Inclusion of these covariates considerably improved the small area estimates.

**Table 13.2** Nutrition related covariates

| | **Males** | | |
|---|---|---|---|
| **S. no.** | **Variable** | **Correlation** | **$R^2$** |
| 1 | Vitamin A | −0.416* | 0.173056 |
| 2 | Vitamin C | −0.566** | 0.320356 |
| | **Females** | | |
| 1 | % of marginal cultivators (with <1.00 ha) to total cultivators | 0.363* | 0.131769 |
| 2 | Distribution (%) of household according to consumption of vitamin A <50 % of RDA | 0.389* | 0.151321 |
| 3 | Fat | −0.421* | 0.177241 |
| 4 | Vitamin A | −0.464** | 0.215296 |
| 5 | Thiamin | −0.396* | 0.156816 |
| 6 | Riboflavin | −0.415* | 0.172225 |
| 7 | Free_folic | −0.434* | 0.188356 |

*Contd...*

*Contd...*

| | Total | | |
|---|---|---|---|
| 1 | % of marginal cultivators (with <1.00 ha) to total cultivators | 0.407* | 0.165649 |
| 2 | Distribution (%) of household according to consumption of vitamin A <50 % of RDA | 0.359* | 0.128881 |
| 3 | Fat | −0.414* | 0.171396 |
| 4 | Iron | −0.353* | 0.124609 |
| 5 | Vitamin A | −0.547** | 0.299209 |
| 6 | Thiamin | −0.395* | 0,156025 |
| 7 | Riboflavin | −0.425* | 0.180625 |
| 8 | Vitamin C | −0.454** | 0.206116 |
| 9 | Free_folic | −0.434* | 0.188356 |

*Source of data on above covariates:* Nutrition Profile of Community: Uttar Pradesh, NIN & IASDS, 2004

*significant at 5% level; **significant at 1% level.

### 13.2.4 Results and discussion

It is clear that selection of covariates is crucial to derive small area estimates. Tables 13.3–13.5 give SAEs of CED of male, female and total population respectively with percent improvement over direct estimate. Also reported is the coefficient of variation for each estimate. It can be seen that in general improvement over direct estimate for male and female population is appreciable, while for total population improvement is not up to that level.

**Table 13.3** Small area estimates of percentage of male population with CED

| | | Percentage of population with CED (Male) | | |
|---|---|---|---|---|
| **S. no.** | **District** | **Direct Estimate** | **Estimate (SAE)** | **% improvement over direct estimate** |
| 1 | Aligarh | 34.6 (8.03) | 34.7(7.07) | 11.96 |
| 2 | Allahabad | 33.1 (9.00) | 33.1(8.65) | 3.89 |
| 3 | Ambedkar Nagar | 37.2 (9.03) | 37.1 (8.58) | 4.98 |
| 4 | Auraiya | 11.3 (23.63) | 13.0 (20.42) | 13.58 |
| 5 | Baghpat | 54.8 (6.82) | 52.5 (6.86) | Nil |
| 6 | Bahriach | 45.1 (6.54) | 44.3 (6.44) | 1.53 |

*Contd...*

*Contd...*

| Percentage of population with CED (Male) | | | | |
|---|---|---|---|---|
| **S. no.** | **District** | **Direct Estimate** | **Estimate (SAE)** | **% improvement over direct estimate** |
| 7 | Balrampur | 40.0 (9.68) | 39.5 (9.14) | 5.58 |
| 8 | Banda | 36.8 (9.48) | 36.7 (9.03) | 4.75 |
| 9 | Basti | 43.2 (7.06) | 42.3 (6.95) | 1.56 |
| 10 | Bulandshahr | 33.8 (7.99) | 33.9 (7.68) | 3.88 |
| 11 | Chandauli | 26.2 (14.92) | 27.2 (13.47) | 9.72 |
| 12 | Chitrakut | 32.7 (11.50) | 33.3 (10.62) | 7.65 |
| 13 | Deoria | 31.1 (11.19) | 31.8 (10.38) | 7.24 |
| 14 | Etawah | 18.6 ( 16.72) | 20.2 (14.99) | 10.35 |
| 15 | Faizabad | 40.4 (10.05) | 39.7(9.56) | 4.88 |
| 16 | Farrukkhabad | 34.6 (9.60) | 34.7 (9.05) | 5.73 |
| 17 | Gautam Budh Nagar | 18.3 (17.70) | 20.2 (15.62) | 11.75 |
| 18 | Ghaziabad | 32.6 (8.34) | 32.9 (7.98) | 4.32 |
| 19 | Gonda | 38.2 (7.59) | 37.8 (7.38) | 2.77 |
| 20 | Hamirpur | 27.0 (10.56) | 27.8 (9.92) | 6.06 |
| 21 | Hathras | 39.9 (10.45) | 38.7 (10.01) | 4.21 |
| 22 | Jyotiba Phule Nagar | 48.3 (9.51) | 46.2 (9.27) | 2.52 |
| 23 | Kannauj | 38.9 (9.69) | 38.6 (9.13) | 5.78 |
| 24 | Kaushambi | 38.6 (19.02) | 37.8 (15.63) | 17.82 |
| 25 | Kushinágar | 35.7 (9.33) | 35.3 (9.02) | 3.32 |
| 26 | Mahoba | 24.2 (14.13) | 25.5 (12.78) | 9.55 |
| 27 | Mathura | 37.5 (6.75) | 37.3 (6.57) | 2.67 |
| 28 | Meerut | 45.8 (7.05) | 44.8 (6.89) | 2.27 |
| 29 | Moradabad | 43.7 (6.52) | 43.1 (6.38) | 2.15 |
| 30 | Sant Kabir Nagar | 52.5 (8.61) | 49.0 (8.72) | −1.28 |
| 31 | Sant Ravidas Nagar | 19.2 (20.10) | 21.00 (17.56) | 12.64 |
| 32 | Shravasti | 48.3 (10.97) | 45.2 (10.51) | 4.19 |
| 33 | Varanasi | 27.2 (14.63) | 27.9 (13.40) | 8.41 |

Figures in parentheses indicate cv

**Table 13.4** Small area estimates of percentage of female population with CED

| Percentage of population with CED (Female) | | | | |
|---|---|---|---|---|
| **S. no.** | **District** | **Direct Estimate** | **Estimate (SAE)** | **% improvement over direct estimate** |
| 1 | Aligarh | 28.0 (9.32) | 27.9 (9.00) | 3.43 |
| 2 | Allahabad | 34.0 (7.74) | 34.3 (7.39) | 4.52 |
| 3 | Ambedkar Nagar | 29.3 (9.15) | 29.9 (8.72) | 4.70 |
| 4 | Auraiya | 14.9 (15.91) | 15.6(14.92) | 6.22 |
| 5 | Baghpat | 51.4 (8.09) | 48.2 (8.36) | −3.33 |
| 6 | Bahriach | 48.5 (5.57) | 46.8 (5.73) | −2.87 |
| 7 | Balrampur | 29.5 (11.19) | 30.1(10.50) | 6.17 |
| 8 | Banda | 30.9 (10.39) | 30.4(10.12) | 2.60 |
| 9 | Basti | 41.7 (6.47) | 40.4 (6.54) | −1.08 |
| 10 | Bulandshahr | 54.2 (4.82) | 53.5 (4.75) | 1.45 |
| 11 | Chandauli | 24.7 (12.55) | 25.1(11.79) | 6.06 |
| 12 | Chitrakut | 29.3 (11.54) | 30.3(10.59) | 8.23 |
| 13 | Deoria | 28.4 (10.49) | 28.2(10.04) | 4.29 |
| 14 | Etawah | 15.4 (15.52) | 16.5(14.34) | 7.60 |
| 15 | Faizabad | 32.0 (9.63) | 31.4 (9.44) | 1.98 |
| 16 | Farrukkhabad | 25.5 (10.82) | 24.7(10.91) | Nil |
| 17 | Gautam Budh Nagar | 22.0 (13.77) | 23.3(12.57) | 8.71 |
| 18 | Ghaziabad | 27.4 (8.65) | 27.8 (8.31) | 3.93 |
| 19 | Gonda | 37.8 (6.75) | 37.7 (6.55) | 2.96 |
| 20 | Hamirpur | 19.1 (12.15) | 19.8(11.49) | 5.43 |
| 21 | Hathras | 27.5 (12.00) | 28.8(10.92) | 9.00 |
| 22 | Jyotiba Phule Nagar | 36.1 (11.52) | 36.2(10.56) | 8.33 |
| 23 | Kannauj | 23.2 (12.63) | 23.9(11.69) | 7.44 |
| 24 | Kaushambi | 38.0 (18.05) | 37.4(15.37) | 14.85 |
| 25 | Kushinagar | 35.9 (7.94) | 35.4 (7.69) | 3.15 |
| 26 | Mahoba | 12.5 (19.12) | 12.8(18.22) | 4.70 |
| 27 | Mathura | 29.2 (7.74) | 28.9 (7.66) | 1.03 |
| 28 | Meerut | 37.2 (7.85) | 36.9 (7.65) | 2.55 |
| 29 | Moradabad | 33.0 (8.45) | 32.8 (8.22) | 2.72 |
| 30 | Sant Kabir Nagar | 45.9 (9.41) | 43.9 (9.10) | 3.29 |
| 31 | Sant Ravidas Nagar | 26.7 (15.13) | 27.4(13.44) | 11.17 |
| 32 | Shravasti | 50.0 (9.30) | 49.1 (8.60) | 7.53 |
| 33 | Varanasi | 27.5 (11.67) | 27.9(10.84) | 7.11 |

Figures in parentheses indicate cv

**Table 13.5** Small area estimates of percentage of total population with CED

| Percentage of population with CED (Total) | | | | |
|---|---|---|---|---|
| **S. no.** | **District** | **Direct Estimate** | **Estimate (SAE)** | **% improvement over direct estimate** |
| 1 | Aligarh | 31.3 (6.07) | 31.3(5.96) | 1.81 |
| 2 | Allahabad | 33.6 (5.89) | 33.5 (5.83) | 1.02 |
| 3 | Ambedkar Nagar | 32.6 (6.44) | 32.7 (6.32) | 1.86 |
| 4 | Auraiya | 13.6 (13.16) | 14.0 (12.64) | 3.95 |
| 5 | Baghpat | 53.3 (5.23) | 51.8 (5.36) | −2.49 |
| 6 | Bahriach | 47.0 (4.26) | 46.4 (4.27) | Nil |
| 7 | Balrampur | 34.3 (7.38) | 34.5 (7.17) | 2.85 |
| 8 | Banda | 33.8 (7.01) | 33.6 (6.91) | 1.43 |
| 9 | Basti | 42.4 (4.79) | 41.8 (4.80) | Nil |
| 10 | Bulandshahr | 30.0 (5.87) | 30.4 (5.74) | 2.21 |
| 11 | Chandauli | 25.3 (9.60) | 25.6 (9.27) | 3.44 |
| 12 | Chitrakut | 30.9 (8.12) | 31.4 (7.80) | 3.94 |
| 13 | Deoria | 29.6 (7.64) | 29.7 (7.42) | 2.88 |
| 14 | Etawah | 19.3 (10.52) | 20.0 (10.08) | 4.18 |
| 15 | Faizabad | 35.3 (7.00) | 35.0 (6.91) | 1.29 |
| 16 | Farrukkhabad | 29.6 (7.26) | 29.3 (7.24) | Nil |
| 17 | Gautam Budh Nagar | 20.4 (10.98) | 21.2 (10.44) | 4.92 |
| 18 | Ghaziabad | 29.8 (6.00) | 30.0 (5.89) | 1.83 |
| 19 | Gonda | 38.0 (5.05) | 38.0 (4.97) | 1.58 |
| 20 | Hamirpur | 22.7 (8.02) | 23.0 (7.83) | 2.37 |
| 21 | Hathras | 32.8 (8.02) | 32.8 (7.86) | 2.37 |
| 22 | Jyotiba Phule Nagar | 41.8 (7.49) | 41.4 (7.26) | 3.07 |
| 23 | Kannuaj | 30.2 (7.85) | 30.4 (7.58) | 3.60 |
| 24 | Kaushambi | 38.3 (13.08) | 37.6 (12.26) | 6.27 |
| 25 | Kushinagar | 35.8 (6.06) | 35.6 (5.98) | 1.32 |
| 26 | Mahoba | 17.8 (11.52) | 18.1 (11.19) | 2.86 |
| 27 | Mathura | 33.2 (5.12) | 32.9 (5.11) | Nil |
| 28 | Meerut | 41.2 (5.27) | 41.0 (5.21) | 1.14 |
| 29 | Moradabad | 38.5 (5.27) | 38.1 (5.26) | Nil |
| 30 | Sant Kabir Nagar | 49.0 (6.39) | 47.9 (6.33) | Nil |
| 31 | Sant Ravidas Nagar | 23.2 (12.20) | 24.0 (11.47) | 5.98 |
| 32 | Shravasti | 49.3 (7.08) | 48.3 (6.91) | 2.40 |
| 33 | Varanasi | 27.4 (9.09) | 27.7 (8.76) | 3.63 |

Figures in parentheses indicate cv

## (i) Details of old and new districts in U.P.

Table (i) in Annexure gives details of these newly created districts and their blocks.

**Table (i)** Details of old and new districts in U.P.

| S. no. | Districts surveyed in NIN according to 1991 census | No. of blocks | | Districts to be covered in the present project | Current no. of blocks |
|---|---|---|---|---|---|
| | Old districts | Total | Surveyed in NIN, IASDS study | | |
| 1 | Agra | 15 | 15 | Agra | 15 |
| 2 | Aligarh | 17 | 17 | Aligarh | 12 |
| 3 | Allahabad | 28 | 20 | Allahabad | 20 |
| 4 | Azamgarh | 21 | 19 | Azamgarh | 22 |
| 5 | Bahriach | 19 | 19 | Bahriach | 14 |
| 6 | Ballia | 17 | 17 | Ballia | 17 |
| 7 | Banda | 13 | 14 | Banda | 8 |
| 8 | Barabanki | 17 | 16 | Barabanki | 15 |
| 9 | Bareilly | 15 | 15 | Bareilly | 15 |
| 10 | Basti | 19 | 19 | Basti | 14 |
| 11 | Bijnour | 11 | 11 | Bijnour | 11 |
| 12 | Badaun | 18 | 18 | Badaun | 18 |
| 13 | Bulandshahr | 17 | 17 | Bulandshahr | 16 |
| 14 | Deoria | 15 | 20 | Deoria | 16 |
| 15 | Etah | 15 | 15 | Etah | 15 |
| 16 | Etawah | 15 | 14 | Etawah | 8 |
| 17 | Faizabad | 18 | 18 | Faizabad | 11 |
| 18 | Farrukkhabad | 14 | 14 | Farrukkhabad | 7 |
| 19 | Fatehpur | 13 | 13 | Fatehpur | 13 |
| 20 | Firozabad | 9 | 9 | Firozabad | 9 |
| 21 | Gaziabad | 10 | 10 | Gaziabad | 8 |
| 22 | Ghazipur | 16 | 16 | Ghazipur | 16 |
| 23 | Gonda | 25 | 20 | Gonda | 16 |
| 24 | Gorakhpur | 19 | 20 | Gorakhpur | 19 |
| 25 | Hamirpur | 11 | 11 | Hamirpur | 7 |
| 26 | Hardoi | 19 | 19 | Hardoi | 19 |
| 27 | Jalaun | 9 | 9 | Jalaun | 9 |
| 28 | Jaunpur | 20 | 20 | Jaunpur | 21 |
| 29 | Jhansi | 8 | 8 | Jhansi | 8 |
| 30 | Kanpur Rural | 17 | 17 | Kanpur Rural | 10 |
| 31 | Kanpur Urban | 3 | 3 | Kanpur Urban | 10 |
| 32 | Lakhimpur | 15 | 15 | Lakhimpur | 15 |
| 33 | Lalitpur | 7 | 7 | Lalitpur | 6 |
| 34 | Lucknow | 8 | 8 | Lucknow | 8 |

*Contd...*

*Contd...*

| S. no. | Districts surveyed in NIN according to 1991 census | No. of blocks | | Districts to be covered in the present project | Current no. of blocks |
|---|---|---|---|---|---|
| | **Old districts** | **Total** | **Surveyed in NIN, IASDS study** | | |
| 35 | Maharajganj | 13 | 13 | Maharajganj | 12 |
| 36 | Mainpuri | 9 | 9 | Mainpuri | 9 |
| 37 | Mathura | 12 | 12 | Mathura | 10 |
| 38 | Maunathbhanjan | 9 | 9 | Maunathbhanjan | 9 |
| 39 | Meerut | 18 | 18 | Meerut | 12 |
| 40 | Mirzapur | 12 | 12 | Mirzapur | 12 |
| 41 | Moradabad | 19 | 19 | Moradabad | 13 |
| 42 | Muzaffarnagar | 14 | 14 | Muzaffarnagar | 14 |
| 43 | Pilibhit | 7 | 7 | Pilibhit | 7 |
| 44 | Prathapgarh | 15 | 15 | Prathapgarh | 17 |
| 45 | Rae Bareli | 19 | 19 | Rae Bareli | 21 |
| 46 | Rampur | 6 | 6 | Rampur | 6 |
| 47 | Saharanpur | 11 | 11 | Saharanpur | 11 |
| 48 | Shahjahanpur | 14 | 14 | Shahjahanpur | 15 |
| 49 | Sidharthnagar | 14 | 15 | Sidharthnagar | 14 |
| 50 | Sitapur | 19 | 19 | Sitapur | 19 |
| 51 | Sonbhadra | 8 | 8 | Sonbhadra | 8 |
| 52 | Sultanpur | 22 | 20 | Sultanpur | 23 |
| 53 | Unnao | 16 | 12 | Unnao | 16 |
| 54 | Varanasi | 20 | 20 | Varanasi | 8 |
| | | | | **New Districts** | |
| 55 | | | | Ambedkarnagar | |
| 56 | | | | Auraiya | |
| 57 | | | | Baghpat | |
| 58 | | | | Balrampur | |
| 59 | | | | Chandauli | |
| 60 | | | | Chitrakut | |
| 61 | | | | Gautam Budh Nagar | |
| 62 | | | | Hathras | |
| 63 | | | | Jyotiba Phule Nagar | |
| 64 | | | | Kannauj | |
| 65 | | | | Kaushambi | |
| 66 | | | | Kushinagar | |
| 67 | | | | Mahoba | |
| 68 | | | | Sant Kabir Nagar | |
| 69 | | | | Sant Ravidas Nagar | |
| 70 | | | | Shravasti | |

**Table (ii)** Blocks coverage under NIN-IASDS (2002) and new districts

| District Covered Under Nin-lasds (2002) | Block Covered Under Nin-lasds (2002) | New District Other Than Nin-lasds (2002) | Block Under New District |
|---|---|---|---|
| Moradabad | Thakurdwara | Jyotiba Phule Nagar | Amroha |
| | Dilari | | Hasanpur |
| | Amroha | | Gajraula |
| | Chhajlet | | Dhanaura |
| | Joya | | Joya |
| | Dhanaura | | Gangeshwari |
| | Gajraula | | |
| | Hasanpur | | |
| | Gangeshwari | | |
| | Asmauli | | |
| | Sambhal | | |
| | Panwasa | | |
| | Bhagatpur Tanda | | |
| | Moradabad | | |
| | Munda Pandey | | |
| | Dingarpur | | |
| | Baniyakhera | | |
| | Bilari | | |
| | Behjaoi | | |
| Farrukhabad | Barahpur | Kannauj | Chhibramau |
| | Kamalganj | | Saurikh |
| | Mohamdabad | | Hasheran |
| | Kayamganj | | Mugrapur |
| | Nawabganj | | Jalabad |
| | Shamsabad | | Kannauj |
| | Rajepur | | Umarda |
| | Chhibramau | | Talgaon |
| | Saurikh | | |
| | Hasheran | | |
| | Mugrapur | | |
| | Jalabad | | |
| | Kannauj | | |
| | Umarda | | |
| | Talgaon | | |

*Contd...*

*Contd...*

| District Covered Under Nin-lasds (2002) | Block Covered Under Nin-lasds (2002) | New District Other Than Nin-lasds (2002) | Block Under New District |
|---|---|---|---|
| Hamirpur | Kurara | Mahoba | Panwari |
| | Sumairpur | | Jaitpur |
| | Sarila | | Charkhari |
| | Gohand | | Kabrai |
| | Raat | | |
| | Muscara | | |
| | Modha | | |
| | Panwari | | |
| | Jaitpur | | |
| | Charkhari | | |
| | Kabrai | | |
| Varanasi | Badagaon | Chandauli | Barahani |
| | Pindra | | Chahania |
| | Cholapur | | Chakia |
| | Chiraigaon | | Chandali |
| | Harhua | | Sakaldeeha |
| | Sevapuri | | Sahabganj |
| | Araziline | | Nayamtabad |
| | Kashi Vidyapeeth | | Dhanepur |
| | Barahani | | Naogarh |
| | Chahania | | |
| | Chakia | | |
| | Chandali | | |
| | Sakaldeeha | | |
| | Sahabganj | | |
| | Nayamtabad | | |
| | Dhanepur | | |
| | Naogarh | | |
| Gonda | Rupaidiha | Balrampur | Haraiya Satgarhwa |
| | Itia Thok | | Balrampur |
| | Pandri Kirpal | | Tulsipur |
| | Jhanjhari | | Gaisadi |
| | Mujehna | | Panchpedwa |
| | Katra Bazaar | | Sriduttganj |
| | Haldharmau | | Utraula |

*Contd...*

*Contd...*

| District Covered Under Nin-lasds (2002) | Block Covered Under Nin-lasds (2002) | New District Other Than Nin-lasds (2002) | Block Under New District |
|---|---|---|---|
| | Paraspur | | Gaidas Buzurg |
| | Belsar | | Rehra Bazaar |
| | Tarehganj | | |
| | Wazirganj | | |
| | Nawabganj | | |
| | Mankapur | | |
| | Babhanjot | | |
| | Chhapiya | | |
| | Karnailganj | | |
| | Haraiya Satgarhwa | | |
| | Balrampur | | |
| | Tulsipur | | |
| | Gaisari | | |
| | Panchpedwa | | |
| | Sriduttganj | | |
| | Utraula | | |
| | Gaidas Buzurg | | |
| | Rehra Bazaar | | |
| Aligarh | Tappal | | |
| | Chandaus | | |
| | Khair | | |
| | Jawan | | |
| | Lodha | | |
| | Dhanipur | | |
| | Gonda | | |
| | Iglas | | |
| | Atrauli | | |
| | Bijauli | | |
| | Gangiri | | |
| | Akrabad | | |
| | Hathras | Hathras | Hathras |
| | Sikandrarau | | Sikandrarau |
| | Sasni | | Sasni |
| | Hasayan | | Hasayan |
| | Mursan | | Mursan |

*Contd...*

*Contd...*

| District Covered Under Nin-lasds (2002) | Block Covered Under Nin-lasds (2002) | New District Other Than Nin-lasds (2002) | Block Under New District |
|---|---|---|---|
| Mathura | Nandgaon | | Sahpau |
| | Chhata | | Sadabad |
| | Chaumuha | | |
| | Govardhan | | |
| | Mathura | | |
| | Farah | | |
| | Nohjhil | | |
| | Mat | | |
| | Raya | | |
| | Baldeo | | |
| | Sahpau | | |
| | Sadabad | | |
| Meerut | Chhaprauli | Baghpat | Chhaprauli |
| | Baraut | | Barrot |
| | Baghpat | | Baghpat |
| | Pilana | | Pilana |
| | Khekra | | Khekra |
| | Binauli | | Binauli |
| | Sarurpur Khurd | | |
| | Sardhana | | |
| | Daurala | | |
| | Mawana Kalan | | |
| | Hastinapur | | |
| | Parikshitgarh | | |
| | Machra | | |
| | Rohta | | |
| | Janikhurd | | |
| | Meerut | | |
| | Rajpura | | |
| | Kharkhoda | | |
| Faizabad | Suhawal | Ambedkar Nagar | Bhiti |
| | Masodha | | Katehri |
| | Pura Bazaar | | Akabarpur |
| | Maya Bazaar | | Tanda |
| | Amani Ganj | | Baskhari |

*Contd...*

*Contd...*

| District Covered Under Nin-lasds (2002) | Block Covered Under Nin-lasds (2002) | New District Other Than Nin-lasds (2002) | Block Under New District |
|---|---|---|---|
| | Milkipur | | Ramnagr |
| | Haringtan Ganj | | Jahangir Ganj |
| | Bikapur | | Jalalpur |
| | Tarun | | Bhiyawan |
| | Bhiti | | |
| | Katehari | | |
| | Akabarpur | | |
| | Tanda | | |
| | Baskhari | | |
| | Ramnagr | | |
| | Jahangir Ganj | | |
| | Jalalpur | | |
| | Bhiyaon | | |

## (ii) Methodology for SAE

### Direct estimator

Let there be D districts (in this case D = 33)

Let $Y_d$ be the proportion of persons in a district with BMI < 18.5; d = 1,2,…,D. An estimator of $Y_d$ is denoted by $Y_d$ where

$$y_d = \frac{n_{1d}}{n_d};$$

$n_{1d}$ = Number of persons in the sample in the d-th district having BMI<18.5

$n_d$ = Sample size in the d-th district

Assuming that the sample of size $n_d$ is selected by simple random sampling with replacement (srswr), then

$$SE(y_d) = \sqrt{\frac{y_d(1-y_d)}{n_d}}$$

### Small area estimation

For the purpose of using small area estimation technique, the approach used was one of mixed models involving random area-specific effects. The 'area level random effects model' is due to Fay and Herriot (1979) and has two components.

(i) The direct survey estimate of the parameter based on sampling design is expressed as

$$y_d = Y_d + e_d, \ d = 1, ..., D \quad (1)$$

where ,

D = Total number of small areas (in our case D = 33, number of districts) that constitute the finite population

$Y_d$ = Parameter of interest

$y_d$ = Observed direct survey estimators (in our case proportion of persons having BMI < 18.5)

$e_d$ = Independent sampling errors of survey estimate with $E(e_d/y_d) = 0$ $V(e_d/y_d) = vd$

(1) is a sampling model and vd is sampling variance.

(ii) The second component is a linking model

$$Y_d = z'_d\beta + u_d,\ d = 1, ..., D \tag{2}$$

where

$z_d$ = p – vector of district level covariates

$\beta$ = p – vector of unknown fixed-effects coefficients

$u_d$ = model errors assumed to be independent and identically distributed with E $(u_d) = 0$ and V $(u_d) = \sigma_u^2$

Combining (1) and (2) we get

$$Y_d = z'_d\beta + u_d + u_d,\ d = 1, ..., D \tag{3}$$

Model (3) is a special case linear mixed model with $u_d$ and $e_d$ as independent random errors. For known variance $\sigma_u^2$ and assuming (3) holds, the Best Linear Unbiased Predictor for $Y_d$ (Henderson 1963) is given by

$$\tilde{y}_d = z'_d\hat{\beta}_{GLS} + \gamma_d(y_d - z'_d\hat{\beta}_{GLS}) = \gamma_d y_d + (1-\gamma_d)z'_d\hat{\beta}_{GLS} \tag{4}$$

Where $\gamma_d = \sigma_u^2/(v_d + \sigma_u^2)$ and $\hat{\beta}_{GLS} = \left(\sum_d (v_d + \sigma_u^2)^{-1} z_d z_d'\right)^{-1}\left(\sum_d (v_d + \sigma_u^2)^{-1} z_d y_d\right)$; $\hat{\beta}_{GLS}$ being generalised least square estimate of $\beta$. Usually $\sigma_u^2$ is unkown and these are replaced by sample esimates in (4) and $\hat{\beta}_{GLS}$. This gives rise to empirical BLUP (EBLUP) denoted by $\hat{y}_d$.

Prasad and Rao (1990) gave approximate true prediction MSE of the EBLUP under normality of two errors and for the case where $\sigma_u^2$ is estimated by the ANOVA (fitting of constants) method as

$$MSE\left(\hat{y}_d\left(\hat{\sigma}_u^2, \hat{\beta}_{GLS}\right)\right) = g_{id} + g_{2d} + g_{3d} \tag{5}$$

Where

$$g_{1d} = \gamma_d v_d = Var\left[\tilde{y}_d\left(\sigma_u^2\right)\right]$$

$$g_{2d} = (1-\gamma_d)^2 z'_d Var\left(\hat{\beta}_{GLS}\right) z_d,\ \text{with}\ Var\left(\hat{\beta}_{GLS}\right) = \left(\Sigma_d\left(v_d + \sigma_u^2\right)^{-1} z'_d z'\right)^{-1}$$

is in exess in MSE due to estimation of $\beta$.

$g_{3d} = \left[ v_d^2 / \left( v_d + \sigma_u^2 \right)^3 \right] \times \text{Var}\left(\sigma_u^2\right)$ is the excess in estimation of $\sigma_u^2$. Prasad and Rao (1990) derived a MSE estimator of (5) with bias of order (1/D) as,

$$\text{mse}\left[ \hat{y}_d\left(\hat{\sigma}_u^2, \hat{b}_{GLS}\right)\right] = g_{1d}\left(\hat{\sigma}_u^2\right) + g_{2d}\left(\hat{\sigma}_u^2\right) + 2g_{3d}\left(\hat{\sigma}_u^2\right) \quad (6)$$

Where $g_{kd}\left(\hat{\sigma}_u^2\right)$ is obtained from $g_{kd}$ by substituting for $\hat{\sigma}_u^2$ for $\sigma_u^2$, for $k = 1,2,3$.

# References


Abul-Ela, Abdel-Latif A, Greenberg BG, and Horvitz DG (1967). A multi-proportions RR model. *Journal of American Statistical Association,* 62, 990–1008.

AbouZahr C and Wardlaw T (2004). Maternal Mortality in 2000: *Estimates developed by WHO, UNICEF and UNFPA, WHO, Geneva.*

AbouZahr C, Wardlaw T and Hill K (2001). Maternal mortality in 1995: *Estimates developed by WHO, UNICEF and UNFPA, WHO, Geneva.*

ACC/SCN (2004). *Fifth Report on the World Nutrition Situation. Geneva.*

Adhikari T, Vir S, Yadav RJ, Pandey A (2015). Undernutrition among children under-two years in India: An examination of determinants, *Journal of Statistics and Applications.* Special Issue on statistical concerns in child health and nutrition, Volume 13, Nos. 1&2, (New Series), 25–38.

Andrew OT, Schoenfield PY, Hopewell PC, Humphries MH (1980). Tuberculosis in patients with end stage renal disease. *American Journal of Medicine,* 68, 59–65.

Andrews KM, Brouillette DB and Brouillette RT (2008). Mortality, infant. *Encyclopedia of Infant and Early Childhood Development.* Elsevier, 343–59.

Angeles AI, Schultink W, Sastramidjojo S, Grass R, Karyadi D (1997). Weekly iron supplementation build iron stores in female Indonesian adolescents. *American Journal of Clinical Nutrition,* 66, 177–83.

Annual Health Survey Bulletin (2011–12). India.

Annual Health Survey Bulletin (2011–12). Uttar Pradesh, India.

Annual Health Survey Bulletin (2012–13). Uttar Pradesh, India.

Antunes JLF and Waldman EA. (2001). Impact of AIDS, immigration, and housing overcrowding on tuberculosis deaths in São Paulo, Brazil, 1994–1998. *Social Science Medicine,* 52, 1071–80.

Assessment of maternal and infant survival in Madhya Pradesh (2005). *Project report* of Institute of Applied Statistics and Development Studies for CARE India.

Bang AT et al. (1999). Effect of home-based neonatal care and management of sepsis on neonatal mortality. *Lancet,* 354, 1955–61.

Baseline survey of impact assessment of ICDS food fortification in district Kanpur Dehat (2002). *Project report* of Institute for Research in Medical Statistics and Institute of Applied Statistics and Development Studies for World Food Program.

Baseline survey of impact assessment of ICDS food fortification in district Kanpur Dehat (2003). *Project report* of Institute for Research in Medical Statistics and Institute of Applied Statistics and Development Studies for World Food Program.

Baseline survey of impact assessment of ICDS food fortification in Dehradun district (2003). *Project report* of Institute for Research in Medical Statistics and Institute of Applied Statistics and Development Studies for World Food Program.

Baseline survey of impact assessment of ICDS food fortification in Nahan district (2004). *Project report* of Institute for Research in Medical Statistics and Institute of Applied Statistics and Development Studies for World Food Program.

Baseline survey of impact assessments of nutrition interventions through food for education in Madhya Pradesh, Uttarakhand & Chhattisgarh (2004). *Project reports* of Institute of Applied Statistics and Development Studies for United Nations World Food Program.

Beaton G and McGabe G (1999). Efficacy of intermittent iron supplementation in the control of iron deficiency anemia in developing countries. *The Micronutrient Initiative, Ottawa, Canada.*

Belcon MC, Smith EKM, Kahana LM, Shimuzu AG (1982). Tuberculosis in dialysis patients. *Clinical Nephrology,* 17, 14–18.

Bifani PJ, Mathema B, Liu Z, Moghazeh SL, Shopsin B, Tempalski B, et al. (1999). Identification of a W-variant outbreak of mycobacterium tuberculosis via population based molecular epidemiology. *Journal of American Medical Association,* 282, 2321–27.

Bisai S, Sen A, Mahalanabis D, Datta N and Bose K (2006). The effect of maternal age and parity on birthweight among Bengalese of Kolkata, India. *Human Ecology,* 14, 139–43.

Bishai D, Opuni M and Poon A (2007). Does the level of infant mortality affect the rate of decline? Time series data from 21 countries. *Economics and Human Biology,* 5 (1): 74–81.

Bishai WR, Graham NMH, Harrington S, Pope DS, Hooper N, Astemborski J, et al. (1998). Molecular and geographic patterns of tuberculosis transmission after 15 years of directly observed therapy. *Journal of American Medical Association,* 280, 1679–84.

Carlough (2005). IJGO.

Census of India (2001).

Census of India (2011).

Chadha VK, Vaidyanathan PS, Jagannatha PS, Unnikrishnan KP, Mini PA (2002). Annual risk of tuberculosis infection in the northern zone of India. *Bulletin of World Health Organization* 81, 572–81.

Chadha VK, Vaidyanathan PS, Jagannatha PS, Unnikrishnan KP, Savanur SJ, Mini PA (2003). Annual risk of tuberculosis infection in the western zone of India. *International Journal of Tuberculosis Lung Disease,* 7, 536–42.

Chadha VK, Kumar P, Gupta J, Jagannatha PS, Magesh V, Singh S, Lakshminarayan, Ahmed J, Srivastava RK, Prasad N, Vaidyanathan PS (2004). Annual risk of tuberculosis infection in the eastern zone of India. *International Journal of Tuberculosis Lung Disease,* 8, 537–44.

Chaput EK, Meek JI, Heimer R (2002). Spatial analysis of human granulocytic ehrlichiosis near Lyme, Connecticut. *Emerging Infectious Diseases,* 943–48.

Chaudhuri A and Mukerjee R (1988). *Randomized response: theory and techniques, Marcel Dekker, New York.*

Child Sex Ratio in India, Census (2011).

Clasen et al. (2006). Interventions to improve water quality for preventing diarrhea. (A Cochrane Review). *In: The Cochrane Library, Issue 3, 2006. Oxford: Update Software.*

Cochran WG (1963). Sampling Techniques, *John Wiley, New York.*

Cochran WG (1977). Sampling Techniques, *John Wiley, New York.*

Comstock GW, Livesay VT and Woolpert SF (1974). The prognosis of a positive tuberculin reaction in childhood and adolescence. *American Journal of Epidemiology,* 99, 131–38.

Cornell JA (2002). Experiments with Mixtures, Design, Models and Analysis of Mixture Data, *John Wiley, New York.*

Cousens S, Smith PG, Ward H, Everington D, Knight RSG (2001). Geographical distribution of variant Creutzfeldt-Jakob disease in Great Britain, 1994–2000. *Lancet.* 357: 1002–07.

Curtis A (1999). Using a spatial filter and a geographic information system to improve rabies surveillance data. *Emerging Infectious Diseases,* 603–06.

Curtis and Cairncross (2003). Effect of washing hands with soap on diarrhea risk in the community: A systematic review. *Lancet,* 3, 275–81.

Data validation and coverage evaluation survey for vitamin A coverage for BSPM round in two urban cities Agra and Meerut in Uttar Pradesh (2014-15). *Project report* of Institute of Applied Statistics and Development Studies for Micronutrient Initiative.

Dwass M (1957). Modified randomization tests for non-parametric hypothesis. *Annals of Mathematical Statistics,* 28, 181–87.

Establishing adolescent friendly health services at Safdarjung hospital; end of term report (2005). *Safdarjung Hospital Adolescent Healthcare Network.* New Delhi, 2005.

Fact Sheet Jharkhand (2005-06). NFHS-3 Provisional Data: Government of India.

FANTA (Food and Nutrition Technical Assistance Project) I, II, III (2002-2017) supported by USAID.

FAST (Food Access Survey Tools), Bangladesh (2003). Measuring food insecurity: Going beyond indicators of income and anthropometry.

Fay RE and Herriot RA (1979). Estimates of income for small places: an application of James-Stein procedures to census data. *Journal of American Statistical Association,* 74, 269–77.

Fewtrell et al. (2005). Water, sanitation, and hygiene interventions to reduce diarrhea in less developed countries. A systematic review and meta-analysis. *Lancet: Infectious Diseases* 5(1), 42–52.

Food insecurity atlas of rural Uttar Pradesh using small area estimates (2010). *Project report* of Institute of Applied Statistics and Development Studies for Central Statistical Office.

Gender bias in intra household food consumption: dietary intakes and patterns (2006). *Project report* of Institute of Applied Statistics & Development Studies for Indian Council of Medical Research.

Gender inequality in intra-houschold consumption expenditure. Development of methodology in Eastern Uttar Pradesh (2003). *Project report* of Institute of Applied Statistics & Development Studies for Central Statistical Office, New Delhi.

Gerty JLM, Levenselt-Mulders, Hox JJ and Peter GM Van Der Heijden (2005). How to improve randomized response design. *Quality and Quantity,* 39, 253–65.

Ginsberg J, Mohebbi MH, Patel RS, Brammer L, Smolinski MS and Brilliant L (2009). Detecting influenza epidemics using search engine query data, *Nature,* 457, 19.

Gomez F, Rammos-Galvan R, et al. (1956). Mortality in second and third degree undernutrition. *Journal of Tropical Pediatrics,* 2, 77–83.

Government of India (2005). Guidelines for antenatal care and skilled birth attendance at birth by ANMs and LHVs.

Government of India (2006). Implementation guide on RCH-II adolescent reproductive sexual health strategy.

Graham W, Brass W and Snow RW (1989). Indirect estimation of maternal mortality: the sisterhood method. *Studies in Family Planning,* 20,125–35.

Graham WJ, Filippi VG and Ronsmans C (1996). Demonstrating programme impact on maternal mortality. *Health Policy and Planning,* 11, 16–20.

Graham W, Bell JS, and Bullough CHW (2001). Can skilled attendance at delivery reduce maternal mortality in developing countries? *Studies in HSO&P.* 17, 97–129.

Green C, Hoppa RD, Young TK, Blanchard JF (2003). Geographic analysis of diabetes prevalence in an urban area. *Journal of Social Science and Medicine,* 57: 551–60.

Greenberg B, Abdul-Ela A, Simmons W and Horvitz D (1969). The unrelated question randomized response model: theoretical framework. *Journal of the American Statistical Association,* 64, 520–39.

Gross R, Angeles-Agdeppa I, Schutlink W, Dillon D, Sastroamidjojo S (1997). Daily versus weekly iron supplementation: programmatic and economic implications for Indonesia. *Food & Nutrition Bulletin,* 18, 64–70.

Gupta SD (2003). Adolescent reproductive health in India: status, policies, programs, and issues. *Futures Group International Policy, USAID;* Washington, DC.

Henderson CR (1963). Selection index and expected genetic advance, in *Statistical Genetics and Plant Breeding,* eds. W.D. Hanson and HF Robinson, *National Academic of Sciences- National Research Council,* Washington, DC, 141–63.

Household survey for the assessment of nutrition and education status (2012). *Project report* of Institute of Applied Statistics and Development Studies for Welthungehilfe for its 'fight hunger first' initiative.

Impact assessments of ICDS food fortification in Madhya Pradesh, Uttar Pradesh and Uttarakhand (2005). *Project reports* of Institute for Research in Medical Statistics and Institute of Applied Statistics and Development Studies for World Food Program.

Impact assessments of nutrition interventions through food for education in Madhya Pradesh, Uttarakhand & Chhattisgarh (2005). *Project reports* of Institute of Applied Statistics and Development Studies for United Nations World Food Program.

Indian Council of Medical Research (1981). *Recommended dietary intakes for Indians.*

Indian Council of Medical Research (1990). *Nutrient requirement and recommended dietary allowances for Indians,* Report of the Expert Group.

International Institute for Population Sciences (IIPS) and ORC Macro. *National Family Health Survey (NFHS)-1,* 1992–93, India.

International Institute for Population Sciences (IIPS) and ORC Macro. 2000. *National Family Health Survey (NFHS)-2,* 1998–99, India.

International Institute for Population Sciences (IIPS) and ORC Macro. 2000. *National Family Health Survey (NFHS)-3*, 2005–06, India.

International Institute for Population Sciences. *District Level Household and Facility Survey (DLHS-3),* 2007–08: India.

James WP, Ferro-Luzi Anna and Waterlow JC (1988). Definition of chronic energy deficiency in adults. Report of a working party of the International Dietary Energy Consultative Group. *European Journal of Clinical Nutrition,* 42(12): 969–81.

Jejeebhoy SJ and Santhya KG (2011). Sexual and reproductive health of young people in India: A review of policies, laws and programmes, *Population Council, India.*

Jolliffe IT (2002). *Principal Component Analysis,* Springer Series.

Kanani SJ and Poojara RH (2000). Supplementation with iron and folic acid enhances growth in adolescent Indian girls. *Journal of Nutrition.* 130: 452–55.

Kish Leslie (1965). Survey sampling, *John Wiley, New York.*

Kochupillai N (1986). Iodised injections in Goiter prophylaxis: possible impact on the newborn. *Nutrition Foundation of India Bulletin.*

Kolappan C, Gopi PG, Subramani R, Chadha VK, Kumar P, Prasad VV, Appegowda BN, Rao RSN, Shashidharan N, Ganesan N, Santha T and Narayanan PR (2004). Estimation of annual risk of tuberculosis infection among children aged one to nine years in the south zone of India. *International Journal of Tuberculosis and Lung Diseases,* 8, 418–23.

Kulkarni PM (2007). Estimation of missing girls at birth and juvenile ages in India, Paper prepared for United Nations Population Fund and also presented *at the XXIX the Annual Conference of the Indian Association for the Study of Population,* Banaras Hindu University, Banaras, India.

Kulldorff M (1997). A spatial scan statistic. *Communications in Statistics: Theory and Methods,* 26, 1481–96.

Kulldorff M (2006). Information Management Services, Inc. *SaTScan$^{TM}$ v6.1 Software for the spatial and space-time scan statistics.*

Kulldorff M, Athas WF, Feuer EJ, Miller BA and Key CR (1998). Evaluating cluster alarms: A space-time scan statistic and brain cancer in Los Alamos, New Mexico. *American Journal of Public Health,* 88, 1377–80.

Kumar V, Mohanty S, Kumar A, et al. (2008). Effect of community-based behavior change management on neonatal mortality in Shivgarh, Uttar Pradesh, India: A cluster randomized controlled trial. *Lancet,* 372, 1151–62.

Lamba R, Misra SK and Rana R (2014). A study on the effect of iron folic acid supplementation and deworming among college going adolescent girls in urban Agra. *Indian Journal of Community Health* 26 (2).

Lawless HT and Heymann H (2010). Sensory evaluation of food. *Springer Series.*

Luby et al. (2011). The Effect of hand washing at recommended times with water alone and with soap on child diarrhea in rural Bangladesh: an observational study. *PLOS Medicine,* 8(6).

Lynch SR (2000). The potential impact of iron supplementation during adolescence on iron status in pregnancy. *Journal of Nutrition,* 130 (Supplement), 452–55.

MacDorman MF and Mathews TJ (2009). The challenge of infant mortality: have we reached a plateau? *Public Health Reports,* 124 (5): 670–81.

Mari Bhat PN (2002). Maternal mortality in India: an update. *Studies in Family Planning,* 33, 227–36.

Mari Bhat PN, Navaneethan K and Rajan SI. (1995). Maternal mortality in India: estimates from a regression Model" *Studies in Family Planning,* 26(4): 217–32.

Freeman MC, Stocks ME, Cumming O, Jeandron A, et al. (2014). Systematic review: hygiene and health: systematic review of hand washing practices worldwide and update of health effects. *Tropical Medicine & International Health.* 19, 906–16.

McIntyre P (2003). Adolescent friendly health services: an agenda for change. *World Health Organization;* Geneva.

Michelozzi P, Capon A, Kirchmayer U, Forastiere F, Biggeri A., et al. (2002). Adult and childhood leukemia near a high power radio station in Rome, Italy. *American Journal of Epidemiology,* 155, 1096–103.

Mid-term assessment of communication initiative for ARSH in Bihar and Jharkhand (2006), *Project Report* of Institute of Applied Statistics and Development Studies for National Foundation of India.

Mishra S, Pandey CM, Chaubey YP and Singh U (2015). Determinants of child malnutrition in empowered action group (EAG) states of India, *Journal of Statistics and Applications.* Special Issue on statistical concerns in child health and nutrition, Volume 13, Nos. 1&2, (New Series), 1–10.

MS Swaminathan Research Foundation (2001). *Food insecurity atlas of rural India.* World Food Program, India.

MS Swaminathan Research Foundation (2002). *Food insecurity atlas of urban India.* World Food Program, India.

MS Swaminathan Research Foundation (2004). *Atlas of the sustainability of food security in India.* World Food Program, India.

Nair MKC (2004). Adolescent sexual and reproductive health. *Indian Pediatrics,* 41(1), 7–13.

Narayanan S, Das S, Garg R, Hari L, Rao VB, Frieden TR, Narayanan PR (2002). Molecular epidemiology of tuberculosis in a rural area of high prevalence in South India: Implications for disease control and prevention. *Journal of Clinical Microbiology,* 40, 4785–88.

National Institute of Nutrition (1999). *Nutritive value of Indian foods.*

Nigam AK (2001). Analysis of undernutrition data - revisited. *Invited talk at the International Conference on Statistics, Combinatorics and Related Areas* held at Wollongong, Australia.

Nigam AK (2003). Determining grades of undernutrition in children: standard deviation classification and alternative. *Demography India,* 32, 137–55.

Nigam AK (2004). Strengthening of NNMB surveys. *Biostatistical aspects of health and population,* edited by Arvind Pandey, 155–60.

Nigam AK (2005). Managing severely undernourished children: clue from analysis of nutrition survey data. *Demography India,* 34, 53–61.

Nigam AK (2008). Large scale surveys on nutrition in India: an appraisal. *Demography India,* Supplement, 129–34.

Nigam AK, Singh, MK, Saxena R, Tewari PP and Shukla S (2010). Intra-household gender inequality in food intakes and efficacy of food intakes and patterns. *Indian Journal of Nutrition and Dietetics,* March issue.

Nigam AK and Singh P (2011). Research methods in public health nutrition: common critical factors, Chapter 11 in the book – Public Health Nutrition in Developing Countries. *Edited by Sheila Vir. WPI Publication.*

Nigam AK, Singh MK, Tiwari PP, Saxena R and Shukla S (2013). Alternative method for analyzing multiple overlapping responses, *International NGO Journal,* Vol 8.

Nigam AK, Srivastava R, Tiwari PP, Saxena R and Shukla S (2014). District level food insecurity atlas of rural Uttar Pradesh, *Journal of Indian Society of Agricultural Statistics,* 68(3), 417–27.

Nunes C (2007). Tuberculosis incidence in Portugal: spatiotemporal clustering. *International Journal of Health Geographics,* 6, 30.

Nutritional status of women and children in Uttar Pradesh. (1995). *Project report* by Institute of Applied Statistics and Development Studies for UNICEF.

Nutritional status of women and children in Uttar Pradesh. (1999). *Publication of* Department of Women and Child Development, Government of Uttar Pradesh and UNICEF.

Nutrition Profile of Community in Uttar Pradesh (2002). *District level reports* of National Institute of Nutrition and Institute of Applied Statistics and Development Studies for Department of Women and Child Development/Food and Nutrition Board, Government of India.

Nutrition Sub-Committee of the Indian Academy of Pediatrics (1972). Report. *Indian Pediatrics,* 9, 60.

Odoi A, Martin SW, Michel P, Middleton D, Holt J, Wilson J (2004). Investigation of clusters of giardiasis using GIS and spatial scan statistic. *International Journal of Health Geographics,* 3:11.

Operations research protocol for field-testing of select maternal and newborn health interventions on Skilled Birth Attendance (SBA) in Dumka district, Jharkhand: *CEDPA/India.*

Opsahl R, Riddervold HO, Wessel AT (1961). Pulmonary tuberculosis in mitral stenosis and diabetes mellitus. *Acta Tuberculosis Scandevia,* 40, 290–96.

Office of Registrar General, Government of India (2012). *India SRS Statistical Report.*

Office of Registrar General, Government of India. (2013). A presentation on maternal mortality levels (2010–12).

Osel JD (2008). "Being (born) black in America: perceived discrimination & African-American infant mortality". *SSRN Electronic Journal.*

Pal M, Bharati P, Vasulu TS, Chaudhuri A, Bhattacharya BN, Das RN and Ghosh R (2002). "Maternal Mortality in Rural North 24-Praganas, West Bengal: Estimation of its rate and Identifications of underlying Causes" *Demography India* 31(2): 253–58.

Panda M (2015). Nutritional and food security in India, *Dr. Rajendra Prasad Memorial Lecture,* Indian Society of Agricultural Statistics, New Delhi.

Pandav CS, Yadav K, Srivastava R, Pandav R and Karmarkar MG (2013). Iodine deficiency disorders (IDD) control in India. *Indian Journal of Medicinal Research,* 138(3): 418–33.

Pandey RM (2009). Approaches to sample size calculation in comparative studies. *Indian Journal of Pediatrics,* 66 (4), 533–38.

Pandey RS and Vir S (2011). Essential new-born care and child survival. Chapter 6 in the book – Public Health Nutrition in Developing Countries. Edited by Sheila Vir. *WPI Publication.*

Paul R (1961). Silicisis in northern Rhodesia copper miners. *Archives of Environmental Health,* 2, 96–109.

Sorcar P (2010). A new approach to global HIV/AIDS education. *The Huffington Post.*

Prasad NGN and Rao JNK (1990). The estimation of the mean squared error of small area estimators. *Journal of the American Statistical Association,* 85, 163–71.

Promoting adolescent reproductive health in Uttarakhand and Uttar Pradesh, (2012). *IFPS Technical Assistance Project,* Futures Group, India.

Rajaretnam T and Jyoti S (2000). Determinants of nutritional status of young children in India: an analysis of 1992-93 NFHS data. *Demography India,* 126.

Rao JNK (2003). Small Area Estimation. *John Wiley & Sons,* New Jersey.

Report on estimates of maternal mortality in five States of India (2002). Institute for Research in Medical Statistics *(Indian Council of Medical Research)*. 33.

Sabel CE, Boyle PJ, Loytonen M, Gatrell AC and Jokelainen M (2003). Spatial clustering of amyotrophic lateral sclerosis in Finland at place of birth and place of death. *American Journal of Epidemiology,* 157: 898–905.

Sachan B, Idris MZ, Jain S, Kumari R and Singh A (2012). Age at menarche and menstrual problems among school-going adolescent girls of a North Indian district. *Journal of Basic Clinical Reproductive Science.* 1, 56–59.

Sample Registration System (2006).

Sample Registration System (2013). SRS Statistical Report 2012.

Save the children (2001).

Sari Locker (2001). The real dirt on everything from sex to school. *HarperCollins:* New York.

Sari M, S de Pee, Martini E, Herman S, Sugiatmi, Bloem MW, et al. (2001). Estimating the prevalence of anemia: a comparison of three methods. *Bulletin of the World Health Organization* 79(6), 506–11.

Schutlink W (1996). Iron supplementation programs: compliance of target groups and frequency of tablet intake. *Food & Nutrition Bulletin,* 17, 22–26.

Sen A (2001). Many faces of gender inequality. (2001). *Frontline,* 18(22), 1–17.

Sen A and Kanani SJ (2006). Deleterious functional impact of anemia on young adolescent school girls. *Indian Pediatrics.* 43(3): 219–26.

Sen A and Kanani SJ (2012). Intermittent iron folate supplementation: impact on hematinic status and growth of school girls. *ISRN Hematology* Volume 2012, Article ID 482153, 6 pages.

Seshadri S (2008). Nutrition survey methodologies with special reference to anemia. *Demography India,* 37 (Supplement), 125–31.

Seshadri S and Gopaldas T (1989). Impact of iron supplementation on cognitive functions in preschool and school-aged children: the Indian experience. *American Journal of Clinical Nutrition,* 50: 675–86.

Shah D and Sachdev HPS (2011). Measuring undernutrition and overnutrition in children. Chapter 5 in the book – Public Health Nutrition in Developing Countries. Edited by Sheila Vir. *WPI Publication.*

Sherif NA (2004). Balanced protein supplementation during pregnancy for the prevention of IUGR in Postgraduate training course in reproductive health 2004 at *Geneva Foundation for Medical Education and Research.*

Singh Padam, Pandey A and Aggarwal A (2007). House-to-house survey vs. snowball technique for capturing maternal deaths in India: A search for a cost-effective method, *Indian Journal of Medical Research,* 125, 550–56.

Singh and Tuteja (2003). Micronutrient Profile of Women and Children in India. *MOST-USAID Publication.*

Situational analysis: anemia and vitamin A deficiency in rural population of Uttar Pradesh (2002). *Project report* by Institute of Applied Statistics and Development Studies and King George Medical University for MOST-USAID.

Snedecor and Cochran (1989). Statistical Methods, *John Wiley, Iowa.*

SRIJAN, a KAPB study (2003). *Project report* by Vastalya for GTZ.

Srivastava VK and Nigam AK (2004) Micronutrient Profile of Women and Children in Uttar Pradesh, India. *MOST-USAID Publication.*

Srivastava VK, Nigam AK and Mishra RP (2015). Diarrhea in rural children – some environmental correlates, *Journal of Statistics and Applications.* Special Issue on statistical concerns in child health and nutrition, Volume 13, Nos. 1&2, (New Series), 59–63.

Srivastava R, Nigam AK and Neelam Singh (2015). Application of randomized response technique in socio-economic surveys. *Journal of Statistics and Applications.* Special Issue on statistical concerns in child health and nutrition, Volume 13, Nos. 1&2, (New Series), 39-47.

Stanton C, Nouureddine A and Kenneth H (2000). An assessment of DHS maternal mortality indicators. *Studies in Family Planning* 3(2).

Status of mid day meal in Madhya Pradesh (2005). *Project report* of Institute of Applied Statistics and Development Studies for United Nations World Food Program.

State level study on status of assessment of child sexual abuse in Uttar Pradesh (2012). *Project report* of Vatsalya with support from Institute of Applied Statistics and Development Studies for PLAN India

Study on child abuse in India (2007). *Ministry of Women and Child Development, Government of India.*

Sudre P, Pfyffer GE, Bodmer T, Prod'hom G, Furrer H, Basetti S, Bernasconi E, et al. (1999). Molecular epidemiology of tuberculosis among HIV-infected persons in Switzerland: A countrywide 9-year cohort study. *Infection,* 27, 323–30.

Targeted intervention among truck operators in Lucknow district to increase the levels of STD/HIV/AIDS information and awareness and distribution of condoms (1997). *Project Report* of Institute of Applied Statistics and Development Studies for World Bank.

Tee ES, Kandial M, Awin N, Chong SM, Satgunasingam N, Kamarudin L, Milani S, Dugdala AE, Viteri F (1999). School administered weekly iron folate supplements improve hemoglobin and ferritin concentration in Malaysian adolescent girls. *American Journal of Clinical Nutrition,* 69, 1249–56.

Thorn PA, Brookes VS, Waterhouse JAH (1956). Peptic ulcer, partial gastrectomy, and pulmonary tuberculosis. *British Medical Journal,* 1, 603–08.

Tiwari N, Adhikari CMS, Tewari A, Kandpal V (2006). Investigation of geo-spatial hotspots for the occurrence of tuberculosis in Almora district, India, using GIS and spatial scan statistic. *International Journal of Health Geographics,* 5, 33.

Tiwari N, Kandpal V, Tewari A, Ram Mohan Rao K and Tolia VS (2010). Investigation of tuberculosis clusters in Dehradun city of India. *Asian Pacific Journal of Tropical Medicine,* 3, 486–90.

Tiwari N, Joshi J and Upreti PK (2012). Investigation of geo-spatial hotspots for the occurrence of tuberculosis. *Lambert Academic Publishing, Germany* (ISBN: 978-3-8484-0806-1).

Tuberculosis in India-a sample survey 1955-58. Special Report, Series No. 34, *Indian Council of Medical Research.*

Tupper KW (2013). Sex, Drugs and the Honour Roll: The Perennial Challenges of Addressing Moral Purity Issues in Schools. *Critical Public Health* 24(2): 115–31.

Turnbull BW, Iwano EJ, Burnett WS, Howe HL, Clark LC (1990). Monitoring for clusters of disease: application to leukemia incidence in upstate New York. *American Journal of Epidemiology,* 132: S136–S143.

Tuteja GS, Singh Padam, Dhillon BS, Saxsena BN, Ahmed FU, Singh RP, P Balendu, Vijayraghvan K, Singh Y, Rauf A, Sarma UC, Gandhi S, Behl L, Mukherjee K, Swami SS, Viu M, Chandra Prakash, Chandrawati, and Mohan Uday (2006). Prevalence of anemia among pregnant women and adolescent girls in 16 districts of India. *Food & Nutrition Bulletin,* 27, no. 4.

UNICEF (2004). State of the World's Children Report.

UNICEF (2010). State of the World's Children Report

UNICEF (2011). State of the World's Children Report.

UNICEF (2012). Progress for Children: a report card on adolescents.

UNICEF and WHO (2010). Implementation completion report (CPL-40560; SCL-4056A), World Bank, 2003.

Viel JF, Arveux P, Baverel J, Cahn JY (2000). Soft-tissue sarcoma and non-Hodgkin's lymphoma clusters around a municipal solid waste incinerator with high dioxin emission levels. *American Journal of Epidemiology,* 152, 13–19.

Vijayaraghavan K (2008). Nutritional deficiency disorders in India—large scale surveys, design and implementation. *Demography India,* 37 (supplement): 111–23.

Vir S (1995). Iodine deficiency in India. *Indian Journal of Public Health,* 39,132–35.

Vir S (2015). Stunting, women's nutrition and South Asia. *Power point presentation.*

Vir S and Nigam AK (2001). Nutritional status of children in Uttar Pradesh. *Nutrition Foundation of India Bulletin, 4–6.*

Vir S, Singh N, Nigam AK and Jain R (2008). Weekly iron and folic acid supplementation with counseling reduces anemia in adolescent girls: a large-scale effectiveness study in Uttar Pradesh, India. *Food & Nutrition Bulletin,* 186–93.

VISTAAR-USAID (2007). Lessons Learned from Facilitating Evidence Reviews. *Technical brief for dissemination.*

VISTAAR-USAID (2012). Improving skilled birth attendance in Jharkhand. *Technical brief for dissemination.*

Warner SL (1965). Randomized response: a survey technique for eliminating evasive answer bias. *Journal of the American Statistical Association* 60, 63–69.

Wikipedia (http://en.wikipedia.org /wiki/Child_sexual_abuse – cite_note-levitan-8).

World Bank (2003). Implementation completion report (CPL-40560; SCL-4056A), 2003.

World Health Organization (1987). Reproductive age mortality surveys.

World Health Organization (1994). Indicators for assessing iodine deficiency disorders and their control through salt iodination, 1–35.

World Health Organization (2004). International classification of diseases, 10th Revision, WHO, *Geneva.*

World Health Organization (2006a). Data limitations in computing MMR.

World Health Organization (2006b). Child growth standards: weight-for-age, length/height-for-age, weight-for-height and BMI-for-age: methods & development, WHO, Geneva. *http://www.who.int/childgrowth/en/-.*

World Health Organization (2007). BMI-for-age (5-19years), WHO, Geneva. *http://www.who.int/entity/growthref/who2007_bmi_for_age/en/-.*

WHO, UNICEF and UNFPA (2003). Maternal mortality in 2000: Estimates developed by AbouZahar C, Wardlaw T (Eds). WHO. *Geneva.*

WHO, UNICEF and UNFPA (2009). Estimates of maternal mortality in 1995. WHO. *Geneva.*

# WHO growth standards tables

(i) z-scores for age, weight, height and BMI for children up to 5 years [*Source:* http://www.who.int/childgrowth/standards/en/]

**Weight-for-age for boys, age in years and months**

| | | Z-scores (weight in kg) | | | | | | |
|---|---|---|---|---|---|---|---|---|
| **Year: Month** | **Month** | **-3 SD** | **-2 SD** | **-1 SD** | **Median** | **1 SD** | **2 SD** | **3 SD** |
| **0: 0** | **0** | 2.1 | 2.5 | 2.9 | 3.3 | 3.9 | 4.4 | 5.0 |
| **0: 1** | **1** | 2.9 | 3.4 | 3.9 | 4.5 | 5.1 | 5.8 | 6.6 |
| **0: 2** | **2** | 3.8 | 4.3 | 4.9 | 5.6 | 6.3 | 7.1 | 8.0 |
| **0: 3** | **3** | 4.4 | 5.0 | 5.7 | 6.4 | 7.2 | 8.0 | 9.0 |
| **0: 4** | **4** | 4.9 | 5.6 | 6.2 | 7.0 | 7.8 | 8.7 | 9.7 |
| **0: 5** | **5** | 5.3 | 6.0 | 6.7 | 7.5 | 8.4 | 9.3 | 10.4 |
| **0: 6** | **6** | 5.7 | 6.4 | 7.1 | 7.9 | 8.8 | 9.8 | 10.9 |
| **0: 7** | **7** | 5.9 | 6.7 | 7.4 | 8.3 | 9.2 | 10.3 | 11.4 |
| **0: 8** | **8** | 6.2 | 6.9 | 7.7 | 8.6 | 9.6 | 10.7 | 11.9 |
| **0: 9** | **9** | 6.4 | 7.1 | 8.0 | 8.9 | 9.9 | 11.0 | 12.3 |
| **0:10** | **10** | 6.6 | 7.4 | 8.2 | 9.2 | 10.2 | 11.4 | 12.7 |
| **0:11** | **11** | 6.8 | 7.6 | 8.4 | 9.4 | 10.5 | 11.7 | 13.0 |
| **1: 0** | **12** | 6.9 | 7.7 | 8.6 | 9.6 | 10.8 | 12.0 | 13.3 |
| **1: 1** | **13** | 7.1 | 7.9 | 8.8 | 9.9 | 11.0 | 12.3 | 13.7 |
| **1: 2** | **14** | 7.2 | 8.1 | 9.0 | 10.1 | 11.3 | 12.6 | 14.0 |
| **1: 3** | **15** | 7.4 | 8.3 | 9.2 | 10.3 | 11.5 | 12.8 | 14.3 |
| **1: 4** | **16** | 7.5 | 8.4 | 9.4 | 10.5 | 11.7 | 13.1 | 14.6 |
| **1: 5** | **17** | 7.7 | 8.6 | 9.6 | 10.7 | 12.0 | 13.4 | 14.9 |
| **1: 6** | **18** | 7.8 | 8.8 | 9.8 | 10.9 | 12.2 | 13.7 | 15.3 |
| **1: 7** | **19** | 8.0 | 8.9 | 10.0 | 11.1 | 12.5 | 13.9 | 15.6 |
| **1: 8** | **20** | 8.1 | 9.1 | 10.1 | 11.3 | 12.7 | 14.2 | 15.9 |
| **1: 9** | **21** | 8.2 | 9.2 | 10.3 | 11.5 | 12.9 | 14.5 | 16.2 |
| **1:10** | **22** | 8.4 | 9.4 | 10.5 | 11.8 | 13.2 | 14.7 | 16.5 |
| **1:11** | **23** | 8.5 | 9.5 | 10.7 | 12.0 | 13.4 | 15.0 | 16.8 |
| **2: 0** | **24** | 8.6 | 9.7 | 10.8 | 12.2 | 13.6 | 15.3 | 17.1 |

**Weight-for-age for boys, age in years and months (continued)**

| | | Z-scores (weight in kg) | | | | | | |
|---|---|---|---|---|---|---|---|---|
| **Year: Month** | **Month** | **-3 SD** | **-2 SD** | **-1 SD** | **Median** | **1 SD** | **2 SD** | **3 SD** |
| 2: 1 | 25 | 8.8 | 9.8 | 11.0 | 12.4 | 13.9 | 15.5 | 17.5 |
| 2: 2 | 26 | 8.9 | 10.0 | 11.2 | 12.5 | 14.1 | 15.8 | 17.8 |
| 2: 3 | 27 | 9.0 | 10.1 | 11.3 | 12.7 | 14.3 | 16.1 | 18.1 |
| 2: 4 | 28 | 9.1 | 10.2 | 11.5 | 12.9 | 14.5 | 16.3 | 18.4 |
| 2: 5 | 29 | 9.2 | 10.4 | 11.7 | 13.1 | 14.8 | 16.6 | 18.7 |
| 2: 6 | 30 | 9.4 | 10.5 | 11.8 | 13.3 | 15.0 | 16.9 | 19.0 |
| 2: 7 | 31 | 9.5 | 10.7 | 12.0 | 13.5 | 15.2 | 17.1 | 19.3 |
| 2: 8 | 32 | 9.6 | 10.8 | 12.1 | 13.7 | 15.4 | 17.4 | 19.6 |
| 2: 9 | 33 | 9.7 | 10.9 | 12.3 | 13.8 | 15.6 | 17.6 | 19.9 |
| 2:10 | 34 | 9.8 | 11.0 | 12.4 | 14.0 | 15.8 | 17.8 | 20.2 |
| 2:11 | 35 | 9.9 | 11.2 | 12.6 | 14.2 | 16.0 | 18.1 | 20.4 |
| 3: 0 | 36 | 10.0 | 11.3 | 12.7 | 14.3 | 16.2 | 18.3 | 20.7 |
| 3: 1 | 37 | 10.1 | 11.4 | 12.9 | 14.5 | 16.4 | 18.6 | 21.0 |
| 3: 2 | 38 | 10.2 | 11.5 | 13.0 | 14.7 | 16.6 | 18.8 | 21.3 |
| 3: 3 | 39 | 10.3 | 11.6 | 13.1 | 14.8 | 16.8 | 19.0 | 21.6 |
| 3: 4 | 40 | 10.4 | 11.8 | 13.3 | 15.0 | 17.0 | 19.3 | 21.9 |
| 3: 5 | 41 | 10.5 | 11.9 | 13.4 | 15.2 | 17.2 | 19.5 | 22.1 |
| 3: 6 | 42 | 10.6 | 12.0 | 13.6 | 15.3 | 17.4 | 19.7 | 22.4 |
| 3: 7 | 43 | 10.7 | 12.1 | 13.7 | 15.5 | 17.6 | 20.0 | 22.7 |
| 3: 8 | 44 | 10.8 | 12.2 | 13.8 | 15.7 | 17.8 | 20.2 | 23.0 |
| 3: 9 | 45 | 10.9 | 12.4 | 14.0 | 15.8 | 18.0 | 20.5 | 23.3 |
| 3:10 | 46 | 11.0 | 12.5 | 14.1 | 16.0 | 18.2 | 20.7 | 23.6 |
| 3:11 | 47 | 11.1 | 12.6 | 14.3 | 16.2 | 18.4 | 20.9 | 23.9 |
| 4: 0 | 48 | 11.2 | 12.7 | 14.4 | 16.3 | 18.6 | 21.2 | 24.2 |

**Weight-for-age for boys, age in years and months (continued)**

| | | Z-scores (weight in kg) | | | | | | |
|---|---|---|---|---|---|---|---|---|
| **Year: Month** | **Month** | **-3 SD** | **-2 SD** | **-1 SD** | **Median** | **1 SD** | **2 SD** | **3 SD** |
| 4: 1 | 49 | 11.3 | 12.8 | 14.5 | 16.5 | 18.8 | 21.4 | 24.5 |
| 4: 2 | 50 | 11.4 | 12.9 | 14.7 | 16.7 | 19.0 | 21.7 | 24.8 |
| 4: 3 | 51 | 11.5 | 13.1 | 14.8 | 16.8 | 19.2 | 21.9 | 25.1 |
| 4: 4 | 52 | 11.6 | 13.2 | 15.0 | 17.0 | 19.4 | 22.2 | 25.4 |
| 4: 5 | 53 | 11.7 | 13.3 | 15.1 | 17.2 | 19.6 | 22.4 | 25.7 |
| 4: 6 | 54 | 11.8 | 13.4 | 15.2 | 17.3 | 19.8 | 22.7 | 26.0 |
| 4: 7 | 55 | 11.9 | 13.5 | 15.4 | 17.5 | 20.0 | 22.9 | 26.3 |
| 4: 8 | 56 | 12.0 | 13.6 | 15.5 | 17.7 | 20.2 | 23.2 | 26.6 |
| 4: 9 | 57 | 12.1 | 13.7 | 15.6 | 17.8 | 20.4 | 23.4 | 26.9 |
| 4:10 | 58 | 12.2 | 13.8 | 15.8 | 18.0 | 20.6 | 23.7 | 27.2 |
| 4:11 | 59 | 12.3 | 14.0 | 15.9 | 18.2 | 20.8 | 23.9 | 27.6 |
| 5: 0 | 60 | 12.4 | 14.1 | 16.0 | 18.3 | 21.0 | 24.2 | 27.9 |

**Weight-for-age for girls, age in years and months**

| | | Z-scores (weight in kg) | | | | | | |
|---|---|---|---|---|---|---|---|---|
| **Year: Month** | **Month** | **-3 SD** | **-2 SD** | **-1 SD** | **Median** | **1 SD** | **2 SD** | **3 SD** |
| 0: 0 | 0 | 2.0 | 2.4 | 2.8 | 3.2 | 3.7 | 4.2 | 4.8 |
| 0: 1 | 1 | 2.7 | 3.2 | 3.6 | 4.2 | 4.8 | 5.5 | 6.2 |
| 0: 2 | 2 | 3.4 | 3.9 | 4.5 | 5.1 | 5.8 | 6.6 | 7.5 |
| 0: 3 | 3 | 4.0 | 4.5 | 5.2 | 5.8 | 6.6 | 7.5 | 8.5 |
| 0: 4 | 4 | 4.4 | 5.0 | 5.7 | 6.4 | 7.3 | 8.2 | 9.3 |
| 0: 5 | 5 | 4.8 | 5.4 | 6.1 | 6.9 | 7.8 | 8.8 | 10.0 |
| 0: 6 | 6 | 5.1 | 5.7 | 6.5 | 7.3 | 8.2 | 9.3 | 10.6 |
| 0: 7 | 7 | 5.3 | 6.0 | 6.8 | 7.6 | 8.6 | 9.8 | 11.1 |
| 0: 8 | 8 | 5.6 | 6.3 | 7.0 | 7.9 | 9.0 | 10.2 | 11.6 |
| 0: 9 | 9 | 5.8 | 6.5 | 7.3 | 8.2 | 9.3 | 10.5 | 12.0 |
| 0:10 | 10 | 5.9 | 6.7 | 7.5 | 8.5 | 9.6 | 10.9 | 12.4 |
| 0:11 | 11 | 6.1 | 6.9 | 7.7 | 8.7 | 9.9 | 11.2 | 12.8 |
| 1: 0 | 12 | 6.3 | 7.0 | 7.9 | 8.9 | 10.1 | 11.5 | 13.1 |
| 1: 1 | 13 | 6.4 | 7.2 | 8.1 | 9.2 | 10.4 | 11.8 | 13.5 |
| 1: 2 | 14 | 6.6 | 7.4 | 8.3 | 9.4 | 10.6 | 12.1 | 13.8 |
| 1: 3 | 15 | 6.7 | 7.6 | 8.5 | 9.6 | 10.9 | 12.4 | 14.1 |
| 1: 4 | 16 | 6.9 | 7.7 | 8.7 | 9.8 | 11.1 | 12.6 | 14.5 |
| 1: 5 | 17 | 7.0 | 7.9 | 8.9 | 10.0 | 11.4 | 12.9 | 14.8 |
| 1: 6 | 18 | 7.2 | 8.1 | 9.1 | 10.2 | 11.6 | 13.2 | 15.1 |
| 1: 7 | 19 | 7.3 | 8.2 | 9.2 | 10.4 | 11.8 | 13.5 | 15.4 |
| 1: 8 | 20 | 7.5 | 8.4 | 9.4 | 10.6 | 12.1 | 13.7 | 15.7 |
| 1: 9 | 21 | 7.6 | 8.6 | 9.6 | 10.9 | 12.3 | 14.0 | 16.0 |
| 1:10 | 22 | 7.8 | 8.7 | 9.8 | 11.1 | 12.5 | 14.3 | 16.4 |
| 1:11 | 23 | 7.9 | 8.9 | 10.0 | 11.3 | 12.8 | 14.6 | 16.7 |
| 2: 0 | 24 | 8.1 | 9.0 | 10.2 | 11.5 | 13.0 | 14.8 | 17.0 |

**Weight-for-age for girls, age in years and months (continued)**

| | | Z-scores (weight in kg) | | | | | | |
|---|---|---|---|---|---|---|---|---|
| **Year: Month** | **Month** | **-3 SD** | **-2 SD** | **-1 SD** | **Median** | **1 SD** | **2 SD** | **3 SD** |
| 2: 1 | 25 | 8.2 | 9.2 | 10.3 | 11.7 | 13.3 | 15.1 | 17.3 |
| 2: 2 | 26 | 8.4 | 9.4 | 10.5 | 11.9 | 13.5 | 15.4 | 17.7 |
| 2: 3 | 27 | 8.5 | 9.5 | 10.7 | 12.1 | 13.7 | 15.7 | 18.0 |
| 2: 4 | 28 | 8.6 | 9.7 | 10.9 | 12.3 | 14.0 | 16.0 | 18.3 |
| 2: 5 | 29 | 8.8 | 9.8 | 11.1 | 12.5 | 14.2 | 16.2 | 18.7 |
| 2: 6 | 30 | 8.9 | 10.0 | 11.2 | 12.7 | 14.4 | 16.5 | 19.0 |
| 2: 7 | 31 | 9.0 | 10.1 | 11.4 | 12.9 | 14.7 | 16.8 | 19.3 |
| 2: 8 | 32 | 9.1 | 10.3 | 11.6 | 13.1 | 14.9 | 17.1 | 19.6 |
| 2: 9 | 33 | 9.3 | 10.4 | 11.7 | 13.3 | 15.1 | 17.3 | 20.0 |
| 2:10 | 34 | 9.4 | 10.5 | 11.9 | 13.5 | 15.4 | 17.6 | 20.3 |
| 2:11 | 35 | 9.5 | 10.7 | 12.0 | 13.7 | 15.6 | 17.9 | 20.6 |
| 3: 0 | 36 | 9.6 | 10.8 | 12.2 | 13.9 | 15.8 | 18.1 | 20.9 |
| 3: 1 | 37 | 9.7 | 10.9 | 12.4 | 14.0 | 16.0 | 18.4 | 21.3 |
| 3: 2 | 38 | 9.8 | 11.1 | 12.5 | 14.2 | 16.3 | 18.7 | 21.6 |
| 3: 3 | 39 | 9.9 | 11.2 | 12.7 | 14.4 | 16.5 | 19.0 | 22.0 |
| 3: 4 | 40 | 10.1 | 11.3 | 12.8 | 14.6 | 16.7 | 19.2 | 22.3 |
| 3: 5 | 41 | 10.2 | 11.5 | 13.0 | 14.8 | 16.9 | 19.5 | 22.7 |
| 3: 6 | 42 | 10.3 | 11.6 | 13.1 | 15.0 | 17.2 | 19.8 | 23.0 |
| 3: 7 | 43 | 10.4 | 11.7 | 13.3 | 15.2 | 17.4 | 20.1 | 23.4 |
| 3: 8 | 44 | 10.5 | 11.8 | 13.4 | 15.3 | 17.6 | 20.4 | 23.7 |
| 3: 9 | 45 | 10.6 | 12.0 | 13.6 | 15.5 | 17.8 | 20.7 | 24.1 |
| 3:10 | 46 | 10.7 | 12.1 | 13.7 | 15.7 | 18.1 | 20.9 | 24.5 |
| 3:11 | 47 | 10.8 | 12.2 | 13.9 | 15.9 | 18.3 | 21.2 | 24.8 |
| 4: 0 | 48 | 10.9 | 12.3 | 14.0 | 16.1 | 18.5 | 21.5 | 25.2 |

**Weight-for-age for girls, age in years and months (continued)**

| Year: Month | Month | Z-scores (weight in kg) -3 SD | -2 SD | -1 SD | Median | 1 SD | 2 SD | 3 SD |
|---|---|---|---|---|---|---|---|---|
| 4: 1 | 49 | 11.0 | 12.4 | 14.2 | 16.3 | 18.8 | 21.8 | 25.5 |
| 4: 2 | 50 | 11.1 | 12.6 | 14.3 | 16.4 | 19.0 | 22.1 | 25.9 |
| 4: 3 | 51 | 11.2 | 12.7 | 14.5 | 16.6 | 19.2 | 22.4 | 26.3 |
| 4: 4 | 52 | 11.3 | 12.8 | 14.6 | 16.8 | 19.4 | 22.6 | 26.6 |
| 4: 5 | 53 | 11.4 | 12.9 | 14.8 | 17.0 | 19.7 | 22.9 | 27.0 |
| 4: 6 | 54 | 11.5 | 13.0 | 14.9 | 17.2 | 19.9 | 23.2 | 27.4 |
| 4: 7 | 55 | 11.6 | 13.2 | 15.1 | 17.3 | 20.1 | 23.5 | 27.7 |
| 4: 8 | 56 | 11.7 | 13.3 | 15.2 | 17.5 | 20.3 | 23.8 | 28.1 |
| 4: 9 | 57 | 11.8 | 13.4 | 15.3 | 17.7 | 20.6 | 24.1 | 28.5 |
| 4:10 | 58 | 11.9 | 13.5 | 15.5 | 17.9 | 20.8 | 24.4 | 28.8 |
| 4:11 | 59 | 12.0 | 13.6 | 15.6 | 18.0 | 21.0 | 24.6 | 29.2 |
| 5: 0 | 60 | 12.1 | 13.7 | 15.8 | 18.2 | 21.2 | 24.9 | 29.5 |

**Weight-for-length for boys**

| Length (cm) | Z-scores (weight in kg) -3 SD | -2 SD | -1 SD | Median | 1 SD | 2 SD | 3 SD |
|---|---|---|---|---|---|---|---|
| 45.0 | 1.9 | 2.0 | 2.2 | 2.4 | 2.7 | 3.0 | 3.3 |
| 45.5 | 1.9 | 2.1 | 2.3 | 2.5 | 2.8 | 3.1 | 3.4 |
| 46.0 | 2.0 | 2.2 | 2.4 | 2.6 | 2.9 | 3.1 | 3.5 |
| 46.5 | 2.1 | 2.3 | 2.5 | 2.7 | 3.0 | 3.2 | 3.6 |
| 47.0 | 2.1 | 2.3 | 2.5 | 2.8 | 3.0 | 3.3 | 3.7 |
| 47.5 | 2.2 | 2.4 | 2.6 | 2.9 | 3.1 | 3.4 | 3.8 |
| 48.0 | 2.3 | 2.5 | 2.7 | 2.9 | 3.2 | 3.6 | 3.9 |
| 48.5 | 2.3 | 2.6 | 2.8 | 3.0 | 3.3 | 3.7 | 4.0 |
| 49.0 | 2.4 | 2.6 | 2.9 | 3.1 | 3.4 | 3.8 | 4.2 |
| 49.5 | 2.5 | 2.7 | 3.0 | 3.2 | 3.5 | 3.9 | 4.3 |
| 50.0 | 2.6 | 2.8 | 3.0 | 3.3 | 3.6 | 4.0 | 4.4 |
| 50.5 | 2.7 | 2.9 | 3.1 | 3.4 | 3.8 | 4.1 | 4.5 |
| 51.0 | 2.7 | 3.0 | 3.2 | 3.5 | 3.9 | 4.2 | 4.7 |
| 51.5 | 2.8 | 3.1 | 3.3 | 3.6 | 4.0 | 4.4 | 4.8 |
| 52.0 | 2.9 | 3.2 | 3.5 | 3.8 | 4.1 | 4.5 | 5.0 |
| 52.5 | 3.0 | 3.3 | 3.6 | 3.9 | 4.2 | 4.6 | 5.1 |
| 53.0 | 3.1 | 3.4 | 3.7 | 4.0 | 4.4 | 4.8 | 5.3 |
| 53.5 | 3.2 | 3.5 | 3.8 | 4.1 | 4.5 | 4.9 | 5.4 |
| 54.0 | 3.3 | 3.6 | 3.9 | 4.3 | 4.7 | 5.1 | 5.6 |
| 54.5 | 3.4 | 3.7 | 4.0 | 4.4 | 4.8 | 5.3 | 5.8 |
| 55.0 | 3.6 | 3.8 | 4.2 | 4.5 | 5.0 | 5.4 | 6.0 |
| 55.5 | 3.7 | 4.0 | 4.3 | 4.7 | 5.1 | 5.6 | 6.1 |
| 56.0 | 3.8 | 4.1 | 4.4 | 4.8 | 5.3 | 5.8 | 6.3 |
| 56.5 | 3.9 | 4.2 | 4.6 | 5.0 | 5.4 | 5.9 | 6.5 |
| 57.0 | 4.0 | 4.3 | 4.7 | 5.1 | 5.6 | 6.1 | 6.7 |
| 57.5 | 4.1 | 4.5 | 4.9 | 5.3 | 5.7 | 6.3 | 6.9 |
| 58.0 | 4.3 | 4.6 | 5.0 | 5.4 | 5.9 | 6.4 | 7.1 |
| 58.5 | 4.4 | 4.7 | 5.1 | 5.6 | 6.1 | 6.6 | 7.2 |
| 59.0 | 4.5 | 4.8 | 5.3 | 5.7 | 6.2 | 6.8 | 7.4 |
| 59.5 | 4.6 | 5.0 | 5.4 | 5.9 | 6.4 | 7.0 | 7.6 |

**Weight-for-length for boys (continued)**

| | Z-scores (weight in kg) | | | | | | |
|---|---|---|---|---|---|---|---|
| **Length (cm)** | **-3 SD** | **-2 SD** | **-1 SD** | **Median** | **1 SD** | **2 SD** | **3 SD** |
| **60.0** | 4.7 | 5.1 | 5.5 | 6.0 | 6.5 | 7.1 | 7.8 |
| **60.5** | 4.8 | 5.2 | 5.6 | 6.1 | 6.7 | 7.3 | 8.0 |
| **61.0** | 4.9 | 5.3 | 5.8 | 6.3 | 6.8 | 7.4 | 8.1 |
| **61.5** | 5.0 | 5.4 | 5.9 | 6.4 | 7.0 | 7.6 | 8.3 |
| **62.0** | 5.1 | 5.6 | 6.0 | 6.5 | 7.1 | 7.7 | 8.5 |
| **62.5** | 5.2 | 5.7 | 6.1 | 6.7 | 7.2 | 7.9 | 8.6 |
| **63.0** | 5.3 | 5.8 | 6.2 | 6.8 | 7.4 | 8.0 | 8.8 |
| **63.5** | 5.4 | 5.9 | 6.4 | 6.9 | 7.5 | 8.2 | 8.9 |
| **64.0** | 5.5 | 6.0 | 6.5 | 7.0 | 7.6 | 8.3 | 9.1 |
| **64.5** | 5.6 | 6.1 | 6.6 | 7.1 | 7.8 | 8.5 | 9.3 |
| **65.0** | 5.7 | 6.2 | 6.7 | 7.3 | 7.9 | 8.6 | 9.4 |
| **65.5** | 5.8 | 6.3 | 6.8 | 7.4 | 8.0 | 8.7 | 9.6 |
| **66.0** | 5.9 | 6.4 | 6.9 | 7.5 | 8.2 | 8.9 | 9.7 |
| **66.5** | 6.0 | 6.5 | 7.0 | 7.6 | 8.3 | 9.0 | 9.9 |
| **67.0** | 6.1 | 6.6 | 7.1 | 7.7 | 8.4 | 9.2 | 10.0 |
| **67.5** | 6.2 | 6.7 | 7.2 | 7.9 | 8.5 | 9.3 | 10.2 |
| **68.0** | 6.3 | 6.8 | 7.3 | 8.0 | 8.7 | 9.4 | 10.3 |
| **68.5** | 6.4 | 6.9 | 7.5 | 8.1 | 8.8 | 9.6 | 10.5 |
| **69.0** | 6.5 | 7.0 | 7.6 | 8.2 | 8.9 | 9.7 | 10.6 |
| **69.5** | 6.6 | 7.1 | 7.7 | 8.3 | 9.0 | 9.8 | 10.8 |
| **70.0** | 6.6 | 7.2 | 7.8 | 8.4 | 9.2 | 10.0 | 10.9 |
| **70.5** | 6.7 | 7.3 | 7.9 | 8.5 | 9.3 | 10.1 | 11.1 |
| **71.0** | 6.8 | 7.4 | 8.0 | 8.6 | 9.4 | 10.2 | 11.2 |
| **71.5** | 6.9 | 7.5 | 8.1 | 8.8 | 9.5 | 10.4 | 11.3 |
| **72.0** | 7.0 | 7.6 | 8.2 | 8.9 | 9.6 | 10.5 | 11.5 |
| **72.5** | 7.1 | 7.6 | 8.3 | 9.0 | 9.8 | 10.6 | 11.6 |
| **73.0** | 7.2 | 7.7 | 8.4 | 9.1 | 9.9 | 10.8 | 11.8 |
| **73.5** | 7.2 | 7.8 | 8.5 | 9.2 | 10.0 | 10.9 | 11.9 |
| **74.0** | 7.3 | 7.9 | 8.6 | 9.3 | 10.1 | 11.0 | 12.1 |
| **74.5** | 7.4 | 8.0 | 8.7 | 9.4 | 10.2 | 11.2 | 12.2 |

**Weight-for-length for boys (continued)**

| | Z-scores (weight in kg) | | | | | | |
|---|---|---|---|---|---|---|---|
| **Length (cm)** | **-3 SD** | **-2 SD** | **-1 SD** | **Median** | **1 SD** | **2 SD** | **3 SD** |
| **75.0** | 7.5 | 8.1 | 8.8 | 9.5 | 10.3 | 11.3 | 12.3 |
| **75.5** | 7.6 | 8.2 | 8.8 | 9.6 | 10.4 | 11.4 | 12.5 |
| **76.0** | 7.6 | 8.3 | 8.9 | 9.7 | 10.6 | 11.5 | 12.6 |
| **76.5** | 7.7 | 8.3 | 9.0 | 9.8 | 10.7 | 11.6 | 12.7 |
| **77.0** | 7.8 | 8.4 | 9.1 | 9.9 | 10.8 | 11.7 | 12.8 |
| **77.5** | 7.9 | 8.5 | 9.2 | 10.0 | 10.9 | 11.9 | 13.0 |
| **78.0** | 7.9 | 8.6 | 9.3 | 10.1 | 11.0 | 12.0 | 13.1 |
| **78.5** | 8.0 | 8.7 | 9.4 | 10.2 | 11.1 | 12.1 | 13.2 |
| **79.0** | 8.1 | 8.7 | 9.5 | 10.3 | 11.2 | 12.2 | 13.3 |
| **79.5** | 8.2 | 8.8 | 9.5 | 10.4 | 11.3 | 12.3 | 13.4 |
| **80.0** | 8.2 | 8.9 | 9.6 | 10.4 | 11.4 | 12.4 | 13.6 |
| **80.5** | 8.3 | 9.0 | 9.7 | 10.5 | 11.5 | 12.5 | 13.7 |
| **81.0** | 8.4 | 9.1 | 9.8 | 10.6 | 11.6 | 12.6 | 13.8 |
| **81.5** | 8.5 | 9.1 | 9.9 | 10.7 | 11.7 | 12.7 | 13.9 |
| **82.0** | 8.5 | 9.2 | 10.0 | 10.8 | 11.8 | 12.8 | 14.0 |
| **82.5** | 8.6 | 9.3 | 10.1 | 10.9 | 11.9 | 13.0 | 14.2 |
| **83.0** | 8.7 | 9.4 | 10.2 | 11.0 | 12.0 | 13.1 | 14.3 |
| **83.5** | 8.8 | 9.5 | 10.3 | 11.2 | 12.1 | 13.2 | 14.4 |
| **84.0** | 8.9 | 9.6 | 10.4 | 11.3 | 12.2 | 13.3 | 14.6 |
| **84.5** | 9.0 | 9.7 | 10.5 | 11.4 | 12.4 | 13.5 | 14.7 |
| **85.0** | 9.1 | 9.8 | 10.6 | 11.5 | 12.5 | 13.6 | 14.9 |
| **85.5** | 9.2 | 9.9 | 10.7 | 11.6 | 12.6 | 13.7 | 15.0 |
| **86.0** | 9.3 | 10.0 | 10.8 | 11.7 | 12.8 | 13.9 | 15.2 |
| **86.5** | 9.4 | 10.1 | 11.0 | 11.9 | 12.9 | 14.0 | 15.3 |
| **87.0** | 9.5 | 10.2 | 11.1 | 12.0 | 13.0 | 14.2 | 15.5 |
| **87.5** | 9.6 | 10.4 | 11.2 | 12.1 | 13.2 | 14.3 | 15.6 |
| **88.0** | 9.7 | 10.5 | 11.3 | 12.2 | 13.3 | 14.5 | 15.8 |
| **88.5** | 9.8 | 10.6 | 11.4 | 12.4 | 13.4 | 14.6 | 15.9 |
| **89.0** | 9.9 | 10.7 | 11.5 | 12.5 | 13.5 | 14.7 | 16.1 |
| **89.5** | 10.0 | 10.8 | 11.6 | 12.6 | 13.7 | 14.9 | 16.2 |

Weight-for-length for boys (continued)

| | Z-scores (weight in kg) | | | | | | |
|---|---|---|---|---|---|---|---|
| Length (cm) | -3 SD | -2 SD | -1 SD | Median | 1 SD | 2 SD | 3 SD |
| 90.0 | 10.1 | 10.9 | 11.8 | 12.7 | 13.8 | 15.0 | 16.4 |
| 90.5 | 10.2 | 11.0 | 11.9 | 12.8 | 13.9 | 15.1 | 16.5 |
| 91.0 | 10.3 | 11.1 | 12.0 | 13.0 | 14.1 | 15.3 | 16.7 |
| 91.5 | 10.4 | 11.2 | 12.1 | 13.1 | 14.2 | 15.4 | 16.8 |
| 92.0 | 10.5 | 11.3 | 12.2 | 13.2 | 14.3 | 15.6 | 17.0 |
| 92.5 | 10.6 | 11.4 | 12.3 | 13.3 | 14.4 | 15.7 | 17.1 |
| 93.0 | 10.7 | 11.5 | 12.4 | 13.4 | 14.6 | 15.8 | 17.3 |
| 93.5 | 10.7 | 11.6 | 12.5 | 13.5 | 14.7 | 16.0 | 17.4 |
| 94.0 | 10.8 | 11.7 | 12.6 | 13.7 | 14.8 | 16.1 | 17.6 |
| 94.5 | 10.9 | 11.8 | 12.7 | 13.8 | 14.9 | 16.3 | 17.7 |
| 95.0 | 11.0 | 11.9 | 12.8 | 13.9 | 15.1 | 16.4 | 17.9 |
| 95.5 | 11.1 | 12.0 | 12.9 | 14.0 | 15.2 | 16.5 | 18.0 |
| 96.0 | 11.2 | 12.1 | 13.1 | 14.1 | 15.3 | 16.7 | 18.2 |
| 96.5 | 11.3 | 12.2 | 13.2 | 14.3 | 15.5 | 16.8 | 18.4 |
| 97.0 | 11.4 | 12.3 | 13.3 | 14.4 | 15.6 | 17.0 | 18.5 |
| 97.5 | 11.5 | 12.4 | 13.4 | 14.5 | 15.7 | 17.1 | 18.7 |
| 98.0 | 11.6 | 12.5 | 13.5 | 14.6 | 15.9 | 17.3 | 18.9 |
| 98.5 | 11.7 | 12.6 | 13.6 | 14.8 | 16.0 | 17.5 | 19.1 |
| 99.0 | 11.8 | 12.7 | 13.7 | 14.9 | 16.2 | 17.6 | 19.2 |
| 99.5 | 11.9 | 12.8 | 13.9 | 15.0 | 16.3 | 17.8 | 19.4 |
| 100.0 | 12.0 | 12.9 | 14.0 | 15.2 | 16.5 | 18.0 | 19.6 |
| 100.5 | 12.1 | 13.0 | 14.1 | 15.3 | 16.6 | 18.1 | 19.8 |
| 101.0 | 12.2 | 13.2 | 14.2 | 15.4 | 16.8 | 18.3 | 20.0 |
| 101.5 | 12.3 | 13.3 | 14.4 | 15.6 | 16.9 | 18.5 | 20.2 |
| 102.0 | 12.4 | 13.4 | 14.5 | 15.7 | 17.1 | 18.7 | 20.4 |
| 102.5 | 12.5 | 13.5 | 14.6 | 15.9 | 17.3 | 18.8 | 20.6 |
| 103.0 | 12.6 | 13.6 | 14.8 | 16.0 | 17.4 | 19.0 | 20.8 |
| 103.5 | 12.7 | 13.7 | 14.9 | 16.2 | 17.6 | 19.2 | 21.0 |
| 104.0 | 12.8 | 13.9 | 15.0 | 16.3 | 17.8 | 19.4 | 21.2 |
| 104.5 | 12.9 | 14.0 | 15.2 | 16.5 | 17.9 | 19.6 | 21.5 |

Weight-for-length for boys (continued)

| | Z-scores (weight in kg) | | | | | | |
|---|---|---|---|---|---|---|---|
| Length (cm) | -3 SD | -2 SD | -1 SD | Median | 1 SD | 2 SD | 3 SD |
| 105.0 | 13.0 | 14.1 | 15.3 | 16.6 | 18.1 | 19.8 | 21.7 |
| 105.5 | 13.2 | 14.2 | 15.4 | 16.8 | 18.3 | 20.0 | 21.9 |
| 106.0 | 13.3 | 14.4 | 15.6 | 16.9 | 18.5 | 20.2 | 22.1 |
| 106.5 | 13.4 | 14.5 | 15.7 | 17.1 | 18.6 | 20.4 | 22.4 |
| 107.0 | 13.5 | 14.6 | 15.9 | 17.3 | 18.8 | 20.6 | 22.6 |
| 107.5 | 13.6 | 14.7 | 16.0 | 17.4 | 19.0 | 20.8 | 22.8 |
| 108.0 | 13.7 | 14.9 | 16.2 | 17.6 | 19.2 | 21.0 | 23.1 |
| 108.5 | 13.8 | 15.0 | 16.3 | 17.8 | 19.4 | 21.2 | 23.3 |
| 109.0 | 14.0 | 15.1 | 16.5 | 17.9 | 19.6 | 21.4 | 23.6 |
| 109.5 | 14.1 | 15.3 | 16.6 | 18.1 | 19.8 | 21.7 | 23.8 |
| 110.0 | 14.2 | 15.4 | 16.8 | 18.3 | 20.0 | 21.9 | 24.1 |

**Weight-for-length for girls**

| | Z-scores (weight in kg) | | | | | | |
|---|---|---|---|---|---|---|---|
| Length (cm) | -3 SD | -2 SD | -1 SD | Median | 1 SD | 2 SD | 3 SD |
| **45.0** | 1.9 | 2.1 | 2.3 | 2.5 | 2.7 | 3.0 | 3.3 |
| **45.5** | 2.0 | 2.1 | 2.3 | 2.5 | 2.8 | 3.1 | 3.4 |
| **46.0** | 2.0 | 2.2 | 2.4 | 2.6 | 2.9 | 3.2 | 3.5 |
| **46.5** | 2.1 | 2.3 | 2.5 | 2.7 | 3.0 | 3.3 | 3.6 |
| **47.0** | 2.2 | 2.4 | 2.6 | 2.8 | 3.1 | 3.4 | 3.7 |
| **47.5** | 2.2 | 2.4 | 2.6 | 2.9 | 3.2 | 3.5 | 3.8 |
| **48.0** | 2.3 | 2.5 | 2.7 | 3.0 | 3.3 | 3.6 | 4.0 |
| **48.5** | 2.4 | 2.6 | 2.8 | 3.1 | 3.4 | 3.7 | 4.1 |
| **49.0** | 2.4 | 2.6 | 2.9 | 3.2 | 3.5 | 3.8 | 4.2 |
| **49.5** | 2.5 | 2.7 | 3.0 | 3.3 | 3.6 | 3.9 | 4.3 |
| **50.0** | 2.6 | 2.8 | 3.1 | 3.4 | 3.7 | 4.0 | 4.5 |
| **50.5** | 2.7 | 2.9 | 3.2 | 3.5 | 3.8 | 4.2 | 4.6 |
| **51.0** | 2.8 | 3.0 | 3.3 | 3.6 | 3.9 | 4.3 | 4.8 |
| **51.5** | 2.8 | 3.1 | 3.4 | 3.7 | 4.0 | 4.4 | 4.9 |
| **52.0** | 2.9 | 3.2 | 3.5 | 3.8 | 4.2 | 4.6 | 5.1 |
| **52.5** | 3.0 | 3.3 | 3.6 | 3.9 | 4.3 | 4.7 | 5.2 |
| **53.0** | 3.1 | 3.4 | 3.7 | 4.0 | 4.4 | 4.9 | 5.4 |
| **53.5** | 3.2 | 3.5 | 3.8 | 4.2 | 4.6 | 5.0 | 5.5 |
| **54.0** | 3.3 | 3.6 | 3.9 | 4.3 | 4.7 | 5.2 | 5.7 |
| **54.5** | 3.4 | 3.7 | 4.0 | 4.4 | 4.8 | 5.3 | 5.9 |
| **55.0** | 3.5 | 3.8 | 4.2 | 4.5 | 5.0 | 5.5 | 6.1 |
| **55.5** | 3.6 | 3.9 | 4.3 | 4.7 | 5.1 | 5.7 | 6.3 |
| **56.0** | 3.7 | 4.0 | 4.4 | 4.8 | 5.3 | 5.8 | 6.4 |
| **56.5** | 3.8 | 4.1 | 4.5 | 5.0 | 5.4 | 6.0 | 6.6 |
| **57.0** | 3.9 | 4.3 | 4.6 | 5.1 | 5.6 | 6.1 | 6.8 |
| **57.5** | 4.0 | 4.4 | 4.8 | 5.2 | 5.7 | 6.3 | 7.0 |
| **58.0** | 4.1 | 4.5 | 4.9 | 5.4 | 5.9 | 6.5 | 7.1 |
| **58.5** | 4.2 | 4.6 | 5.0 | 5.5 | 6.0 | 6.6 | 7.3 |
| **59.0** | 4.3 | 4.7 | 5.1 | 5.6 | 6.2 | 6.8 | 7.5 |
| **59.5** | 4.4 | 4.8 | 5.3 | 5.7 | 6.3 | 6.9 | 7.7 |

**Weight-for-length for girls (continued)**

| | Z-scores (weight in kg) | | | | | | |
|---|---|---|---|---|---|---|---|
| **Length (cm)** | **-3 SD** | **-2 SD** | **-1 SD** | **Median** | **1 SD** | **2 SD** | **3 SD** |
| **60.0** | 4.5 | 4.9 | 5.4 | 5.9 | 6.4 | 7.1 | 7.8 |
| **60.5** | 4.6 | 5.0 | 5.5 | 6.0 | 6.6 | 7.3 | 8.0 |
| **61.0** | 4.7 | 5.1 | 5.6 | 6.1 | 6.7 | 7.4 | 8.2 |
| **61.5** | 4.8 | 5.2 | 5.7 | 6.3 | 6.9 | 7.6 | 8.4 |
| **62.0** | 4.9 | 5.3 | 5.8 | 6.4 | 7.0 | 7.7 | 8.5 |
| **62.5** | 5.0 | 5.4 | 5.9 | 6.5 | 7.1 | 7.8 | 8.7 |
| **63.0** | 5.1 | 5.5 | 6.0 | 6.6 | 7.3 | 8.0 | 8.8 |
| **63.5** | 5.2 | 5.6 | 6.2 | 6.7 | 7.4 | 8.1 | 9.0 |
| **64.0** | 5.3 | 5.7 | 6.3 | 6.9 | 7.5 | 8.3 | 9.1 |
| **64.5** | 5.4 | 5.8 | 6.4 | 7.0 | 7.6 | 8.4 | 9.3 |
| **65.0** | 5.5 | 5.9 | 6.5 | 7.1 | 7.8 | 8.6 | 9.5 |
| **65.5** | 5.5 | 6.0 | 6.6 | 7.2 | 7.9 | 8.7 | 9.6 |
| **66.0** | 5.6 | 6.1 | 6.7 | 7.3 | 8.0 | 8.8 | 9.8 |
| **66.5** | 5.7 | 6.2 | 6.8 | 7.4 | 8.1 | 9.0 | 9.9 |
| **67.0** | 5.8 | 6.3 | 6.9 | 7.5 | 8.3 | 9.1 | 10.0 |
| **67.5** | 5.9 | 6.4 | 7.0 | 7.6 | 8.4 | 9.2 | 10.2 |
| **68.0** | 6.0 | 6.5 | 7.1 | 7.7 | 8.5 | 9.4 | 10.3 |
| **68.5** | 6.1 | 6.6 | 7.2 | 7.9 | 8.6 | 9.5 | 10.5 |
| **69.0** | 6.1 | 6.7 | 7.3 | 8.0 | 8.7 | 9.6 | 10.6 |
| **69.5** | 6.2 | 6.8 | 7.4 | 8.1 | 8.8 | 9.7 | 10.7 |
| **70.0** | 6.3 | 6.9 | 7.5 | 8.2 | 9.0 | 9.9 | 10.9 |
| **70.5** | 6.4 | 6.9 | 7.6 | 8.3 | 9.1 | 10.0 | 11.0 |
| **71.0** | 6.5 | 7.0 | 7.7 | 8.4 | 9.2 | 10.1 | 11.1 |
| **71.5** | 6.5 | 7.1 | 7.7 | 8.5 | 9.3 | 10.2 | 11.3 |
| **72.0** | 6.6 | 7.2 | 7.8 | 8.6 | 9.4 | 10.3 | 11.4 |
| **72.5** | 6.7 | 7.3 | 7.9 | 8.7 | 9.5 | 10.5 | 11.5 |
| **73.0** | 6.8 | 7.4 | 8.0 | 8.8 | 9.6 | 10.6 | 11.7 |
| **73.5** | 6.9 | 7.4 | 8.1 | 8.9 | 9.7 | 10.7 | 11.8 |
| **74.0** | 6.9 | 7.5 | 8.2 | 9.0 | 9.8 | 10.8 | 11.9 |
| **74.5** | 7.0 | 7.6 | 8.3 | 9.1 | 9.9 | 10.9 | 12.0 |

**Weight-for-length for girls (continued)**

| | Z-scores (weight in kg) | | | | | | |
|---|---|---|---|---|---|---|---|
| **Length (cm)** | **-3 SD** | **-2 SD** | **-1 SD** | **Median** | **1 SD** | **2 SD** | **3 SD** |
| **75.0** | 7.1 | 7.7 | 8.4 | 9.1 | 10.0 | 11.0 | 12.2 |
| **75.5** | 7.1 | 7.8 | 8.5 | 9.2 | 10.1 | 11.1 | 12.3 |
| **76.0** | 7.2 | 7.8 | 8.5 | 9.3 | 10.2 | 11.2 | 12.4 |
| **76.5** | 7.3 | 7.9 | 8.6 | 9.4 | 10.3 | 11.4 | 12.5 |
| **77.0** | 7.4 | 8.0 | 8.7 | 9.5 | 10.4 | 11.5 | 12.6 |
| **77.5** | 7.4 | 8.1 | 8.8 | 9.6 | 10.5 | 11.6 | 12.8 |
| **78.0** | 7.5 | 8.2 | 8.9 | 9.7 | 10.6 | 11.7 | 12.9 |
| **78.5** | 7.6 | 8.2 | 9.0 | 9.8 | 10.7 | 11.8 | 13.0 |
| **79.0** | 7.7 | 8.3 | 9.1 | 9.9 | 10.8 | 11.9 | 13.1 |
| **79.5** | 7.7 | 8.4 | 9.1 | 10.0 | 10.9 | 12.0 | 13.3 |
| **80.0** | 7.8 | 8.5 | 9.2 | 10.1 | 11.0 | 12.1 | 13.4 |
| **80.5** | 7.9 | 8.6 | 9.3 | 10.2 | 11.2 | 12.3 | 13.5 |
| **81.0** | 8.0 | 8.7 | 9.4 | 10.3 | 11.3 | 12.4 | 13.7 |
| **81.5** | 8.1 | 8.8 | 9.5 | 10.4 | 11.4 | 12.5 | 13.8 |
| **82.0** | 8.1 | 8.8 | 9.6 | 10.5 | 11.5 | 12.6 | 13.9 |
| **82.5** | 8.2 | 8.9 | 9.7 | 10.6 | 11.6 | 12.8 | 14.1 |
| **83.0** | 8.3 | 9.0 | 9.8 | 10.7 | 11.8 | 12.9 | 14.2 |
| **83.5** | 8.4 | 9.1 | 9.9 | 10.9 | 11.9 | 13.1 | 14.4 |
| **84.0** | 8.5 | 9.2 | 10.1 | 11.0 | 12.0 | 13.2 | 14.5 |
| **84.5** | 8.6 | 9.3 | 10.2 | 11.1 | 12.1 | 13.3 | 14.7 |
| **85.0** | 8.7 | 9.4 | 10.3 | 11.2 | 12.3 | 13.5 | 14.9 |
| **85.5** | 8.8 | 9.5 | 10.4 | 11.3 | 12.4 | 13.6 | 15.0 |
| **86.0** | 8.9 | 9.7 | 10.5 | 11.5 | 12.6 | 13.8 | 15.2 |
| **86.5** | 9.0 | 9.8 | 10.6 | 11.6 | 12.7 | 13.9 | 15.4 |
| **87.0** | 9.1 | 9.9 | 10.7 | 11.7 | 12.8 | 14.1 | 15.5 |
| **87.5** | 9.2 | 10.0 | 10.9 | 11.8 | 13.0 | 14.2 | 15.7 |
| **88.0** | 9.3 | 10.1 | 11.0 | 12.0 | 13.1 | 14.4 | 15.9 |
| **88.5** | 9.4 | 10.2 | 11.1 | 12.1 | 13.2 | 14.5 | 16.0 |
| **89.0** | 9.5 | 10.3 | 11.2 | 12.2 | 13.4 | 14.7 | 16.2 |
| **89.5** | 9.6 | 10.4 | 11.3 | 12.3 | 13.5 | 14.8 | 16.4 |

**Weight-for-length for girls (continued)**

| | Z-scores (weight in kg) | | | | | | |
|---|---|---|---|---|---|---|---|
| **Length (cm)** | **-3 SD** | **-2 SD** | **-1 SD** | **Median** | **1 SD** | **2 SD** | **3 SD** |
| **90.0** | 9.7 | 10.5 | 11.4 | 12.5 | 13.7 | 15.0 | 16.5 |
| **90.5** | 9.8 | 10.6 | 11.5 | 12.6 | 13.8 | 15.1 | 16.7 |
| **91.0** | 9.9 | 10.7 | 11.7 | 12.7 | 13.9 | 15.3 | 16.9 |
| **91.5** | 10.0 | 10.8 | 11.8 | 12.8 | 14.1 | 15.5 | 17.0 |
| **92.0** | 10.1 | 10.9 | 11.9 | 13.0 | 14.2 | 15.6 | 17.2 |
| **92.5** | 10.1 | 11.0 | 12.0 | 13.1 | 14.3 | 15.8 | 17.4 |
| **93.0** | 10.2 | 11.1 | 12.1 | 13.2 | 14.5 | 15.9 | 17.5 |
| **93.5** | 10.3 | 11.2 | 12.2 | 13.3 | 14.6 | 16.1 | 17.7 |
| **94.0** | 10.4 | 11.3 | 12.3 | 13.5 | 14.7 | 16.2 | 17.9 |
| **94.5** | 10.5 | 11.4 | 12.4 | 13.6 | 14.9 | 16.4 | 18.0 |
| **95.0** | 10.6 | 11.5 | 12.6 | 13.7 | 15.0 | 16.5 | 18.2 |
| **95.5** | 10.7 | 11.6 | 12.7 | 13.8 | 15.2 | 16.7 | 18.4 |
| **96.0** | 10.8 | 11.7 | 12.8 | 14.0 | 15.3 | 16.8 | 18.6 |
| **96.5** | 10.9 | 11.8 | 12.9 | 14.1 | 15.4 | 17.0 | 18.7 |
| **97.0** | 11.0 | 12.0 | 13.0 | 14.2 | 15.6 | 17.1 | 18.9 |
| **97.5** | 11.1 | 12.1 | 13.1 | 14.4 | 15.7 | 17.3 | 19.1 |
| **98.0** | 11.2 | 12.2 | 13.3 | 14.5 | 15.9 | 17.5 | 19.3 |
| **98.5** | 11.3 | 12.3 | 13.4 | 14.6 | 16.0 | 17.6 | 19.5 |
| **99.0** | 11.4 | 12.4 | 13.5 | 14.8 | 16.2 | 17.8 | 19.6 |
| **99.5** | 11.5 | 12.5 | 13.6 | 14.9 | 16.3 | 18.0 | 19.8 |
| **100.0** | 11.6 | 12.6 | 13.7 | 15.0 | 16.5 | 18.1 | 20.0 |
| **100.5** | 11.7 | 12.7 | 13.9 | 15.2 | 16.6 | 18.3 | 20.2 |
| **101.0** | 11.8 | 12.8 | 14.0 | 15.3 | 16.8 | 18.5 | 20.4 |
| **101.5** | 11.9 | 13.0 | 14.1 | 15.5 | 17.0 | 18.7 | 20.6 |
| **102.0** | 12.0 | 13.1 | 14.3 | 15.6 | 17.1 | 18.9 | 20.8 |
| **102.5** | 12.1 | 13.2 | 14.4 | 15.8 | 17.3 | 19.0 | 21.0 |
| **103.0** | 12.3 | 13.3 | 14.5 | 15.9 | 17.5 | 19.2 | 21.3 |
| **103.5** | 12.4 | 13.5 | 14.7 | 16.1 | 17.6 | 19.4 | 21.5 |
| **104.0** | 12.5 | 13.6 | 14.8 | 16.2 | 17.8 | 19.6 | 21.7 |
| **104.5** | 12.6 | 13.7 | 15.0 | 16.4 | 18.0 | 19.8 | 21.9 |

**Weight-for-length for girls (continued)**

| | Z-scores (weight in kg) | | | | | | |
|---|---|---|---|---|---|---|---|
| **Length (cm)** | **-3 SD** | **-2 SD** | **-1 SD** | **Median** | **1 SD** | **2 SD** | **3 SD** |
| **105.0** | 12.7 | 13.8 | 15.1 | 16.5 | 18.2 | 20.0 | 22.2 |
| **105.5** | 12.8 | 14.0 | 15.3 | 16.7 | 18.4 | 20.2 | 22.4 |
| **106.0** | 13.0 | 14.1 | 15.4 | 16.9 | 18.5 | 20.5 | 22.6 |
| **106.5** | 13.1 | 14.3 | 15.6 | 17.1 | 18.7 | 20.7 | 22.9 |
| **107.0** | 13.2 | 14.4 | 15.7 | 17.2 | 18.9 | 20.9 | 23.1 |
| **107.5** | 13.3 | 14.5 | 15.9 | 17.4 | 19.1 | 21.1 | 23.4 |
| **108.0** | 13.5 | 14.7 | 16.0 | 17.6 | 19.3 | 21.3 | 23.6 |
| **108.5** | 13.6 | 14.8 | 16.2 | 17.8 | 19.5 | 21.6 | 23.9 |
| **109.0** | 13.7 | 15.0 | 16.4 | 18.0 | 19.7 | 21.8 | 24.2 |
| **109.5** | 13.9 | 15.1 | 16.5 | 18.1 | 20.0 | 22.0 | 24.4 |
| **110.0** | 14.0 | 15.3 | 16.7 | 18.3 | 20.2 | 22.3 | 24.7 |

**Weight-for-height for boys**

| | Z-scores (weight in kg) | | | | | | |
|---|---|---|---|---|---|---|---|
| **Height (cm)** | **-3 SD** | **-2 SD** | **-1 SD** | **Median** | **1 SD** | **2 SD** | **3 SD** |
| **65.0** | 5.9 | 6.3 | 6.9 | 7.4 | 8.1 | 8.8 | 9.6 |
| **65.5** | 6.0 | 6.4 | 7.0 | 7.6 | 8.2 | 8.9 | 9.8 |
| **66.0** | 6.1 | 6.5 | 7.1 | 7.7 | 8.3 | 9.1 | 9.9 |
| **66.5** | 6.1 | 6.6 | 7.2 | 7.8 | 8.5 | 9.2 | 10.1 |
| **67.0** | 6.2 | 6.7 | 7.3 | 7.9 | 8.6 | 9.4 | 10.2 |
| **67.5** | 6.3 | 6.8 | 7.4 | 8.0 | 8.7 | 9.5 | 10.4 |
| **68.0** | 6.4 | 6.9 | 7.5 | 8.1 | 8.8 | 9.6 | 10.5 |
| **68.5** | 6.5 | 7.0 | 7.6 | 8.2 | 9.0 | 9.8 | 10.7 |
| **69.0** | 6.6 | 7.1 | 7.7 | 8.4 | 9.1 | 9.9 | 10.8 |
| **69.5** | 6.7 | 7.2 | 7.8 | 8.5 | 9.2 | 10.0 | 11.0 |
| **70.0** | 6.8 | 7.3 | 7.9 | 8.6 | 9.3 | 10.2 | 11.1 |
| **70.5** | 6.9 | 7.4 | 8.0 | 8.7 | 9.5 | 10.3 | 11.3 |
| **71.0** | 6.9 | 7.5 | 8.1 | 8.8 | 9.6 | 10.4 | 11.4 |
| **71.5** | 7.0 | 7.6 | 8.2 | 8.9 | 9.7 | 10.6 | 11.6 |
| **72.0** | 7.1 | 7.7 | 8.3 | 9.0 | 9.8 | 10.7 | 11.7 |
| **72.5** | 7.2 | 7.8 | 8.4 | 9.1 | 9.9 | 10.8 | 11.8 |
| **73.0** | 7.3 | 7.9 | 8.5 | 9.2 | 10.0 | 11.0 | 12.0 |
| **73.5** | 7.4 | 7.9 | 8.6 | 9.3 | 10.2 | 11.1 | 12.1 |
| **74.0** | 7.4 | 8.0 | 8.7 | 9.4 | 10.3 | 11.2 | 12.2 |
| **74.5** | 7.5 | 8.1 | 8.8 | 9.5 | 10.4 | 11.3 | 12.4 |
| **75.0** | 7.6 | 8.2 | 8.9 | 9.6 | 10.5 | 11.4 | 12.5 |
| **75.5** | 7.7 | 8.3 | 9.0 | 9.7 | 10.6 | 11.6 | 12.6 |
| **76.0** | 7.7 | 8.4 | 9.1 | 9.8 | 10.7 | 11.7 | 12.8 |
| **76.5** | 7.8 | 8.5 | 9.2 | 9.9 | 10.8 | 11.8 | 12.9 |
| **77.0** | 7.9 | 8.5 | 9.2 | 10.0 | 10.9 | 11.9 | 13.0 |
| **77.5** | 8.0 | 8.6 | 9.3 | 10.1 | 11.0 | 12.0 | 13.1 |
| **78.0** | 8.0 | 8.7 | 9.4 | 10.2 | 11.1 | 12.1 | 13.3 |
| **78.5** | 8.1 | 8.8 | 9.5 | 10.3 | 11.2 | 12.2 | 13.4 |
| **79.0** | 8.2 | 8.8 | 9.6 | 10.4 | 11.3 | 12.3 | 13.5 |
| **79.5** | 8.3 | 8.9 | 9.7 | 10.5 | 11.4 | 12.4 | 13.6 |

**Weight-for-height for boys (continued)**

| Height (cm) | Z-scores (weight in kg) | | | | | | |
|---|---|---|---|---|---|---|---|
| | -3 SD | -2 SD | -1 SD | Median | 1 SD | 2 SD | 3 SD |
| **80.0** | 8.3 | 9.0 | 9.7 | 10.6 | 11.5 | 12.6 | 13.7 |
| **80.5** | 8.4 | 9.1 | 9.8 | 10.7 | 11.6 | 12.7 | 13.8 |
| **81.0** | 8.5 | 9.2 | 9.9 | 10.8 | 11.7 | 12.8 | 14.0 |
| **81.5** | 8.6 | 9.3 | 10.0 | 10.9 | 11.8 | 12.9 | 14.1 |
| **82.0** | 8.7 | 9.3 | 10.1 | 11.0 | 11.9 | 13.0 | 14.2 |
| **82.5** | 8.7 | 9.4 | 10.2 | 11.1 | 12.1 | 13.1 | 14.4 |
| **83.0** | 8.8 | 9.5 | 10.3 | 11.2 | 12.2 | 13.3 | 14.5 |
| **83.5** | 8.9 | 9.6 | 10.4 | 11.3 | 12.3 | 13.4 | 14.6 |
| **84.0** | 9.0 | 9.7 | 10.5 | 11.4 | 12.4 | 13.5 | 14.8 |
| **84.5** | 9.1 | 9.9 | 10.7 | 11.5 | 12.5 | 13.7 | 14.9 |
| **85.0** | 9.2 | 10.0 | 10.8 | 11.7 | 12.7 | 13.8 | 15.1 |
| **85.5** | 9.3 | 10.1 | 10.9 | 11.8 | 12.8 | 13.9 | 15.2 |
| **86.0** | 9.4 | 10.2 | 11.0 | 11.9 | 12.9 | 14.1 | 15.4 |
| **86.5** | 9.5 | 10.3 | 11.1 | 12.0 | 13.1 | 14.2 | 15.5 |
| **87.0** | 9.6 | 10.4 | 11.2 | 12.2 | 13.2 | 14.4 | 15.7 |
| **87.5** | 9.7 | 10.5 | 11.3 | 12.3 | 13.3 | 14.5 | 15.8 |
| **88.0** | 9.8 | 10.6 | 11.5 | 12.4 | 13.5 | 14.7 | 16.0 |
| **88.5** | 9.9 | 10.7 | 11.6 | 12.5 | 13.6 | 14.8 | 16.1 |
| **89.0** | 10.0 | 10.8 | 11.7 | 12.6 | 13.7 | 14.9 | 16.3 |
| **89.5** | 10.1 | 10.9 | 11.8 | 12.8 | 13.9 | 15.1 | 16.4 |
| **90.0** | 10.2 | 11.0 | 11.9 | 12.9 | 14.0 | 15.2 | 16.6 |
| **90.5** | 10.3 | 11.1 | 12.0 | 13.0 | 14.1 | 15.3 | 16.7 |
| **91.0** | 10.4 | 11.2 | 12.1 | 13.1 | 14.2 | 15.5 | 16.9 |
| **91.5** | 10.5 | 11.3 | 12.2 | 13.2 | 14.4 | 15.6 | 17.0 |
| **92.0** | 10.6 | 11.4 | 12.3 | 13.4 | 14.5 | 15.8 | 17.2 |
| **92.5** | 10.7 | 11.5 | 12.4 | 13.5 | 14.6 | 15.9 | 17.3 |
| **93.0** | 10.8 | 11.6 | 12.6 | 13.6 | 14.7 | 16.0 | 17.5 |
| **93.5** | 10.9 | 11.7 | 12.7 | 13.7 | 14.9 | 16.2 | 17.6 |
| **94.0** | 11.0 | 11.8 | 12.8 | 13.8 | 15.0 | 16.3 | 17.8 |
| **94.5** | 11.1 | 11.9 | 12.9 | 13.9 | 15.1 | 16.5 | 17.9 |

**Weight-for-height for boys (continued)**

| Height (cm) | Z-scores (weight in kg) | | | | | | |
|---|---|---|---|---|---|---|---|
| | -3 SD | -2 SD | -1 SD | Median | 1 SD | 2 SD | 3 SD |
| 95.0 | 11.1 | 12.0 | 13.0 | 14.1 | 15.3 | 16.6 | 18.1 |
| 95.5 | 11.2 | 12.1 | 13.1 | 14.2 | 15.4 | 16.7 | 18.3 |
| 96.0 | 11.3 | 12.2 | 13.2 | 14.3 | 15.5 | 16.9 | 18.4 |
| 96.5 | 11.4 | 12.3 | 13.3 | 14.4 | 15.7 | 17.0 | 18.6 |
| 97.0 | 11.5 | 12.4 | 13.4 | 14.6 | 15.8 | 17.2 | 18.8 |
| 97.5 | 11.6 | 12.5 | 13.6 | 14.7 | 15.9 | 17.4 | 18.9 |
| 98.0 | 11.7 | 12.6 | 13.7 | 14.8 | 16.1 | 17.5 | 19.1 |
| 98.5 | 11.8 | 12.8 | 13.8 | 14.9 | 16.2 | 17.7 | 19.3 |
| 99.0 | 11.9 | 12.9 | 13.9 | 15.1 | 16.4 | 17.9 | 19.5 |
| 99.5 | 12.0 | 13.0 | 14.0 | 15.2 | 16.5 | 18.0 | 19.7 |
| 100.0 | 12.1 | 13.1 | 14.2 | 15.4 | 16.7 | 18.2 | 19.9 |
| 100.5 | 12.2 | 13.2 | 14.3 | 15.5 | 16.9 | 18.4 | 20.1 |
| 101.0 | 12.3 | 13.3 | 14.4 | 15.6 | 17.0 | 18.5 | 20.3 |
| 101.5 | 12.4 | 13.4 | 14.5 | 15.8 | 17.2 | 18.7 | 20.5 |
| 102.0 | 12.5 | 13.6 | 14.7 | 15.9 | 17.3 | 18.9 | 20.7 |
| 102.5 | 12.6 | 13.7 | 14.8 | 16.1 | 17.5 | 19.1 | 20.9 |
| 103.0 | 12.8 | 13.8 | 14.9 | 16.2 | 17.7 | 19.3 | 21.1 |
| 103.5 | 12.9 | 13.9 | 15.1 | 16.4 | 17.8 | 19.5 | 21.3 |
| 104.0 | 13.0 | 14.0 | 15.2 | 16.5 | 18.0 | 19.7 | 21.6 |
| 104.5 | 13.1 | 14.2 | 15.4 | 16.7 | 18.2 | 19.9 | 21.8 |
| 105.0 | 13.2 | 14.3 | 15.5 | 16.8 | 18.4 | 20.1 | 22.0 |
| 105.5 | 13.3 | 14.4 | 15.6 | 17.0 | 18.5 | 20.3 | 22.2 |
| 106.0 | 13.4 | 14.5 | 15.8 | 17.2 | 18.7 | 20.5 | 22.5 |
| 106.5 | 13.5 | 14.7 | 15.9 | 17.3 | 18.9 | 20.7 | 22.7 |
| 107.0 | 13.7 | 14.8 | 16.1 | 17.5 | 19.1 | 20.9 | 22.9 |
| 107.5 | 13.8 | 14.9 | 16.2 | 17.7 | 19.3 | 21.1 | 23.2 |
| 108.0 | 13.9 | 15.1 | 16.4 | 17.8 | 19.5 | 21.3 | 23.4 |
| 108.5 | 14.0 | 15.2 | 16.5 | 18.0 | 19.7 | 21.5 | 23.7 |
| 109.0 | 14.1 | 15.3 | 16.7 | 18.2 | 19.8 | 21.8 | 23.9 |
| 109.5 | 14.3 | 15.5 | 16.8 | 18.3 | 20.0 | 22.0 | 24.2 |

**Weight-for-height for boys (continued)**

| Height (cm) | Z-scores (weight in kg) | | | | | | |
|---|---|---|---|---|---|---|---|
| | -3 SD | -2 SD | -1 SD | Median | 1 SD | 2 SD | 3 SD |
| **110.0** | 14.4 | 15.6 | 17.0 | 18.5 | 20.2 | 22.2 | 24.4 |
| **110.5** | 14.5 | 15.8 | 17.1 | 18.7 | 20.4 | 22.4 | 24.7 |
| **111.0** | 14.6 | 15.9 | 17.3 | 18.9 | 20.7 | 22.7 | 25.0 |
| **111.5** | 14.8 | 16.0 | 17.5 | 19.1 | 20.9 | 22.9 | 25.2 |
| **112.0** | 14.9 | 16.2 | 17.6 | 19.2 | 21.1 | 23.1 | 25.5 |
| **112.5** | 15.0 | 16.3 | 17.8 | 19.4 | 21.3 | 23.4 | 25.8 |
| **113.0** | 15.2 | 16.5 | 18.0 | 19.6 | 21.5 | 23.6 | 26.0 |
| **113.5** | 15.3 | 16.6 | 18.1 | 19.8 | 21.7 | 23.9 | 26.3 |
| **114.0** | 15.4 | 16.8 | 18.3 | 20.0 | 21.9 | 24.1 | 26.6 |
| **114.5** | 15.6 | 16.9 | 18.5 | 20.2 | 22.1 | 24.4 | 26.9 |
| **115.0** | 15.7 | 17.1 | 18.6 | 20.4 | 22.4 | 24.6 | 27.2 |
| **115.5** | 15.8 | 17.2 | 18.8 | 20.6 | 22.6 | 24.9 | 27.5 |
| **116.0** | 16.0 | 17.4 | 19.0 | 20.8 | 22.8 | 25.1 | 27.8 |
| **116.5** | 16.1 | 17.5 | 19.2 | 21.0 | 23.0 | 25.4 | 28.0 |
| **117.0** | 16.2 | 17.7 | 19.3 | 21.2 | 23.3 | 25.6 | 28.3 |
| **117.5** | 16.4 | 17.9 | 19.5 | 21.4 | 23.5 | 25.9 | 28.6 |
| **118.0** | 16.5 | 18.0 | 19.7 | 21.6 | 23.7 | 26.1 | 28.9 |
| **118.5** | 16.7 | 18.2 | 19.9 | 21.8 | 23.9 | 26.4 | 29.2 |
| **119.0** | 16.8 | 18.3 | 20.0 | 22.0 | 24.1 | 26.6 | 29.5 |
| **119.5** | 16.9 | 18.5 | 20.2 | 22.2 | 24.4 | 26.9 | 29.8 |
| **120.0** | 17.1 | 18.6 | 20.4 | 22.4 | 24.6 | 27.2 | 30.1 |

**Weight-for-height for girls**

| Height (cm) | Z-scores (weight in kg) | | | | | | |
|---|---|---|---|---|---|---|---|
| | -3 SD | -2 SD | -1 SD | Median | 1 SD | 2 SD | 3 SD |
| 65.0 | 5.6 | 6.1 | 6.6 | 7.2 | 7.9 | 8.7 | 9.7 |
| 65.5 | 5.7 | 6.2 | 6.7 | 7.4 | 8.1 | 8.9 | 9.8 |
| 66.0 | 5.8 | 6.3 | 6.8 | 7.5 | 8.2 | 9.0 | 10.0 |
| 66.5 | 5.8 | 6.4 | 6.9 | 7.6 | 8.3 | 9.1 | 10.1 |
| 67.0 | 5.9 | 6.4 | 7.0 | 7.7 | 8.4 | 9.3 | 10.2 |
| 67.5 | 6.0 | 6.5 | 7.1 | 7.8 | 8.5 | 9.4 | 10.4 |
| 68.0 | 6.1 | 6.6 | 7.2 | 7.9 | 8.7 | 9.5 | 10.5 |
| 68.5 | 6.2 | 6.7 | 7.3 | 8.0 | 8.8 | 9.7 | 10.7 |
| 69.0 | 6.3 | 6.8 | 7.4 | 8.1 | 8.9 | 9.8 | 10.8 |
| 69.5 | 6.3 | 6.9 | 7.5 | 8.2 | 9.0 | 9.9 | 10.9 |
| 70.0 | 6.4 | 7.0 | 7.6 | 8.3 | 9.1 | 10.0 | 11.1 |
| 70.5 | 6.5 | 7.1 | 7.7 | 8.4 | 9.2 | 10.1 | 11.2 |
| 71.0 | 6.6 | 7.1 | 7.8 | 8.5 | 9.3 | 10.3 | 11.3 |
| 71.5 | 6.7 | 7.2 | 7.9 | 8.6 | 9.4 | 10.4 | 11.5 |
| 72.0 | 6.7 | 7.3 | 8.0 | 8.7 | 9.5 | 10.5 | 11.6 |
| 72.5 | 6.8 | 7.4 | 8.1 | 8.8 | 9.7 | 10.6 | 11.7 |
| 73.0 | 6.9 | 7.5 | 8.1 | 8.9 | 9.8 | 10.7 | 11.8 |
| 73.5 | 7.0 | 7.6 | 8.2 | 9.0 | 9.9 | 10.8 | 12.0 |
| 74.0 | 7.0 | 7.6 | 8.3 | 9.1 | 10.0 | 11.0 | 12.1 |
| 74.5 | 7.1 | 7.7 | 8.4 | 9.2 | 10.1 | 11.1 | 12.2 |
| 75.0 | 7.2 | 7.8 | 8.5 | 9.3 | 10.2 | 11.2 | 12.3 |
| 75.5 | 7.2 | 7.9 | 8.6 | 9.4 | 10.3 | 11.3 | 12.5 |
| 76.0 | 7.3 | 8.0 | 8.7 | 9.5 | 10.4 | 11.4 | 12.6 |
| 76.5 | 7.4 | 8.0 | 8.7 | 9.6 | 10.5 | 11.5 | 12.7 |
| 77.0 | 7.5 | 8.1 | 8.8 | 9.6 | 10.6 | 11.6 | 12.8 |
| 77.5 | 7.5 | 8.2 | 8.9 | 9.7 | 10.7 | 11.7 | 12.9 |
| 78.0 | 7.6 | 8.3 | 9.0 | 9.8 | 10.8 | 11.8 | 13.1 |
| 78.5 | 7.7 | 8.4 | 9.1 | 9.9 | 10.9 | 12.0 | 13.2 |
| 79.0 | 7.8 | 8.4 | 9.2 | 10.0 | 11.0 | 12.1 | 13.3 |
| 79.5 | 7.8 | 8.5 | 9.3 | 10.1 | 11.1 | 12.2 | 13.4 |

**Weight-for-height for girls (continued)**

| | Z-scores (weight in kg) | | | | | | |
|---|---|---|---|---|---|---|---|
| **Height (cm)** | **-3 SD** | **-2 SD** | **-1 SD** | **Median** | **1 SD** | **2 SD** | **3 SD** |
| **80.0** | 7.9 | 8.6 | 9.4 | 10.2 | 11.2 | 12.3 | 13.6 |
| **80.5** | 8.0 | 8.7 | 9.5 | 10.3 | 11.3 | 12.4 | 13.7 |
| **81.0** | 8.1 | 8.8 | 9.6 | 10.4 | 11.4 | 12.6 | 13.9 |
| **81.5** | 8.2 | 8.9 | 9.7 | 10.6 | 11.6 | 12.7 | 14.0 |
| **82.0** | 8.3 | 9.0 | 9.8 | 10.7 | 11.7 | 12.8 | 14.1 |
| **82.5** | 8.4 | 9.1 | 9.9 | 10.8 | 11.8 | 13.0 | 14.3 |
| **83.0** | 8.5 | 9.2 | 10.0 | 10.9 | 11.9 | 13.1 | 14.5 |
| **83.5** | 8.5 | 9.3 | 10.1 | 11.0 | 12.1 | 13.3 | 14.6 |
| **84.0** | 8.6 | 9.4 | 10.2 | 11.1 | 12.2 | 13.4 | 14.8 |
| **84.5** | 8.7 | 9.5 | 10.3 | 11.3 | 12.3 | 13.5 | 14.9 |
| **85.0** | 8.8 | 9.6 | 10.4 | 11.4 | 12.5 | 13.7 | 15.1 |
| **85.5** | 8.9 | 9.7 | 10.6 | 11.5 | 12.6 | 13.8 | 15.3 |
| **86.0** | 9.0 | 9.8 | 10.7 | 11.6 | 12.7 | 14.0 | 15.4 |
| **86.5** | 9.1 | 9.9 | 10.8 | 11.8 | 12.9 | 14.2 | 15.6 |
| **87.0** | 9.2 | 10.0 | 10.9 | 11.9 | 13.0 | 14.3 | 15.8 |
| **87.5** | 9.3 | 10.1 | 11.0 | 12.0 | 13.2 | 14.5 | 15.9 |
| **88.0** | 9.4 | 10.2 | 11.1 | 12.1 | 13.3 | 14.6 | 16.1 |
| **88.5** | 9.5 | 10.3 | 11.2 | 12.3 | 13.4 | 14.8 | 16.3 |
| **89.0** | 9.6 | 10.4 | 11.4 | 12.4 | 13.6 | 14.9 | 16.4 |
| **89.5** | 9.7 | 10.5 | 11.5 | 12.5 | 13.7 | 15.1 | 16.6 |
| **90.0** | 9.8 | 10.6 | 11.6 | 12.6 | 13.8 | 15.2 | 16.8 |
| **90.5** | 9.9 | 10.7 | 11.7 | 12.8 | 14.0 | 15.4 | 16.9 |
| **91.0** | 10.0 | 10.9 | 11.8 | 12.9 | 14.1 | 15.5 | 17.1 |
| **91.5** | 10.1 | 11.0 | 11.9 | 13.0 | 14.3 | 15.7 | 17.3 |
| **92.0** | 10.2 | 11.1 | 12.0 | 13.1 | 14.4 | 15.8 | 17.4 |
| **92.5** | 10.3 | 11.2 | 12.1 | 13.3 | 14.5 | 16.0 | 17.6 |
| **93.0** | 10.4 | 11.3 | 12.3 | 13.4 | 14.7 | 16.1 | 17.8 |
| **93.5** | 10.5 | 11.4 | 12.4 | 13.5 | 14.8 | 16.3 | 17.9 |
| **94.0** | 10.6 | 11.5 | 12.5 | 13.6 | 14.9 | 16.4 | 18.1 |
| **94.5** | 10.7 | 11.6 | 12.6 | 13.8 | 15.1 | 16.6 | 18.3 |

**Weight-for-height for girls (continued)**

| Height (cm) | Z-scores (weight in kg) | | | | | | |
|---|---|---|---|---|---|---|---|
| | -3 SD | -2 SD | -1 SD | Median | 1 SD | 2 SD | 3 SD |
| **95.0** | 10.8 | 11.7 | 12.7 | 13.9 | 15.2 | 16.7 | 18.5 |
| **95.5** | 10.8 | 11.8 | 12.8 | 14.0 | 15.4 | 16.9 | 18.6 |
| **96.0** | 10.9 | 11.9 | 12.9 | 14.1 | 15.5 | 17.0 | 18.8 |
| **96.5** | 11.0 | 12.0 | 13.1 | 14.3 | 15.6 | 17.2 | 19.0 |
| **97.0** | 11.1 | 12.1 | 13.2 | 14.4 | 15.8 | 17.4 | 19.2 |
| **97.5** | 11.2 | 12.2 | 13.3 | 14.5 | 15.9 | 17.5 | 19.3 |
| **98.0** | 11.3 | 12.3 | 13.4 | 14.7 | 16.1 | 17.7 | 19.5 |
| **98.5** | 11.4 | 12.4 | 13.5 | 14.8 | 16.2 | 17.9 | 19.7 |
| **99.0** | 11.5 | 12.5 | 13.7 | 14.9 | 16.4 | 18.0 | 19.9 |
| **99.5** | 11.6 | 12.7 | 13.8 | 15.1 | 16.5 | 18.2 | 20.1 |
| **100.0** | 11.7 | 12.8 | 13.9 | 15.2 | 16.7 | 18.4 | 20.3 |
| **100.5** | 11.9 | 12.9 | 14.1 | 15.4 | 16.9 | 18.6 | 20.5 |
| **101.0** | 12.0 | 13.0 | 14.2 | 15.5 | 17.0 | 18.7 | 20.7 |
| **101.5** | 12.1 | 13.1 | 14.3 | 15.7 | 17.2 | 18.9 | 20.9 |
| **102.0** | 12.2 | 13.3 | 14.5 | 15.8 | 17.4 | 19.1 | 21.1 |
| **102.5** | 12.3 | 13.4 | 14.6 | 16.0 | 17.5 | 19.3 | 21.4 |
| **103.0** | 12.4 | 13.5 | 14.7 | 16.1 | 17.7 | 19.5 | 21.6 |
| **103.5** | 12.5 | 13.6 | 14.9 | 16.3 | 17.9 | 19.7 | 21.8 |
| **104.0** | 12.6 | 13.8 | 15.0 | 16.4 | 18.1 | 19.9 | 22.0 |
| **104.5** | 12.8 | 13.9 | 15.2 | 16.6 | 18.2 | 20.1 | 22.3 |
| **105.0** | 12.9 | 14.0 | 15.3 | 16.8 | 18.4 | 20.3 | 22.5 |
| **105.5** | 13.0 | 14.2 | 15.5 | 16.9 | 18.6 | 20.5 | 22.7 |
| **106.0** | 13.1 | 14.3 | 15.6 | 17.1 | 18.8 | 20.8 | 23.0 |
| **106.5** | 13.3 | 14.5 | 15.8 | 17.3 | 19.0 | 21.0 | 23.2 |
| **107.0** | 13.4 | 14.6 | 15.9 | 17.5 | 19.2 | 21.2 | 23.5 |
| **107.5** | 13.5 | 14.7 | 16.1 | 17.7 | 19.4 | 21.4 | 23.7 |
| **108.0** | 13.7 | 14.9 | 16.3 | 17.8 | 19.6 | 21.7 | 24.0 |
| **108.5** | 13.8 | 15.0 | 16.4 | 18.0 | 19.8 | 21.9 | 24.3 |
| **109.0** | 13.9 | 15.2 | 16.6 | 18.2 | 20.0 | 22.1 | 24.5 |
| **109.5** | 14.1 | 15.4 | 16.8 | 18.4 | 20.3 | 22.4 | 24.8 |

Weight-for-height for girls (continued)

| Height (cm) | Z-scores (weight in kg) | | | | | | |
|---|---|---|---|---|---|---|---|
| | -3 SD | -2 SD | -1 SD | Median | 1 SD | 2 SD | 3 SD |
| 110.0 | 14.2 | 15.5 | 17.0 | 18.6 | 20.5 | 22.6 | 25.1 |
| 110.5 | 14.4 | 15.7 | 17.1 | 18.8 | 20.7 | 22.9 | 25.4 |
| 111.0 | 14.5 | 15.8 | 17.3 | 19.0 | 20.9 | 23.1 | 25.7 |
| 111.5 | 14.7 | 16.0 | 17.5 | 19.2 | 21.2 | 23.4 | 26.0 |
| 112.0 | 14.8 | 16.2 | 17.7 | 19.4 | 21.4 | 23.6 | 26.2 |
| 112.5 | 15.0 | 16.3 | 17.9 | 19.6 | 21.6 | 23.9 | 26.5 |
| 113.0 | 15.1 | 16.5 | 18.0 | 19.8 | 21.8 | 24.2 | 26.8 |
| 113.5 | 15.3 | 16.7 | 18.2 | 20.0 | 22.1 | 24.4 | 27.1 |
| 114.0 | 15.4 | 16.8 | 18.4 | 20.2 | 22.3 | 24.7 | 27.4 |
| 114.5 | 15.6 | 17.0 | 18.6 | 20.5 | 22.6 | 25.0 | 27.8 |
| 115.0 | 15.7 | 17.2 | 18.8 | 20.7 | 22.8 | 25.2 | 28.1 |
| 115.5 | 15.9 | 17.3 | 19.0 | 20.9 | 23.0 | 25.5 | 28.4 |
| 116.0 | 16.0 | 17.5 | 19.2 | 21.1 | 23.3 | 25.8 | 28.7 |
| 116.5 | 16.2 | 17.7 | 19.4 | 21.3 | 23.5 | 26.1 | 29.0 |
| 117.0 | 16.3 | 17.8 | 19.6 | 21.5 | 23.8 | 26.3 | 29.3 |
| 117.5 | 16.5 | 18.0 | 19.8 | 21.7 | 24.0 | 26.6 | 29.6 |
| 118.0 | 16.6 | 18.2 | 19.9 | 22.0 | 24.2 | 26.9 | 29.9 |
| 118.5 | 16.8 | 18.4 | 20.1 | 22.2 | 24.5 | 27.2 | 30.3 |
| 119.0 | 16.9 | 18.5 | 20.3 | 22.4 | 24.7 | 27.4 | 30.6 |
| 119.5 | 17.1 | 18.7 | 20.5 | 22.6 | 25.0 | 27.7 | 30.9 |
| 120.0 | 17.3 | 18.9 | 20.7 | 22.8 | 25.2 | 28.0 | 31.2 |

## Length-for-age Boys birth to 2 years (z scores)

| Month | -3SD | -2SD | -1SD | Median | 1SD | 2SD | 3SD |
|---|---|---|---|---|---|---|---|
| 0 | 44.2 | 46.1 | 48.0 | 49.9 | 51.8 | 53.7 | 55.6 |
| 1 | 48.9 | 50.8 | 52.8 | 54.7 | 56.7 | 58.6 | 60.6 |
| 2 | 52.4 | 54.4 | 56.4 | 58.4 | 60.4 | 62.4 | 64.4 |
| 3 | 55.3 | 57.3 | 59.4 | 61.4 | 63.5 | 65.5 | 67.6 |
| 4 | 57.6 | 59.7 | 61.8 | 63.9 | 66.0 | 68.0 | 70.1 |
| 5 | 59.6 | 61.7 | 63.8 | 65.9 | 68.0 | 70.1 | 72.2 |
| 6 | 61.2 | 63.3 | 65.5 | 67.6 | 69.8 | 71.9 | 74.0 |
| 7 | 62.7 | 64.8 | 67.0 | 69.2 | 71.3 | 73.5 | 75.7 |
| 8 | 64.0 | 66.2 | 68.4 | 70.6 | 72.8 | 75.0 | 77.2 |
| 9 | 65.2 | 67.5 | 69.7 | 72.0 | 74.2 | 76.5 | 78.7 |
| 10 | 66.4 | 68.7 | 71.0 | 73.3 | 75.6 | 77.9 | 80.1 |
| 11 | 67.6 | 69.9 | 72.2 | 74.5 | 76.9 | 79.2 | 81.5 |
| 12 | 68.6 | 71.0 | 73.4 | 75.7 | 78.1 | 80.5 | 82.9 |
| 13 | 69.6 | 72.1 | 74.5 | 76.9 | 79.3 | 81.8 | 84.2 |
| 14 | 70.6 | 73.1 | 75.6 | 78.0 | 80.5 | 83.0 | 85.5 |
| 15 | 71.6 | 74.1 | 76.6 | 79.1 | 81.7 | 84.2 | 86.7 |
| 16 | 72.5 | 75.0 | 77.6 | 80.2 | 82.8 | 85.4 | 88.0 |
| 17 | 73.3 | 76.0 | 78.6 | 81.2 | 83.9 | 86.5 | 89.2 |
| 18 | 74.2 | 76.9 | 79.6 | 82.3 | 85.0 | 87.7 | 90.4 |
| 19 | 75.0 | 77.7 | 80.5 | 83.2 | 86.0 | 88.8 | 91.5 |
| 20 | 75.8 | 78.6 | 81.4 | 84.2 | 87.0 | 89.8 | 92.6 |
| 21 | 76.5 | 79.4 | 82.3 | 85.1 | 88.0 | 90.9 | 93.8 |
| 22 | 77.2 | 80.2 | 83.1 | 86.0 | 89.0 | 91.9 | 94.9 |
| 23 | 78.0 | 81.0 | 83.9 | 86.9 | 89.9 | 92.9 | 95.9 |
| 24 | 78.7 | 81.7 | 84.8 | 87.8 | 90.9 | 93.9 | 97.0 |

## Length-for-age Girls birth to 2 years (z scores)

| Month | -3SD | -2SD | -1SD | Median | 1SD | 2SD | 3SD |
|---|---|---|---|---|---|---|---|
| 0 | 43.6 | 45.4 | 47.3 | 49.1 | 51.0 | 52.9 | 54.7 |
| 1 | 47.8 | 49.8 | 51.7 | 53.7 | 55.6 | 57.6 | 59.5 |
| 2 | 51.0 | 53.0 | 55.0 | 57.1 | 59.1 | 61.1 | 63.2 |
| 3 | 53.5 | 55.6 | 57.7 | 59.8 | 61.9 | 64.0 | 66.1 |
| 4 | 55.6 | 57.8 | 59.9 | 62.1 | 64.3 | 66.4 | 68.6 |
| 5 | 57.4 | 59.6 | 61.8 | 64.0 | 66.2 | 68.5 | 70.7 |
| 6 | 58.9 | 61.2 | 63.5 | 65.7 | 68.0 | 70.3 | 72.5 |
| 7 | 60.3 | 62.7 | 65.0 | 67.3 | 69.6 | 71.9 | 74.2 |
| 8 | 61.7 | 64.0 | 66.4 | 68.7 | 71.1 | 73.5 | 75.8 |
| 9 | 62.9 | 65.3 | 67.7 | 70.1 | 72.6 | 75.0 | 77.4 |
| 10 | 64.1 | 66.5 | 69.0 | 71.5 | 73.9 | 76.4 | 78.9 |
| 11 | 65.2 | 67.7 | 70.3 | 72.8 | 75.3 | 77.8 | 80.3 |
| 12 | 66.3 | 68.9 | 71.4 | 74.0 | 76.6 | 79.2 | 81.7 |
| 13 | 67.3 | 70.0 | 72.6 | 75.2 | 77.8 | 80.5 | 83.1 |
| 14 | 68.3 | 71.0 | 73.7 | 76.4 | 79.1 | 81.7 | 84.4 |
| 15 | 69.3 | 72.0 | 74.8 | 77.5 | 80.2 | 83.0 | 85.7 |
| 16 | 70.2 | 73.0 | 75.8 | 78.6 | 81.4 | 84.2 | 87.0 |
| 17 | 71.1 | 74.0 | 76.8 | 79.7 | 82.5 | 85.4 | 88.2 |
| 18 | 72.0 | 74.9 | 77.8 | 80.7 | 83.6 | 86.5 | 89.4 |
| 19 | 72.8 | 75.8 | 78.8 | 81.7 | 84.7 | 87.6 | 90.6 |
| 20 | 73.7 | 76.7 | 79.7 | 82.7 | 85.7 | 88.7 | 91.7 |
| 21 | 74.5 | 77.5 | 80.6 | 83.7 | 86.7 | 89.8 | 92.9 |
| 22 | 75.2 | 78.4 | 81.5 | 84.6 | 87.7 | 90.8 | 94.0 |
| 23 | 76.0 | 79.2 | 82.3 | 85.5 | 88.7 | 91.9 | 95.0 |
| 24 | 76.7 | 80.0 | 83.2 | 86.4 | 89.6 | 92.9 | 96.1 |

## Height-for-age Boys 2 to 5 years (z scores)

| Month | -3SD | -2SD | -1SD | Median | 1SD | 2SD | 3SD |
|---|---|---|---|---|---|---|---|
| 24 | 78.0 | 81.0 | 84.1 | 87.1 | 90.2 | 93.2 | 96.3 |
| 25 | 78.6 | 81.7 | 84.9 | 88.0 | 91.1 | 94.2 | 97.3 |
| 26 | 79.3 | 82.5 | 85.6 | 88.8 | 92.0 | 95.2 | 98.3 |
| 27 | 79.9 | 83.1 | 86.4 | 89.6 | 92.9 | 96.1 | 99.3 |
| 28 | 80.5 | 83.8 | 87.1 | 90.4 | 93.7 | 97.0 | 100.3 |
| 29 | 81.1 | 84.5 | 87.8 | 91.2 | 94.5 | 97.9 | 101.2 |
| 30 | 81.7 | 85.1 | 88.5 | 91.9 | 95.3 | 98.7 | 102.1 |
| 31 | 82.3 | 85.7 | 89.2 | 92.7 | 96.1 | 99.6 | 103.0 |

| | | | | | | | |
|---|---|---|---|---|---|---|---|
| 32 | 82.8 | 86.4 | 89.9 | 93.4 | 96.9 | 100.4 | 103.9 |
| 33 | 83.4 | 86.9 | 90.5 | 94.1 | 97.6 | 101.2 | 104.8 |
| 34 | 83.9 | 87.5 | 91.1 | 94.8 | 98.4 | 102.0 | 105.6 |
| 35 | 84.4 | 88.1 | 91.8 | 95.4 | 99.1 | 102.7 | 106.4 |
| 36 | 85.0 | 88.7 | 92.4 | 96.1 | 99.8 | 103.5 | 107.2 |
| 37 | 85.5 | 89.2 | 93.0 | 96.7 | 100.5 | 104.2 | 108.0 |
| 38 | 86.0 | 89.8 | 93.6 | 97.4 | 101.2 | 105.0 | 108.8 |
| 39 | 86.5 | 90.3 | 94.2 | 98.0 | 101.8 | 105.7 | 109.5 |
| 40 | 87.0 | 90.9 | 94.7 | 98.6 | 102.5 | 106.4 | 110.3 |
| 41 | 87.5 | 91.4 | 95.3 | 99.2 | 103.2 | 107.1 | 111.0 |
| 42 | 88.0 | 91.9 | 95.9 | 99.9 | 103.8 | 107.8 | 111.7 |
| 43 | 88.4 | 92.4 | 96.4 | 100.4 | 104.5 | 108.5 | 112.5 |
| 44 | 88.9 | 93.0 | 97.0 | 101.0 | 105.1 | 109.1 | 113.2 |
| 45 | 89.4 | 93.5 | 97.5 | 101.6 | 105.7 | 109.8 | 113.9 |
| 46 | 89.8 | 94.0 | 98.1 | 102.2 | 106.3 | 110.4 | 114.6 |
| 47 | 90.3 | 94.4 | 98.6 | 102.8 | 106.9 | 111.1 | 115.2 |
| 48 | 90.7 | 94.9 | 99.1 | 103.3 | 107.5 | 111.7 | 115.9 |
| 49 | 91.2 | 95.4 | 99.7 | 103.9 | 108.1 | 112.4 | 116.6 |
| 50 | 91.6 | 95.9 | 100.2 | 104.4 | 108.7 | 113.0 | 117.3 |
| 51 | 92.1 | 96.4 | 100.7 | 105.0 | 109.3 | 113.6 | 117.9 |
| 52 | 92.5 | 96.9 | 101.2 | 105.6 | 109.9 | 114.2 | 118.6 |
| 53 | 93.0 | 97.4 | 101.7 | 106.1 | 110.5 | 114.9 | 119.2 |
| 54 | 93.4 | 97.8 | 102.3 | 106.7 | 111.1 | 115.5 | 119.9 |
| 55 | 93.9 | 98.3 | 102.8 | 107.2 | 111.7 | 116.1 | 120.6 |
| 56 | 94.3 | 98.8 | 103.3 | 107.8 | 112.3 | 116.7 | 121.2 |
| 57 | 94.7 | 99.3 | 103.8 | 108.3 | 112.8 | 117.4 | 121.9 |
| 58 | 95.2 | 99.7 | 104.3 | 108.9 | 113.4 | 118.0 | 122.6 |
| 59 | 95.6 | 100.2 | 104.8 | 109.4 | 114.0 | 118.6 | 123.2 |
| 60 | 96.1 | 100.7 | 105.3 | 110.0 | 114.6 | 119.2 | 123.9 |

**Height-for-age Girls 2 to 5 years (z scores)**

| Month | -3SD | -2SD | -1SD | Median | 1SD | 2SD | 3SD |
|---|---|---|---|---|---|---|---|
| 24 | 76.0 | 79.3 | 82.5 | 85.7 | 88.9 | 92.2 | 95.4 |
| 25 | 76.8 | 80.0 | 83.3 | 86.6 | 89.9 | 93.1 | 96.4 |
| 26 | 77.5 | 80.8 | 84.1 | 87.4 | 90.8 | 94.1 | 97.4 |
| 27 | 78.1 | 81.5 | 84.9 | 88.3 | 91.7 | 95.0 | 98.4 |
| 28 | 78.8 | 82.2 | 85.7 | 89.1 | 92.5 | 96.0 | 99.4 |
| 29 | 79.5 | 82.9 | 86.4 | 89.9 | 93.4 | 96.9 | 100.3 |
| 30 | 80.1 | 83.6 | 87.1 | 90.7 | 94.2 | 97.7 | 101.3 |
| 31 | 80.7 | 84.3 | 87.9 | 91.4 | 95.0 | 98.6 | 102.2 |
| 32 | 81.3 | 84.9 | 88.6 | 92.2 | 95.8 | 99.4 | 103.1 |
| 33 | 81.9 | 85.6 | 89.3 | 92.9 | 96.6 | 100.3 | 103.9 |
| 34 | 82.5 | 86.2 | 89.9 | 93.6 | 97.4 | 101.1 | 104.8 |
| 35 | 83.1 | 86.8 | 90.6 | 94.4 | 98.1 | 101.9 | 105.6 |
| 36 | 83.6 | 87.4 | 91.2 | 95.1 | 98.9 | 102.7 | 106.5 |
| 37 | 84.2 | 88.0 | 91.9 | 95.7 | 99.6 | 103.4 | 107.3 |
| 38 | 84.7 | 88.6 | 92.5 | 96.4 | 100.3 | 104.2 | 108.1 |
| 39 | 85.3 | 89.2 | 93.1 | 97.1 | 101.0 | 105.0 | 108.9 |
| 40 | 85.8 | 89.8 | 93.8 | 97.7 | 101.7 | 105.7 | 109.7 |
| 41 | 86.3 | 90.4 | 94.4 | 98.4 | 102.4 | 106.4 | 110.5 |
| 42 | 86.8 | 90.9 | 95.0 | 99.0 | 103.1 | 107.2 | 111.2 |
| 43 | 87.4 | 91.5 | 95.6 | 99.7 | 103.8 | 107.9 | 112.0 |
| 44 | 87.9 | 92.0 | 96.2 | 100.3 | 104.5 | 108.6 | 112.7 |
| 45 | 88.4 | 92.5 | 96.7 | 100.9 | 105.1 | 109.3 | 113.5 |
| 46 | 88.9 | 93.1 | 97.3 | 101.5 | 105.8 | 110.0 | 114.2 |
| 47 | 89.3 | 93.6 | 97.9 | 102.1 | 106.4 | 110.7 | 114.9 |
| 48 | 89.8 | 94.1 | 98.4 | 102.7 | 107.0 | 111.3 | 115.7 |
| 49 | 90.3 | 94.6 | 99.0 | 103.3 | 107.7 | 112.0 | 116.4 |
| 50 | 90.7 | 95.1 | 99.5 | 103.9 | 108.3 | 112.7 | 117.1 |
| 51 | 91.2 | 95.6 | 100.1 | 104.5 | 108.9 | 113.3 | 117.7 |
| 52 | 91.7 | 96.1 | 100.6 | 105.0 | 109.5 | 114.0 | 118.4 |
| 53 | 92.1 | 96.6 | 101.1 | 105.6 | 110.1 | 114.6 | 119.1 |
| 54 | 92.6 | 97.1 | 101.6 | 106.2 | 110.7 | 115.2 | 119.8 |
| 55 | 93.0 | 97.6 | 102.2 | 106.7 | 111.3 | 115.9 | 120.4 |
| 56 | 93.4 | 98.1 | 102.7 | 107.3 | 111.9 | 116.5 | 121.1 |
| 57 | 93.9 | 98.5 | 103.2 | 107.8 | 112.5 | 117.1 | 121.8 |
| 58 | 94.3 | 99.0 | 103.7 | 108.4 | 113.0 | 117.7 | 122.4 |
| 59 | 94.7 | 99.5 | 104.2 | 108.9 | 113.6 | 118.3 | 123.1 |
| 60 | 95.2 | 99.9 | 104.7 | 109.4 | 114.2 | 118.9 | 123.7 |

## BMI-for-Age for boys birth to 5 years (z scores)

| Month | -3SD | -2SD | -1SD | Median | 1SD | 2SD | 3SD |
|---|---|---|---|---|---|---|---|
| 0 | 10.2 | 11.1 | 12.2 | 13.4 | 14.8 | 16.3 | 18.1 |
| 1 | 11.3 | 12.4 | 13.6 | 14.9 | 16.3 | 17.8 | 19.4 |
| 2 | 12.5 | 13.7 | 15.0 | 16.3 | 17.8 | 19.4 | 21.1 |
| 3 | 13.1 | 14.3 | 15.5 | 16.9 | 18.4 | 20.0 | 21.8 |
| 4 | 13.4 | 14.5 | 15.8 | 17.2 | 18.7 | 20.3 | 22.1 |
| 5 | 13.5 | 14.7 | 15.9 | 17.3 | 18.8 | 20.5 | 22.3 |
| 6 | 13.6 | 14.7 | 16.0 | 17.3 | 18.8 | 20.5 | 22.3 |
| 7 | 13.7 | 14.8 | 16.0 | 17.3 | 18.8 | 20.5 | 22.3 |
| 8 | 13.6 | 14.7 | 15.9 | 17.3 | 18.7 | 20.4 | 22.2 |
| 9 | 13.6 | 14.7 | 15.8 | 17.2 | 18.6 | 20.3 | 22.1 |
| 10 | 13.5 | 14.6 | 15.7 | 17.0 | 18.5 | 20.1 | 22.0 |
| 11 | 13.4 | 14.5 | 15.6 | 16.9 | 18.4 | 20.0 | 21.8 |
| 12 | 13.4 | 14.4 | 15.5 | 16.8 | 18.2 | 19.8 | 21.6 |
| 13 | 13.3 | 14.3 | 15.4 | 16.7 | 18.1 | 19.7 | 21.5 |
| 14 | 13.2 | 14.2 | 15.3 | 16.6 | 18.0 | 19.5 | 21.3 |
| 15 | 13.1 | 14.1 | 15.2 | 16.4 | 17.8 | 19.4 | 21.2 |
| 16 | 13.1 | 14.0 | 15.1 | 16.3 | 17.7 | 19.3 | 21.0 |
| 17 | 13.0 | 13.9 | 15.0 | 16.2 | 17.6 | 19.1 | 20.9 |
| 18 | 12.9 | 13.9 | 14.9 | 16.1 | 17.5 | 19.0 | 20.8 |
| 19 | 12.9 | 13.8 | 14.9 | 16.1 | 17.4 | 18.9 | 20.7 |
| 20 | 12.8 | 13.7 | 14.8 | 16.0 | 17.3 | 18.8 | 20.6 |
| 21 | 12.8 | 13.7 | 14.7 | 15.9 | 17.2 | 18.7 | 20.5 |
| 22 | 12.7 | 13.6 | 14.7 | 15.8 | 17.2 | 18.7 | 20.4 |
| 23 | 12.7 | 13.6 | 14.6 | 15.8 | 17.1 | 18.6 | 20.3 |
| 24 | 12.9 | 13.8 | 14.8 | 16.0 | 17.3 | 18.9 | 20.6 |
| 25 | 12.8 | 13.8 | 14.8 | 16.0 | 17.3 | 18.8 | 20.5 |
| 26 | 12.8 | 13.7 | 14.8 | 15.9 | 17.3 | 18.8 | 20.5 |
| 27 | 12.7 | 13.7 | 14.7 | 15.9 | 17.2 | 18.7 | 20.4 |
| 28 | 12.7 | 13.6 | 14.7 | 15.9 | 17.2 | 18.7 | 20.4 |
| 29 | 12.7 | 13.6 | 14.7 | 15.8 | 17.1 | 18.6 | 20.3 |
| 30 | 12.6 | 13.6 | 14.6 | 15.8 | 17.1 | 18.6 | 20.2 |
| 31 | 12.6 | 13.5 | 14.6 | 15.8 | 17.1 | 18.5 | 20.2 |
| 32 | 12.5 | 13.5 | 14.6 | 15.7 | 17.0 | 18.5 | 20.1 |
| 33 | 12.5 | 13.5 | 14.5 | 15.7 | 17.0 | 18.5 | 20.1 |
| 34 | 12.5 | 13.4 | 14.5 | 15.7 | 17.0 | 18.4 | 20.0 |
| 35 | 12.4 | 13.4 | 14.5 | 15.6 | 16.9 | 18.4 | 20.0 |
| 36 | 12.4 | 13.4 | 14.4 | 15.6 | 16.9 | 18.4 | 20.0 |
| 37 | 12.4 | 13.3 | 14.4 | 15.6 | 16.9 | 18.3 | 19.9 |
| 38 | 12.3 | 13.3 | 14.4 | 15.5 | 16.8 | 18.3 | 19.9 |
| 39 | 12.3 | 13.3 | 14.3 | 15.5 | 16.8 | 18.3 | 19.9 |
| 40 | 12.3 | 13.2 | 14.3 | 15.5 | 16.8 | 18.2 | 19.9 |

| 41 | 12.2 | 13.2 | 14.3 | 15.5 | 16.8 | 18.2 | 19.9 |
|---|---|---|---|---|---|---|---|
| 42 | 12.2 | 13.2 | 14.3 | 15.4 | 16.8 | 18.2 | 19.8 |
| 43 | 12.2 | 13.2 | 14.2 | 15.4 | 16.7 | 18.2 | 19.8 |
| 44 | 12.2 | 13.1 | 14.2 | 15.4 | 16.7 | 18.2 | 19.8 |
| 45 | 12.2 | 13.1 | 14.2 | 15.4 | 16.7 | 18.2 | 19.8 |
| 46 | 12.1 | 13.1 | 14.2 | 15.4 | 16.7 | 18.2 | 19.8 |
| 47 | 12.1 | 13.1 | 14.2 | 15.3 | 16.7 | 18.2 | 19.9 |
| 48 | 12.1 | 13.1 | 14.1 | 15.3 | 16.7 | 18.2 | 19.9 |
| 49 | 12.1 | 13.0 | 14.1 | 15.3 | 16.7 | 18.2 | 19.9 |
| 50 | 12.1 | 13.0 | 14.1 | 15.3 | 16.7 | 18.2 | 19.9 |
| 51 | 12.1 | 13.0 | 14.1 | 15.3 | 16.6 | 18.2 | 19.9 |
| 52 | 12.0 | 13.0 | 14.1 | 15.3 | 16.6 | 18.2 | 19.9 |
| 53 | 12.0 | 13.0 | 14.1 | 15.3 | 16.6 | 18.2 | 20.0 |
| 54 | 12.0 | 13.0 | 14.0 | 15.3 | 16.6 | 18.2 | 20.0 |
| 55 | 12.0 | 13.0 | 14.0 | 15.2 | 16.6 | 18.2 | 20.0 |
| 56 | 12.0 | 12.9 | 14.0 | 15.2 | 16.6 | 18.2 | 20.1 |
| 57 | 12.0 | 12.9 | 14.0 | 15.2 | 16.6 | 18.2 | 20.1 |
| 58 | 12.0 | 12.9 | 14.0 | 15.2 | 16.6 | 18.3 | 20.2 |
| 59 | 12.0 | 12.9 | 14.0 | 15.2 | 16.6 | 18.3 | 20.2 |
| 60 | 12.0 | 12.9 | 14.0 | 15.2 | 16.6 | 18.3 | 20.3 |

## BMI-for-Age for girls birth to 5 years (z scores)

| Month | -3SD | -2SD | -1SD | Median | 1SD | 2SD | 3SD |
|---|---|---|---|---|---|---|---|
| 0 | 10.1 | 11.1 | 12.2 | 13.3 | 14.6 | 16.1 | 17.7 |
| 1 | 10.8 | 12.0 | 13.2 | 14.6 | 16.0 | 17.5 | 19.1 |
| 2 | 11.8 | 13.0 | 14.3 | 15.8 | 17.3 | 19.0 | 20.7 |
| 3 | 12.4 | 13.6 | 14.9 | 16.4 | 17.9 | 19.7 | 21.5 |
| 4 | 12.7 | 13.9 | 15.2 | 16.7 | 18.3 | 20.0 | 22.0 |
| 5 | 12.9 | 14.1 | 15.4 | 16.8 | 18.4 | 20.2 | 22.2 |
| 6 | 13.0 | 14.1 | 15.5 | 16.9 | 18.5 | 20.3 | 22.3 |
| 7 | 13.0 | 14.2 | 15.5 | 16.9 | 18.5 | 20.3 | 22.3 |
| 8 | 13.0 | 14.1 | 15.4 | 16.8 | 18.4 | 20.2 | 22.2 |
| 9 | 12.9 | 14.1 | 15.3 | 16.7 | 18.3 | 20.1 | 22.1 |
| 10 | 12.9 | 14.0 | 15.2 | 16.6 | 18.2 | 19.9 | 21.9 |
| 11 | 12.8 | 13.9 | 15.1 | 16.5 | 18.0 | 19.8 | 21.8 |
| 12 | 12.7 | 13.8 | 15.0 | 16.4 | 17.9 | 19.6 | 21.6 |
| 13 | 12.6 | 13.7 | 14.9 | 16.2 | 17.7 | 19.5 | 21.4 |
| 14 | 12.6 | 13.6 | 14.8 | 16.1 | 17.6 | 19.3 | 21.3 |
| 15 | 12.5 | 13.5 | 14.7 | 16.0 | 17.5 | 19.2 | 21.1 |
| 16 | 12.4 | 13.5 | 14.6 | 15.9 | 17.4 | 19.1 | 21.0 |
| 17 | 12.4 | 13.4 | 14.5 | 15.8 | 17.3 | 18.9 | 20.9 |
| 18 | 12.3 | 13.3 | 14.4 | 15.7 | 17.2 | 18.8 | 20.8 |
| 19 | 12.3 | 13.3 | 14.4 | 15.7 | 17.1 | 18.8 | 20.7 |
| 20 | 12.2 | 13.2 | 14.3 | 15.6 | 17.0 | 18.7 | 20.6 |

| 21 | 12.2 | 13.2 | 14.3 | 15.5 | 17.0 | 18.6 | 20.5 |
|---|---|---|---|---|---|---|---|
| 22 | 12.2 | 13.1 | 14.2 | 15.5 | 16.9 | 18.5 | 20.4 |
| 23 | 12.2 | 13.1 | 14.2 | 15.4 | 16.9 | 18.5 | 20.4 |
| 24 | 12.1 | 13.1 | 14.2 | 15.4 | 16.8 | 18.4 | 20.3 |
| 25 | 12.4 | 13.3 | 14.4 | 15.7 | 17.1 | 18.7 | 20.6 |
| 26 | 12.3 | 13.3 | 14.4 | 15.6 | 17.0 | 18.7 | 20.6 |
| 27 | 12.3 | 13.3 | 14.4 | 15.6 | 17.0 | 18.6 | 20.5 |
| 28 | 12.3 | 13.3 | 14.3 | 15.6 | 17.0 | 18.6 | 20.5 |
| 29 | 12.3 | 13.2 | 14.3 | 15.6 | 17.0 | 18.6 | 20.4 |
| 30 | 12.3 | 13.2 | 14.3 | 15.5 | 16.9 | 18.5 | 20.4 |
| 31 | 12.2 | 13.2 | 14.3 | 15.5 | 16.9 | 18.5 | 20.4 |
| 32 | 12.2 | 13.2 | 14.3 | 15.5 | 16.9 | 18.5 | 20.4 |
| 33 | 12.2 | 13.1 | 14.2 | 15.5 | 16.9 | 18.5 | 20.3 |
| 34 | 12.2 | 13.1 | 14.2 | 15.4 | 16.8 | 18.5 | 20.3 |
| 35 | 12.1 | 13.1 | 14.2 | 15.4 | 16.8 | 18.4 | 20.3 |
| 36 | 12.1 | 13.1 | 14.2 | 15.4 | 16.8 | 18.4 | 20.3 |
| 37 | 12.1 | 13.1 | 14.1 | 15.4 | 16.8 | 18.4 | 20.3 |
| 38 | 12.1 | 13.0 | 14.1 | 15.4 | 16.8 | 18.4 | 20.3 |
| 39 | 12.0 | 13.0 | 14.1 | 15.3 | 16.8 | 18.4 | 20.3 |
| 40 | 12.0 | 13.0 | 14.1 | 15.3 | 16.8 | 18.4 | 20.3 |
| 41 | 12.0 | 13.0 | 14.1 | 15.3 | 16.8 | 18.4 | 20.4 |
| 42 | 12.0 | 12.9 | 14.0 | 15.3 | 16.8 | 18.4 | 20.4 |
| 43 | 11.9 | 12.9 | 14.0 | 15.3 | 16.8 | 18.4 | 20.4 |
| 44 | 11.9 | 12.9 | 14.0 | 15.3 | 16.8 | 18.5 | 20.4 |
| 45 | 11.9 | 12.9 | 14.0 | 15.3 | 16.8 | 18.5 | 20.5 |
| 46 | 11.9 | 12.9 | 14.0 | 15.3 | 16.8 | 18.5 | 20.5 |
| 47 | 11.8 | 12.8 | 14.0 | 15.3 | 16.8 | 18.5 | 20.5 |
| 48 | 11.8 | 12.8 | 14.0 | 15.3 | 16.8 | 18.5 | 20.6 |
| 49 | 11.8 | 12.8 | 13.9 | 15.3 | 16.8 | 18.5 | 20.6 |
| 50 | 11.8 | 12.8 | 13.9 | 15.3 | 16.8 | 18.6 | 20.7 |
| 51 | 11.8 | 12.8 | 13.9 | 15.3 | 16.8 | 18.6 | 20.7 |
| 52 | 11.7 | 12.8 | 13.9 | 15.2 | 16.8 | 18.6 | 20.7 |
| 53 | 11.7 | 12.7 | 13.9 | 15.3 | 16.8 | 18.6 | 20.8 |
| 54 | 11.7 | 12.7 | 13.9 | 15.3 | 16.8 | 18.7 | 20.8 |
| 55 | 11.7 | 12.7 | 13.9 | 15.3 | 16.8 | 18.7 | 20.9 |
| 56 | 11.7 | 12.7 | 13.9 | 15.3 | 16.8 | 18.7 | 20.9 |
| 57 | 11.7 | 12.7 | 13.9 | 15.3 | 16.9 | 18.7 | 21.0 |
| 58 | 11.7 | 12.7 | 13.9 | 15.3 | 16.9 | 18.8 | 21.0 |
| 59 | 11.6 | 12.7 | 13.9 | 15.3 | 16.9 | 18.8 | 21.0 |
| 60 | 11.6 | 12.7 | 13.9 | 15.3 | 16.9 | 18.8 | 21.1 |

(ii) z-scores for BMI-for-age for children 5–19 years [Source: http://www.who.int/entity/growthref/who2007_bmi_for_age/en/-]

**BMI-for-age BOYS**

**5 to 19 years (z-scores)**

| | | Z-scores (BMI in kg/m$^2$) | | | | | | |
|---|---|---|---|---|---|---|---|---|
| Year: Month | Month | -3 SD | -2 SD | -1 SD | Median | 1 SD | 2 SD | 3 SD |
| 5: 1 | 61 | 12.1 | 13.0 | 14.1 | 15.3 | 16.6 | 18.3 | 20.2 |
| 5: 2 | 62 | 12.1 | 13.0 | 14.1 | 15.3 | 16.6 | 18.3 | 20.2 |
| 5: 3 | 63 | 12.1 | 13.0 | 14.1 | 15.3 | 16.7 | 18.3 | 20.2 |
| 5: 4 | 64 | 12.1 | 13.0 | 14.1 | 15.3 | 16.7 | 18.3 | 20.3 |
| 5: 5 | 65 | 12.1 | 13.0 | 14.1 | 15.3 | 16.7 | 18.3 | 20.3 |
| 5: 6 | 66 | 12.1 | 13.0 | 14.1 | 15.3 | 16.7 | 18.4 | 20.4 |
| 5: 7 | 67 | 12.1 | 13.0 | 14.1 | 15.3 | 16.7 | 18.4 | 20.4 |
| 5: 8 | 68 | 12.1 | 13.0 | 14.1 | 15.3 | 16.7 | 18.4 | 20.5 |
| 5: 9 | 69 | 12.1 | 13.0 | 14.1 | 15.3 | 16.7 | 18.4 | 20.5 |
| 5:10 | 70 | 12.1 | 13.0 | 14.1 | 15.3 | 16.7 | 18.5 | 20.6 |
| 5:11 | 71 | 12.1 | 13.0 | 14.1 | 15.3 | 16.7 | 18.5 | 20.6 |
| 6: 0 | 72 | 12.1 | 13.0 | 14.1 | 15.3 | 16.8 | 18.5 | 20.7 |
| 6: 1 | 73 | 12.1 | 13.0 | 14.1 | 15.3 | 16.8 | 18.6 | 20.8 |
| 6: 2 | 74 | 12.2 | 13.1 | 14.1 | 15.3 | 16.8 | 18.6 | 20.8 |
| 6: 3 | 75 | 12.2 | 13.1 | 14.1 | 15.3 | 16.8 | 18.6 | 20.9 |
| 6: 4 | 76 | 12.2 | 13.1 | 14.1 | 15.4 | 16.8 | 18.7 | 21.0 |
| 6: 5 | 77 | 12.2 | 13.1 | 14.1 | 15.4 | 16.9 | 18.7 | 21.0 |
| 6: 6 | 78 | 12.2 | 13.1 | 14.1 | 15.4 | 16.9 | 18.7 | 21.1 |
| 6: 7 | 79 | 12.2 | 13.1 | 14.1 | 15.4 | 16.9 | 18.8 | 21.2 |
| 6: 8 | 80 | 12.2 | 13.1 | 14.2 | 15.4 | 16.9 | 18.8 | 21.3 |
| 6: 9 | 81 | 12.2 | 13.1 | 14.2 | 15.4 | 17.0 | 18.9 | 21.3 |
| 6:10 | 82 | 12.2 | 13.1 | 14.2 | 15.4 | 17.0 | 18.9 | 21.4 |
| 6:11 | 83 | 12.2 | 13.1 | 14.2 | 15.5 | 17.0 | 19.0 | 21.5 |
| 7: 0 | 84 | 12.3 | 13.1 | 14.2 | 15.5 | 17.0 | 19.0 | 21.6 |
| 7: 1 | 85 | 12.3 | 13.2 | 14.2 | 15.5 | 17.1 | 19.1 | 21.7 |
| 7: 2 | 86 | 12.3 | 13.2 | 14.2 | 15.5 | 17.1 | 19.1 | 21.8 |

**BMI-for-age BOYS**

**5 to 19 years (z-scores)**

| | | Z-scores (BMI in kg/m$^2$) | | | | | | |
|---|---|---|---|---|---|---|---|---|
| Year: Month | Month | -3 SD | -2 SD | -1 SD | Median | 1 SD | 2 SD | 3 SD |
| 7: 3 | 87 | 12.3 | 13.2 | 14.3 | 15.5 | 17.1 | 19.2 | 21.9 |
| 7: 4 | 88 | 12.3 | 13.2 | 14.3 | 15.6 | 17.2 | 19.2 | 22.0 |
| 7: 5 | 89 | 12.3 | 13.2 | 14.3 | 15.6 | 17.2 | 19.3 | 22.0 |
| 7: 6 | 90 | 12.3 | 13.2 | 14.3 | 15.6 | 17.2 | 19.3 | 22.1 |
| 7: 7 | 91 | 12.3 | 13.2 | 14.3 | 15.6 | 17.3 | 19.4 | 22.2 |
| 7: 8 | 92 | 12.3 | 13.2 | 14.3 | 15.6 | 17.3 | 19.4 | 22.4 |
| 7: 9 | 93 | 12.4 | 13.3 | 14.3 | 15.7 | 17.3 | 19.5 | 22.5 |
| 7:10 | 94 | 12.4 | 13.3 | 14.4 | 15.7 | 17.4 | 19.6 | 22.6 |
| 7:11 | 95 | 12.4 | 13.3 | 14.4 | 15.7 | 17.4 | 19.6 | 22.7 |
| 8: 0 | 96 | 12.4 | 13.3 | 14.4 | 15.7 | 17.4 | 19.7 | 22.8 |
| 8: 1 | 97 | 12.4 | 13.3 | 14.4 | 15.8 | 17.5 | 19.7 | 22.9 |
| 8: 2 | 98 | 12.4 | 13.3 | 14.4 | 15.8 | 17.5 | 19.8 | 23.0 |
| 8: 3 | 99 | 12.4 | 13.3 | 14.4 | 15.8 | 17.5 | 19.9 | 23.1 |
| 8: 4 | 100 | 12.4 | 13.4 | 14.5 | 15.8 | 17.6 | 19.9 | 23.3 |
| 8: 5 | 101 | 12.5 | 13.4 | 14.5 | 15.9 | 17.6 | 20.0 | 23.4 |
| 8: 6 | 102 | 12.5 | 13.4 | 14.5 | 15.9 | 17.7 | 20.1 | 23.5 |
| 8: 7 | 103 | 12.5 | 13.4 | 14.5 | 15.9 | 17.7 | 20.1 | 23.6 |
| 8: 8 | 104 | 12.5 | 13.4 | 14.5 | 15.9 | 17.7 | 20.2 | 23.8 |
| 8: 9 | 105 | 12.5 | 13.4 | 14.6 | 16.0 | 17.8 | 20.3 | 23.9 |
| 8:10 | 106 | 12.5 | 13.5 | 14.6 | 16.0 | 17.8 | 20.3 | 24.0 |
| 8:11 | 107 | 12.5 | 13.5 | 14.6 | 16.0 | 17.9 | 20.4 | 24.2 |
| 9: 0 | 108 | 12.6 | 13.5 | 14.6 | 16.0 | 17.9 | 20.5 | 24.3 |
| 9: 1 | 109 | 12.6 | 13.5 | 14.6 | 16.1 | 18.0 | 20.5 | 24.4 |
| 9: 2 | 110 | 12.6 | 13.5 | 14.7 | 16.1 | 18.0 | 20.6 | 24.6 |
| 9: 3 | 111 | 12.6 | 13.5 | 14.7 | 16.1 | 18.0 | 20.7 | 24.7 |

## BMI-for-age BOYS

**5 to 19 years (z-scores)**

| | | Z-scores (BMI in kg/m²) | | | | | | |
|---|---|---|---|---|---|---|---|---|
| Year: Month | Month | -3 SD | -2 SD | -1 SD | Median | 1 SD | 2 SD | 3 SD |
| 9: 4 | 112 | 12.6 | 13.6 | 14.7 | 16.2 | 18.1 | 20.8 | 24.9 |
| 9: 5 | 113 | 12.6 | 13.6 | 14.7 | 16.2 | 18.1 | 20.8 | 25.0 |
| 9: 6 | 114 | 12.7 | 13.6 | 14.8 | 16.2 | 18.2 | 20.9 | 25.1 |
| 9: 7 | 115 | 12.7 | 13.6 | 14.8 | 16.3 | 18.2 | 21.0 | 25.3 |
| 9: 8 | 116 | 12.7 | 13.6 | 14.8 | 16.3 | 18.3 | 21.1 | 25.5 |
| 9: 9 | 117 | 12.7 | 13.7 | 14.8 | 16.3 | 18.3 | 21.2 | 25.6 |
| 9:10 | 118 | 12.7 | 13.7 | 14.9 | 16.4 | 18.4 | 21.2 | 25.8 |
| 9:11 | 119 | 12.8 | 13.7 | 14.9 | 16.4 | 18.4 | 21.3 | 25.9 |
| 10: 0 | 120 | 12.8 | 13.7 | 14.9 | 16.4 | 18.5 | 21.4 | 26.1 |
| 10: 1 | 121 | 12.8 | 13.8 | 15.0 | 16.5 | 18.5 | 21.5 | 26.2 |
| 10: 2 | 122 | 12.8 | 13.8 | 15.0 | 16.5 | 18.6 | 21.6 | 26.4 |
| 10: 3 | 123 | 12.8 | 13.8 | 15.0 | 16.6 | 18.6 | 21.7 | 26.6 |
| 10: 4 | 124 | 12.9 | 13.8 | 15.0 | 16.6 | 18.7 | 21.7 | 26.7 |
| 10: 5 | 125 | 12.9 | 13.9 | 15.1 | 16.6 | 18.8 | 21.8 | 26.9 |
| 10: 6 | 126 | 12.9 | 13.9 | 15.1 | 16.7 | 18.8 | 21.9 | 27.0 |
| 10: 7 | 127 | 12.9 | 13.9 | 15.1 | 16.7 | 18.9 | 22.0 | 27.2 |
| 10: 8 | 128 | 13.0 | 13.9 | 15.2 | 16.8 | 18.9 | 22.1 | 27.4 |
| 10: 9 | 129 | 13.0 | 14.0 | 15.2 | 16.8 | 19.0 | 22.2 | 27.5 |
| 10:10 | 130 | 13.0 | 14.0 | 15.2 | 16.9 | 19.0 | 22.3 | 27.7 |
| 10:11 | 131 | 13.0 | 14.0 | 15.3 | 16.9 | 19.1 | 22.4 | 27.9 |
| 11: 0 | 132 | 13.1 | 14.1 | 15.3 | 16.9 | 19.2 | 22.5 | 28.0 |
| 11: 1 | 133 | 13.1 | 14.1 | 15.3 | 17.0 | 19.2 | 22.5 | 28.2 |
| 11: 2 | 134 | 13.1 | 14.1 | 15.4 | 17.0 | 19.3 | 22.6 | 28.4 |
| 11: 3 | 135 | 13.1 | 14.1 | 15.4 | 17.1 | 19.3 | 22.7 | 28.5 |

## BMI-for-age BOYS

**5 to 19 years (z-scores)**

| | | Z-scores (BMI in kg/m²) | | | | | | |
|---|---|---|---|---|---|---|---|---|
| Year: Month | Month | -3 SD | -2 SD | -1 SD | Median | 1 SD | 2 SD | 3 SD |
| 11: 4 | 136 | 13.2 | 14.2 | 15.5 | 17.1 | 19.4 | 22.8 | 28.7 |
| 11: 5 | 137 | 13.2 | 14.2 | 15.5 | 17.2 | 19.5 | 22.9 | 28.8 |
| 11: 6 | 138 | 13.2 | 14.2 | 15.5 | 17.2 | 19.5 | 23.0 | 29.0 |
| 11: 7 | 139 | 13.2 | 14.3 | 15.6 | 17.3 | 19.6 | 23.1 | 29.2 |
| 11: 8 | 140 | 13.3 | 14.3 | 15.6 | 17.3 | 19.7 | 23.2 | 29.3 |
| 11: 9 | 141 | 13.3 | 14.3 | 15.7 | 17.4 | 19.7 | 23.3 | 29.5 |
| 11:10 | 142 | 13.3 | 14.4 | 15.7 | 17.4 | 19.8 | 23.4 | 29.6 |
| 11:11 | 143 | 13.4 | 14.4 | 15.7 | 17.5 | 19.9 | 23.5 | 29.8 |
| 12: 0 | 144 | 13.4 | 14.5 | 15.8 | 17.5 | 19.9 | 23.6 | 30.0 |
| 12: 1 | 145 | 13.4 | 14.5 | 15.8 | 17.6 | 20.0 | 23.7 | 30.1 |
| 12: 2 | 146 | 13.5 | 14.5 | 15.9 | 17.6 | 20.1 | 23.8 | 30.3 |
| 12: 3 | 147 | 13.5 | 14.6 | 15.9 | 17.7 | 20.2 | 23.9 | 30.4 |
| 12: 4 | 148 | 13.5 | 14.6 | 16.0 | 17.8 | 20.2 | 24.0 | 30.6 |
| 12: 5 | 149 | 13.6 | 14.6 | 16.0 | 17.8 | 20.3 | 24.1 | 30.7 |
| 12: 6 | 150 | 13.6 | 14.7 | 16.1 | 17.9 | 20.4 | 24.2 | 30.9 |
| 12: 7 | 151 | 13.6 | 14.7 | 16.1 | 17.9 | 20.4 | 24.3 | 31.0 |
| 12: 8 | 152 | 13.7 | 14.8 | 16.2 | 18.0 | 20.5 | 24.4 | 31.1 |
| 12: 9 | 153 | 13.7 | 14.8 | 16.2 | 18.0 | 20.6 | 24.5 | 31.3 |
| 12:10 | 154 | 13.7 | 14.8 | 16.3 | 18.1 | 20.7 | 24.6 | 31.4 |
| 12:11 | 155 | 13.8 | 14.9 | 16.3 | 18.2 | 20.8 | 24.7 | 31.6 |
| 13: 0 | 156 | 13.8 | 14.9 | 16.4 | 18.2 | 20.8 | 24.8 | 31.7 |
| 13: 1 | 157 | 13.8 | 15.0 | 16.4 | 18.3 | 20.9 | 24.9 | 31.8 |
| 13: 2 | 158 | 13.9 | 15.0 | 16.5 | 18.4 | 21.0 | 25.0 | 31.9 |
| 13: 3 | 159 | 13.9 | 15.1 | 16.5 | 18.4 | 21.1 | 25.1 | 32.1 |

## BMI-for-age BOYS

**5 to 19 years (z-scores)**

| | | Z-scores (BMI in kg/m$^2$) | | | | | | |
|---|---|---|---|---|---|---|---|---|
| Year: Month | Month | -3 SD | -2 SD | -1 SD | Median | 1 SD | 2 SD | 3 SD |
| 13: 4 | 160 | 14.0 | 15.1 | 16.6 | 18.5 | 21.1 | 25.2 | 32.2 |
| 13: 5 | 161 | 14.0 | 15.2 | 16.6 | 18.6 | 21.2 | 25.2 | 32.3 |
| 13: 6 | 162 | 14.0 | 15.2 | 16.7 | 18.6 | 21.3 | 25.3 | 32.4 |
| 13: 7 | 163 | 14.1 | 15.2 | 16.7 | 18.7 | 21.4 | 25.4 | 32.6 |
| 13: 8 | 164 | 14.1 | 15.3 | 16.8 | 18.7 | 21.5 | 25.5 | 32.7 |
| 13: 9 | 165 | 14.1 | 15.3 | 16.8 | 18.8 | 21.5 | 25.6 | 32.8 |
| 13:10 | 166 | 14.2 | 15.4 | 16.9 | 18.9 | 21.6 | 25.7 | 32.9 |
| 13:11 | 167 | 14.2 | 15.4 | 17.0 | 18.9 | 21.7 | 25.8 | 33.0 |
| 14: 0 | 168 | 14.3 | 15.5 | 17.0 | 19.0 | 21.8 | 25.9 | 33.1 |
| 14: 1 | 169 | 14.3 | 15.5 | 17.1 | 19.1 | 21.8 | 26.0 | 33.2 |
| 14: 2 | 170 | 14.3 | 15.6 | 17.1 | 19.1 | 21.9 | 26.1 | 33.3 |
| 14: 3 | 171 | 14.4 | 15.6 | 17.2 | 19.2 | 22.0 | 26.2 | 33.4 |
| 14: 4 | 172 | 14.4 | 15.7 | 17.2 | 19.3 | 22.1 | 26.3 | 33.5 |
| 14: 5 | 173 | 14.5 | 15.7 | 17.3 | 19.3 | 22.2 | 26.4 | 33.5 |
| 14: 6 | 174 | 14.5 | 15.7 | 17.3 | 19.4 | 22.2 | 26.5 | 33.6 |
| 14: 7 | 175 | 14.5 | 15.8 | 17.4 | 19.5 | 22.3 | 26.5 | 33.7 |
| 14: 8 | 176 | 14.6 | 15.8 | 17.4 | 19.5 | 22.4 | 26.6 | 33.8 |
| 14: 9 | 177 | 14.6 | 15.9 | 17.5 | 19.6 | 22.5 | 26.7 | 33.9 |
| 14:10 | 178 | 14.6 | 15.9 | 17.5 | 19.6 | 22.5 | 26.8 | 33.9 |
| 14:11 | 179 | 14.7 | 16.0 | 17.6 | 19.7 | 22.6 | 26.9 | 34.0 |
| 15: 0 | 180 | 14.7 | 16.0 | 17.6 | 19.8 | 22.7 | 27.0 | 34.1 |
| 15: 1 | 181 | 14.7 | 16.1 | 17.7 | 19.8 | 22.8 | 27.1 | 34.1 |
| 15: 2 | 182 | 14.8 | 16.1 | 17.8 | 19.9 | 22.8 | 27.1 | 34.2 |
| 15: 3 | 183 | 14.8 | 16.1 | 17.8 | 20.0 | 22.9 | 27.2 | 34.3 |

## BMI-for-age BOYS

**5 to 19 years (z-scores)**

| | | Z-scores (BMI in kg/m$^2$) | | | | | | |
|---|---|---|---|---|---|---|---|---|
| Year: Month | Month | -3 SD | -2 SD | -1 SD | Median | 1 SD | 2 SD | 3 SD |
| 15: 4 | 184 | 14.8 | 16.2 | 17.9 | 20.0 | 23.0 | 27.3 | 34.3 |
| 15: 5 | 185 | 14.9 | 16.2 | 17.9 | 20.1 | 23.0 | 27.4 | 34.4 |
| 15: 6 | 186 | 14.9 | 16.3 | 18.0 | 20.1 | 23.1 | 27.4 | 34.5 |
| 15: 7 | 187 | 15.0 | 16.3 | 18.0 | 20.2 | 23.2 | 27.5 | 34.5 |
| 15: 8 | 188 | 15.0 | 16.3 | 18.1 | 20.3 | 23.3 | 27.6 | 34.6 |
| 15: 9 | 189 | 15.0 | 16.4 | 18.1 | 20.3 | 23.3 | 27.7 | 34.6 |
| 15:10 | 190 | 15.0 | 16.4 | 18.2 | 20.4 | 23.4 | 27.7 | 34.7 |
| 15:11 | 191 | 15.1 | 16.5 | 18.2 | 20.4 | 23.5 | 27.8 | 34.7 |
| 16: 0 | 192 | 15.1 | 16.5 | 18.2 | 20.5 | 23.5 | 27.9 | 34.8 |
| 16: 1 | 193 | 15.1 | 16.5 | 18.3 | 20.6 | 23.6 | 27.9 | 34.8 |
| 16: 2 | 194 | 15.2 | 16.6 | 18.3 | 20.6 | 23.7 | 28.0 | 34.8 |
| 16: 3 | 195 | 15.2 | 16.6 | 18.4 | 20.7 | 23.7 | 28.1 | 34.9 |
| 16: 4 | 196 | 15.2 | 16.7 | 18.4 | 20.7 | 23.8 | 28.1 | 34.9 |
| 16: 5 | 197 | 15.3 | 16.7 | 18.5 | 20.8 | 23.8 | 28.2 | 35.0 |
| 16: 6 | 198 | 15.3 | 16.7 | 18.5 | 20.8 | 23.9 | 28.3 | 35.0 |
| 16: 7 | 199 | 15.3 | 16.8 | 18.6 | 20.9 | 24.0 | 28.3 | 35.0 |
| 16: 8 | 200 | 15.3 | 16.8 | 18.6 | 20.9 | 24.0 | 28.4 | 35.1 |
| 16: 9 | 201 | 15.4 | 16.8 | 18.7 | 21.0 | 24.1 | 28.5 | 35.1 |
| 16:10 | 202 | 15.4 | 16.9 | 18.7 | 21.0 | 24.2 | 28.5 | 35.1 |
| 16:11 | 203 | 15.4 | 16.9 | 18.7 | 21.1 | 24.2 | 28.6 | 35.2 |
| 17: 0 | 204 | 15.4 | 16.9 | 18.8 | 21.1 | 24.3 | 28.6 | 35.2 |
| 17: 1 | 205 | 15.5 | 17.0 | 18.8 | 21.2 | 24.3 | 28.7 | 35.2 |
| 17: 2 | 206 | 15.5 | 17.0 | 18.9 | 21.2 | 24.4 | 28.7 | 35.2 |
| 17: 3 | 207 | 15.5 | 17.0 | 18.9 | 21.3 | 24.4 | 28.8 | 35.3 |

## BMI-for-age BOYS

**5 to 19 years (z-scores)**

| | | Z-scores (BMI in kg/m²) | | | | | | |
|---|---|---|---|---|---|---|---|---|
| **Year: Month** | **Month** | **-3 SD** | **-2 SD** | **-1 SD** | **Median** | **1 SD** | **2 SD** | **3 SD** |
| 17: 4 | 208 | 15.5 | 17.1 | 18.9 | 21.3 | 24.5 | 28.9 | 35.3 |
| 17: 5 | 209 | 15.6 | 17.1 | 19.0 | 21.4 | 24.5 | 28.9 | 35.3 |
| 17: 6 | 210 | 15.6 | 17.1 | 19.0 | 21.4 | 24.6 | 29.0 | 35.3 |
| 17: 7 | 211 | 15.6 | 17.1 | 19.1 | 21.5 | 24.7 | 29.0 | 35.4 |
| 17: 8 | 212 | 15.6 | 17.2 | 19.1 | 21.5 | 24.7 | 29.1 | 35.4 |
| 17: 9 | 213 | 15.6 | 17.2 | 19.1 | 21.6 | 24.8 | 29.1 | 35.4 |
| 17:10 | 214 | 15.7 | 17.2 | 19.2 | 21.6 | 24.8 | 29.2 | 35.4 |
| 17:11 | 215 | 15.7 | 17.3 | 19.2 | 21.7 | 24.9 | 29.2 | 35.4 |
| 18: 0 | 216 | 15.7 | 17.3 | 19.2 | 21.7 | 24.9 | 29.2 | 35.4 |
| 18: 1 | 217 | 15.7 | 17.3 | 19.3 | 21.8 | 25.0 | 29.3 | 35.4 |
| 18: 2 | 218 | 15.7 | 17.3 | 19.3 | 21.8 | 25.0 | 29.3 | 35.5 |
| 18: 3 | 219 | 15.7 | 17.4 | 19.3 | 21.8 | 25.1 | 29.4 | 35.5 |
| 18: 4 | 220 | 15.8 | 17.4 | 19.4 | 21.9 | 25.1 | 29.4 | 35.5 |
| 18: 5 | 221 | 15.8 | 17.4 | 19.4 | 21.9 | 25.1 | 29.5 | 35.5 |
| 18: 6 | 222 | 15.8 | 17.4 | 19.4 | 22.0 | 25.2 | 29.5 | 35.5 |
| 18: 7 | 223 | 15.8 | 17.5 | 19.5 | 22.0 | 25.2 | 29.5 | 35.5 |
| 18: 8 | 224 | 15.8 | 17.5 | 19.5 | 22.0 | 25.3 | 29.6 | 35.5 |
| 18: 9 | 225 | 15.8 | 17.5 | 19.5 | 22.1 | 25.3 | 29.6 | 35.5 |
| 18:10 | 226 | 15.8 | 17.5 | 19.6 | 22.1 | 25.4 | 29.6 | 35.5 |
| 18:11 | 227 | 15.8 | 17.5 | 19.6 | 22.2 | 25.4 | 29.7 | 35.5 |
| 19: 0 | 228 | 15.9 | 17.6 | 19.6 | 22.2 | 25.4 | 29.7 | 35.5 |

## BMI-for-age GIRLS

**5 to 19 years (z-scores)**

| | | Z-scores (BMI in kg/m²) | | | | | | |
|---|---|---|---|---|---|---|---|---|
| **Year: Month** | **Month** | **-3 SD** | **-2 SD** | **-1 SD** | **Median** | **1 SD** | **2 SD** | **3 SD** |
| 5: 1 | 61 | 11.8 | 12.7 | 13.9 | 15.2 | 16.9 | 18.9 | 21.3 |
| 5: 2 | 62 | 11.8 | 12.7 | 13.9 | 15.2 | 16.9 | 18.9 | 21.4 |
| 5: 3 | 63 | 11.8 | 12.7 | 13.9 | 15.2 | 16.9 | 18.9 | 21.5 |
| 5: 4 | 64 | 11.8 | 12.7 | 13.9 | 15.2 | 16.9 | 18.9 | 21.5 |
| 5: 5 | 65 | 11.7 | 12.7 | 13.9 | 15.2 | 16.9 | 19.0 | 21.6 |
| 5: 6 | 66 | 11.7 | 12.7 | 13.9 | 15.2 | 16.9 | 19.0 | 21.7 |
| 5: 7 | 67 | 11.7 | 12.7 | 13.9 | 15.2 | 16.9 | 19.0 | 21.7 |
| 5: 8 | 68 | 11.7 | 12.7 | 13.9 | 15.3 | 17.0 | 19.1 | 21.8 |
| 5: 9 | 69 | 11.7 | 12.7 | 13.9 | 15.3 | 17.0 | 19.1 | 21.9 |
| 5:10 | 70 | 11.7 | 12.7 | 13.9 | 15.3 | 17.0 | 19.1 | 22.0 |
| 5:11 | 71 | 11.7 | 12.7 | 13.9 | 15.3 | 17.0 | 19.2 | 22.1 |
| 6: 0 | 72 | 11.7 | 12.7 | 13.9 | 15.3 | 17.0 | 19.2 | 22.1 |
| 6: 1 | 73 | 11.7 | 12.7 | 13.9 | 15.3 | 17.0 | 19.3 | 22.2 |
| 6: 2 | 74 | 11.7 | 12.7 | 13.9 | 15.3 | 17.0 | 19.3 | 22.3 |
| 6: 3 | 75 | 11.7 | 12.7 | 13.9 | 15.3 | 17.1 | 19.3 | 22.4 |
| 6: 4 | 76 | 11.7 | 12.7 | 13.9 | 15.3 | 17.1 | 19.4 | 22.5 |
| 6: 5 | 77 | 11.7 | 12.7 | 13.9 | 15.3 | 17.1 | 19.4 | 22.6 |
| 6: 6 | 78 | 11.7 | 12.7 | 13.9 | 15.3 | 17.1 | 19.5 | 22.7 |
| 6: 7 | 79 | 11.7 | 12.7 | 13.9 | 15.3 | 17.2 | 19.5 | 22.8 |
| 6: 8 | 80 | 11.7 | 12.7 | 13.9 | 15.3 | 17.2 | 19.6 | 22.9 |
| 6: 9 | 81 | 11.7 | 12.7 | 13.9 | 15.4 | 17.2 | 19.6 | 23.0 |
| 6:10 | 82 | 11.7 | 12.7 | 13.9 | 15.4 | 17.2 | 19.7 | 23.1 |
| 6:11 | 83 | 11.7 | 12.7 | 13.9 | 15.4 | 17.3 | 19.7 | 23.2 |
| 7: 0 | 84 | 11.8 | 12.7 | 13.9 | 15.4 | 17.3 | 19.8 | 23.3 |
| 7: 1 | 85 | 11.8 | 12.7 | 13.9 | 15.4 | 17.3 | 19.8 | 23.4 |
| 7: 2 | 86 | 11.8 | 12.8 | 14.0 | 15.4 | 17.4 | 19.9 | 23.5 |

## BMI-for-age GIRLS

**5 to 19 years (z-scores)**

| | | Z-scores (BMI in kg/m²) | | | | | | |
|---|---|---|---|---|---|---|---|---|
| **Year: Month** | **Month** | **-3 SD** | **-2 SD** | **-1 SD** | **Median** | **1 SD** | **2 SD** | **3 SD** |
| **7: 3** | **87** | 11.8 | 12.8 | 14.0 | 15.5 | 17.4 | 20.0 | 23.6 |
| **7: 4** | **88** | 11.8 | 12.8 | 14.0 | 15.5 | 17.4 | 20.0 | 23.7 |
| **7: 5** | **89** | 11.8 | 12.8 | 14.0 | 15.5 | 17.5 | 20.1 | 23.9 |
| **7: 6** | **90** | 11.8 | 12.8 | 14.0 | 15.5 | 17.5 | 20.1 | 24.0 |
| **7: 7** | **91** | 11.8 | 12.8 | 14.0 | 15.5 | 17.5 | 20.2 | 24.1 |
| **7: 8** | **92** | 11.8 | 12.8 | 14.0 | 15.6 | 17.6 | 20.3 | 24.2 |
| **7: 9** | **93** | 11.8 | 12.8 | 14.1 | 15.6 | 17.6 | 20.3 | 24.4 |
| **7:10** | **94** | 11.9 | 12.9 | 14.1 | 15.6 | 17.6 | 20.4 | 24.5 |
| **7:11** | **95** | 11.9 | 12.9 | 14.1 | 15.7 | 17.7 | 20.5 | 24.6 |
| **8: 0** | **96** | 11.9 | 12.9 | 14.1 | 15.7 | 17.7 | 20.6 | 24.8 |
| **8: 1** | **97** | 11.9 | 12.9 | 14.1 | 15.7 | 17.8 | 20.6 | 24.9 |
| **8: 2** | **98** | 11.9 | 12.9 | 14.2 | 15.7 | 17.8 | 20.7 | 25.1 |
| **8: 3** | **99** | 11.9 | 12.9 | 14.2 | 15.8 | 17.9 | 20.8 | 25.2 |
| **8: 4** | **100** | 11.9 | 13.0 | 14.2 | 15.8 | 17.9 | 20.9 | 25.3 |
| **8: 5** | **101** | 12.0 | 13.0 | 14.2 | 15.8 | 18.0 | 20.9 | 25.5 |
| **8: 6** | **102** | 12.0 | 13.0 | 14.3 | 15.9 | 18.0 | 21.0 | 25.6 |
| **8: 7** | **103** | 12.0 | 13.0 | 14.3 | 15.9 | 18.1 | 21.1 | 25.8 |
| **8: 8** | **104** | 12.0 | 13.0 | 14.3 | 15.9 | 18.1 | 21.2 | 25.9 |
| **8: 9** | **105** | 12.0 | 13.1 | 14.3 | 16.0 | 18.2 | 21.3 | 26.1 |
| **8:10** | **106** | 12.1 | 13.1 | 14.4 | 16.0 | 18.2 | 21.3 | 26.2 |
| **8:11** | **107** | 12.1 | 13.1 | 14.4 | 16.1 | 18.3 | 21.4 | 26.4 |
| **9: 0** | **108** | 12.1 | 13.1 | 14.4 | 16.1 | 18.3 | 21.5 | 26.5 |
| **9: 1** | **109** | 12.1 | 13.2 | 14.5 | 16.1 | 18.4 | 21.6 | 26.7 |
| **9: 2** | **110** | 12.1 | 13.2 | 14.5 | 16.2 | 18.4 | 21.7 | 26.8 |
| **9: 3** | **111** | 12.2 | 13.2 | 14.5 | 16.2 | 18.5 | 21.8 | 27.0 |

## BMI-for-age GIRLS

**5 to 19 years (z-scores)**

| | | Z-scores (BMI in kg/m²) | | | | | | |
|---|---|---|---|---|---|---|---|---|
| **Year: Month** | **Month** | **-3 SD** | **-2 SD** | **-1 SD** | **Median** | **1 SD** | **2 SD** | **3 SD** |
| **9: 4** | **112** | 12.2 | 13.2 | 14.6 | 16.3 | 18.6 | 21.9 | 27.2 |
| **9: 5** | **113** | 12.2 | 13.3 | 14.6 | 16.3 | 18.6 | 21.9 | 27.3 |
| **9: 6** | **114** | 12.2 | 13.3 | 14.6 | 16.3 | 18.7 | 22.0 | 27.5 |
| **9: 7** | **115** | 12.3 | 13.3 | 14.7 | 16.4 | 18.7 | 22.1 | 27.6 |
| **9: 8** | **116** | 12.3 | 13.4 | 14.7 | 16.4 | 18.8 | 22.2 | 27.8 |
| **9: 9** | **117** | 12.3 | 13.4 | 14.7 | 16.5 | 18.8 | 22.3 | 27.9 |
| **9:10** | **118** | 12.3 | 13.4 | 14.8 | 16.5 | 18.9 | 22.4 | 28.1 |
| **9:11** | **119** | 12.4 | 13.4 | 14.8 | 16.6 | 19.0 | 22.5 | 28.2 |
| **10: 0** | **120** | 12.4 | 13.5 | 14.8 | 16.6 | 19.0 | 22.6 | 28.4 |
| **10: 1** | **121** | 12.4 | 13.5 | 14.9 | 16.7 | 19.1 | 22.7 | 28.5 |
| **10: 2** | **122** | 12.4 | 13.5 | 14.9 | 16.7 | 19.2 | 22.8 | 28.7 |
| **10: 3** | **123** | 12.5 | 13.6 | 15.0 | 16.8 | 19.2 | 22.8 | 28.8 |
| **10: 4** | **124** | 12.5 | 13.6 | 15.0 | 16.8 | 19.3 | 22.9 | 29.0 |
| **10: 5** | **125** | 12.5 | 13.6 | 15.0 | 16.9 | 19.4 | 23.0 | 29.1 |
| **10: 6** | **126** | 12.5 | 13.7 | 15.1 | 16.9 | 19.4 | 23.1 | 29.3 |
| **10: 7** | **127** | 12.6 | 13.7 | 15.1 | 17.0 | 19.5 | 23.2 | 29.4 |
| **10: 8** | **128** | 12.6 | 13.7 | 15.2 | 17.0 | 19.6 | 23.3 | 29.6 |
| **10: 9** | **129** | 12.6 | 13.8 | 15.2 | 17.1 | 19.6 | 23.4 | 29.7 |
| **10:10** | **130** | 12.7 | 13.8 | 15.3 | 17.1 | 19.7 | 23.5 | 29.9 |
| **10:11** | **131** | 12.7 | 13.8 | 15.3 | 17.2 | 19.8 | 23.6 | 30.0 |
| **11: 0** | **132** | 12.7 | 13.9 | 15.3 | 17.2 | 19.9 | 23.7 | 30.2 |
| **11: 1** | **133** | 12.8 | 13.9 | 15.4 | 17.3 | 19.9 | 23.8 | 30.3 |
| **11: 2** | **134** | 12.8 | 14.0 | 15.4 | 17.4 | 20.0 | 23.9 | 30.5 |
| **11: 3** | **135** | 12.8 | 14.0 | 15.5 | 17.4 | 20.1 | 24.0 | 30.6 |

## BMI-for-age GIRLS

**5 to 19 years (z-scores)**

| Year: Month | Month | -3 SD | -2 SD | -1 SD | Median | 1 SD | 2 SD | 3 SD |
|---|---|---|---|---|---|---|---|---|
| | | Z-scores (BMI in kg/m²) | | | | | | |
| 11: 4 | 136 | 12.9 | 14.0 | 15.5 | 17.5 | 20.2 | 24.1 | 30.8 |
| 11: 5 | 137 | 12.9 | 14.1 | 15.6 | 17.5 | 20.2 | 24.2 | 30.9 |
| 11: 6 | 138 | 12.9 | 14.1 | 15.6 | 17.6 | 20.3 | 24.3 | 31.1 |
| 11: 7 | 139 | 13.0 | 14.2 | 15.7 | 17.7 | 20.4 | 24.4 | 31.2 |
| 11: 8 | 140 | 13.0 | 14.2 | 15.7 | 17.7 | 20.5 | 24.5 | 31.4 |
| 11: 9 | 141 | 13.0 | 14.3 | 15.8 | 17.8 | 20.6 | 24.7 | 31.5 |
| 11:10 | 142 | 13.1 | 14.3 | 15.8 | 17.9 | 20.6 | 24.8 | 31.6 |
| 11:11 | 143 | 13.1 | 14.3 | 15.9 | 17.9 | 20.7 | 24.9 | 31.8 |
| 12: 0 | 144 | 13.2 | 14.4 | 16.0 | 18.0 | 20.8 | 25.0 | 31.9 |
| 12: 1 | 145 | 13.2 | 14.4 | 16.0 | 18.1 | 20.9 | 25.1 | 32.0 |
| 12: 2 | 146 | 13.2 | 14.5 | 16.1 | 18.1 | 21.0 | 25.2 | 32.2 |
| 12: 3 | 147 | 13.3 | 14.5 | 16.1 | 18.2 | 21.1 | 25.3 | 32.3 |
| 12: 4 | 148 | 13.3 | 14.6 | 16.2 | 18.3 | 21.1 | 25.4 | 32.4 |
| 12: 5 | 149 | 13.3 | 14.6 | 16.2 | 18.3 | 21.2 | 25.5 | 32.6 |
| 12: 6 | 150 | 13.4 | 14.7 | 16.3 | 18.4 | 21.3 | 25.6 | 32.7 |
| 12: 7 | 151 | 13.4 | 14.7 | 16.3 | 18.5 | 21.4 | 25.7 | 32.8 |
| 12: 8 | 152 | 13.5 | 14.8 | 16.4 | 18.5 | 21.5 | 25.8 | 33.0 |
| 12: 9 | 153 | 13.5 | 14.8 | 16.4 | 18.6 | 21.6 | 25.9 | 33.1 |
| 12:10 | 154 | 13.5 | 14.8 | 16.5 | 18.7 | 21.6 | 26.0 | 33.2 |
| 12:11 | 155 | 13.6 | 14.9 | 16.6 | 18.7 | 21.7 | 26.1 | 33.3 |
| 13: 0 | 156 | 13.6 | 14.9 | 16.6 | 18.8 | 21.8 | 26.2 | 33.4 |
| 13: 1 | 157 | 13.6 | 15.0 | 16.7 | 18.9 | 21.9 | 26.3 | 33.6 |
| 13: 2 | 158 | 13.7 | 15.0 | 16.7 | 18.9 | 22.0 | 26.4 | 33.7 |
| 13: 3 | 159 | 13.7 | 15.1 | 16.8 | 19.0 | 22.0 | 26.5 | 33.8 |

## BMI-for-age GIRLS

**5 to 19 years (z-scores)**

| Year: Month | Month | -3 SD | -2 SD | -1 SD | Median | 1 SD | 2 SD | 3 SD |
|---|---|---|---|---|---|---|---|---|
| | | Z-scores (BMI in kg/m²) | | | | | | |
| 13: 4 | 160 | 13.8 | 15.1 | 16.8 | 19.1 | 22.1 | 26.6 | 33.9 |
| 13: 5 | 161 | 13.8 | 15.2 | 16.9 | 19.1 | 22.2 | 26.7 | 34.0 |
| 13: 6 | 162 | 13.8 | 15.2 | 16.9 | 19.2 | 22.3 | 26.8 | 34.1 |
| 13: 7 | 163 | 13.9 | 15.2 | 17.0 | 19.3 | 22.4 | 26.9 | 34.2 |
| 13: 8 | 164 | 13.9 | 15.3 | 17.0 | 19.3 | 22.4 | 27.0 | 34.3 |
| 13: 9 | 165 | 13.9 | 15.3 | 17.1 | 19.4 | 22.5 | 27.1 | 34.4 |
| 13:10 | 166 | 14.0 | 15.4 | 17.1 | 19.4 | 22.6 | 27.1 | 34.5 |
| 13:11 | 167 | 14.0 | 15.4 | 17.2 | 19.5 | 22.7 | 27.2 | 34.6 |
| 14: 0 | 168 | 14.0 | 15.4 | 17.2 | 19.6 | 22.7 | 27.3 | 34.7 |
| 14: 1 | 169 | 14.1 | 15.5 | 17.3 | 19.6 | 22.8 | 27.4 | 34.7 |
| 14: 2 | 170 | 14.1 | 15.5 | 17.3 | 19.7 | 22.9 | 27.5 | 34.8 |
| 14: 3 | 171 | 14.1 | 15.6 | 17.4 | 19.7 | 22.9 | 27.6 | 34.9 |
| 14: 4 | 172 | 14.1 | 15.6 | 17.4 | 19.8 | 23.0 | 27.7 | 35.0 |
| 14: 5 | 173 | 14.2 | 15.6 | 17.5 | 19.9 | 23.1 | 27.7 | 35.1 |
| 14: 6 | 174 | 14.2 | 15.7 | 17.5 | 19.9 | 23.1 | 27.8 | 35.1 |
| 14: 7 | 175 | 14.2 | 15.7 | 17.6 | 20.0 | 23.2 | 27.9 | 35.2 |
| 14: 8 | 176 | 14.3 | 15.7 | 17.6 | 20.0 | 23.3 | 28.0 | 35.3 |
| 14: 9 | 177 | 14.3 | 15.8 | 17.6 | 20.1 | 23.3 | 28.0 | 35.4 |
| 14:10 | 178 | 14.3 | 15.8 | 17.7 | 20.1 | 23.4 | 28.1 | 35.4 |
| 14:11 | 179 | 14.3 | 15.8 | 17.7 | 20.2 | 23.5 | 28.2 | 35.5 |
| 15: 0 | 180 | 14.4 | 15.9 | 17.8 | 20.2 | 23.5 | 28.2 | 35.5 |
| 15: 1 | 181 | 14.4 | 15.9 | 17.8 | 20.3 | 23.6 | 28.3 | 35.6 |
| 15: 2 | 182 | 14.4 | 15.9 | 17.8 | 20.3 | 23.6 | 28.4 | 35.7 |
| 15: 3 | 183 | 14.4 | 16.0 | 17.9 | 20.4 | 23.7 | 28.4 | 35.7 |

## BMI-for-age GIRLS

**5 to 19 years (z-scores)**

| | | Z-scores (BMI in kg/m²) | | | | | | |
|---|---|---|---|---|---|---|---|---|
| Year: Month | Month | -3 SD | -2 SD | -1 SD | Median | 1 SD | 2 SD | 3 SD |
| 15: 4 | 184 | 14.5 | 16.0 | 17.9 | 20.4 | 23.7 | 28.5 | 35.8 |
| 15: 5 | 185 | 14.5 | 16.0 | 17.9 | 20.4 | 23.8 | 28.5 | 35.8 |
| 15: 6 | 186 | 14.5 | 16.0 | 18.0 | 20.5 | 23.8 | 28.6 | 35.8 |
| 15: 7 | 187 | 14.5 | 16.1 | 18.0 | 20.5 | 23.9 | 28.6 | 35.9 |
| 15: 8 | 188 | 14.5 | 16.1 | 18.0 | 20.6 | 23.9 | 28.7 | 35.9 |
| 15: 9 | 189 | 14.5 | 16.1 | 18.1 | 20.6 | 24.0 | 28.7 | 36.0 |
| 15:10 | 190 | 14.6 | 16.1 | 18.1 | 20.6 | 24.0 | 28.8 | 36.0 |
| 15:11 | 191 | 14.6 | 16.2 | 18.1 | 20.7 | 24.1 | 28.8 | 36.0 |
| 16: 0 | 192 | 14.6 | 16.2 | 18.2 | 20.7 | 24.1 | 28.9 | 36.1 |
| 16: 1 | 193 | 14.6 | 16.2 | 18.2 | 20.7 | 24.1 | 28.9 | 36.1 |
| 16: 2 | 194 | 14.6 | 16.2 | 18.2 | 20.8 | 24.2 | 29.0 | 36.1 |
| 16: 3 | 195 | 14.6 | 16.2 | 18.2 | 20.8 | 24.2 | 29.0 | 36.1 |
| 16: 4 | 196 | 14.6 | 16.2 | 18.3 | 20.8 | 24.3 | 29.0 | 36.2 |
| 16: 5 | 197 | 14.6 | 16.3 | 18.3 | 20.9 | 24.3 | 29.1 | 36.2 |
| 16: 6 | 198 | 14.7 | 16.3 | 18.3 | 20.9 | 24.3 | 29.1 | 36.2 |
| 16: 7 | 199 | 14.7 | 16.3 | 18.3 | 20.9 | 24.4 | 29.1 | 36.2 |
| 16: 8 | 200 | 14.7 | 16.3 | 18.3 | 20.9 | 24.4 | 29.2 | 36.2 |
| 16: 9 | 201 | 14.7 | 16.3 | 18.4 | 21.0 | 24.4 | 29.2 | 36.3 |
| 16:10 | 202 | 14.7 | 16.3 | 18.4 | 21.0 | 24.4 | 29.2 | 36.3 |
| 16:11 | 203 | 14.7 | 16.3 | 18.4 | 21.0 | 24.5 | 29.3 | 36.3 |
| 17: 0 | 204 | 14.7 | 16.4 | 18.4 | 21.0 | 24.5 | 29.3 | 36.3 |
| 17: 1 | 205 | 14.7 | 16.4 | 18.4 | 21.1 | 24.5 | 29.3 | 36.3 |
| 17: 2 | 206 | 14.7 | 16.4 | 18.4 | 21.1 | 24.6 | 29.3 | 36.3 |
| 17: 3 | 207 | 14.7 | 16.4 | 18.5 | 21.1 | 24.6 | 29.4 | 36.3 |

## BMI-for-age GIRLS

**5 to 19 years (z-scores)**

| | | Z-scores (BMI in kg/m²) | | | | | | |
|---|---|---|---|---|---|---|---|---|
| Year: Month | Month | -3 SD | -2 SD | -1 SD | Median | 1 SD | 2 SD | 3 SD |
| 17: 4 | 208 | 14.7 | 16.4 | 18.5 | 21.1 | 24.6 | 29.4 | 36.3 |
| 17: 5 | 209 | 14.7 | 16.4 | 18.5 | 21.1 | 24.6 | 29.4 | 36.3 |
| 17: 6 | 210 | 14.7 | 16.4 | 18.5 | 21.2 | 24.6 | 29.4 | 36.3 |
| 17: 7 | 211 | 14.7 | 16.4 | 18.5 | 21.2 | 24.7 | 29.4 | 36.3 |
| 17: 8 | 212 | 14.7 | 16.4 | 18.5 | 21.2 | 24.7 | 29.5 | 36.3 |
| 17: 9 | 213 | 14.7 | 16.4 | 18.5 | 21.2 | 24.7 | 29.5 | 36.3 |
| 17:10 | 214 | 14.7 | 16.4 | 18.5 | 21.2 | 24.7 | 29.5 | 36.3 |
| 17:11 | 215 | 14.7 | 16.4 | 18.6 | 21.2 | 24.8 | 29.5 | 36.3 |
| 18: 0 | 216 | 14.7 | 16.4 | 18.6 | 21.3 | 24.8 | 29.5 | 36.3 |
| 18: 1 | 217 | 14.7 | 16.5 | 18.6 | 21.3 | 24.8 | 29.5 | 36.3 |
| 18: 2 | 218 | 14.7 | 16.5 | 18.6 | 21.3 | 24.8 | 29.6 | 36.3 |
| 18: 3 | 219 | 14.7 | 16.5 | 18.6 | 21.3 | 24.8 | 29.6 | 36.3 |
| 18: 4 | 220 | 14.7 | 16.5 | 18.6 | 21.3 | 24.8 | 29.6 | 36.3 |
| 18: 5 | 221 | 14.7 | 16.5 | 18.6 | 21.3 | 24.9 | 29.6 | 36.2 |
| 18: 6 | 222 | 14.7 | 16.5 | 18.6 | 21.3 | 24.9 | 29.6 | 36.2 |
| 18: 7 | 223 | 14.7 | 16.5 | 18.6 | 21.4 | 24.9 | 29.6 | 36.2 |
| 18: 8 | 224 | 14.7 | 16.5 | 18.6 | 21.4 | 24.9 | 29.6 | 36.2 |
| 18: 9 | 225 | 14.7 | 16.5 | 18.7 | 21.4 | 24.9 | 29.6 | 36.2 |
| 18:10 | 226 | 14.7 | 16.5 | 18.7 | 21.4 | 24.9 | 29.6 | 36.2 |
| 18:11 | 227 | 14.7 | 16.5 | 18.7 | 21.4 | 25.0 | 29.7 | 36.2 |
| 19: 0 | 228 | 14.7 | 16.5 | 18.7 | 21.4 | 25.0 | 29.7 | 36.2 |

## Height-for-age BOYS

**5 to 19 years (z-scores)**

| | | Z-scores (height in cm) | | | | | | |
|---|---|---|---|---|---|---|---|---|
| Year: Month | Month | -3 SD | -2 SD | -1 SD | Median | 1 SD | 2 SD | 3 SD |
| **5: 1** | **61** | 96.5 | 101.1 | 105.7 | 110.3 | 114.9 | 119.4 | 124.0 |
| **5: 2** | **62** | 96.9 | 101.6 | 106.2 | 110.8 | 115.4 | 120.0 | 124.7 |
| **5: 3** | **63** | 97.4 | 102.0 | 106.7 | 111.3 | 116.0 | 120.6 | 125.3 |
| **5: 4** | **64** | 97.8 | 102.5 | 107.2 | 111.9 | 116.5 | 121.2 | 125.9 |
| **5: 5** | **65** | 98.2 | 103.0 | 107.7 | 112.4 | 117.1 | 121.8 | 126.5 |
| **5: 6** | **66** | 98.7 | 103.4 | 108.2 | 112.9 | 117.7 | 122.4 | 127.1 |
| **5: 7** | **67** | 99.1 | 103.9 | 108.7 | 113.4 | 118.2 | 123.0 | 127.8 |
| **5: 8** | **68** | 99.5 | 104.3 | 109.1 | 113.9 | 118.7 | 123.6 | 128.4 |
| **5: 9** | **69** | 99.9 | 104.8 | 109.6 | 114.5 | 119.3 | 124.1 | 129.0 |
| **5:10** | **70** | 100.4 | 105.2 | 110.1 | 115.0 | 119.8 | 124.7 | 129.6 |
| **5:11** | **71** | 100.8 | 105.7 | 110.6 | 115.5 | 120.4 | 125.2 | 130.1 |
| **6: 0** | **72** | 101.2 | 106.1 | 111.0 | 116.0 | 120.9 | 125.8 | 130.7 |
| **6: 1** | **73** | 101.6 | 106.5 | 111.5 | 116.4 | 121.4 | 126.4 | 131.3 |
| **6: 2** | **74** | 102.0 | 107.0 | 111.9 | 116.9 | 121.9 | 126.9 | 131.9 |
| **6: 3** | **75** | 102.4 | 107.4 | 112.4 | 117.4 | 122.4 | 127.5 | 132.5 |
| **6: 4** | **76** | 102.8 | 107.8 | 112.9 | 117.9 | 123.0 | 128.0 | 133.0 |
| **6: 5** | **77** | 103.2 | 108.2 | 113.3 | 118.4 | 123.5 | 128.5 | 133.6 |
| **6: 6** | **78** | 103.6 | 108.7 | 113.8 | 118.9 | 124.0 | 129.1 | 134.2 |
| **6: 7** | **79** | 103.9 | 109.1 | 114.2 | 119.4 | 124.5 | 129.6 | 134.8 |
| **6: 8** | **80** | 104.3 | 109.5 | 114.7 | 119.8 | 125.0 | 130.2 | 135.3 |
| **6: 9** | **81** | 104.7 | 109.9 | 115.1 | 120.3 | 125.5 | 130.7 | 135.9 |
| **6:10** | **82** | 105.1 | 110.3 | 115.6 | 120.8 | 126.0 | 131.2 | 136.5 |
| **6:11** | **83** | 105.5 | 110.8 | 116.0 | 121.3 | 126.5 | 131.8 | 137.0 |
| **7: 0** | **84** | 105.9 | 111.2 | 116.4 | 121.7 | 127.0 | 132.3 | 137.6 |
| **7: 1** | **85** | 106.3 | 111.6 | 116.9 | 122.2 | 127.5 | 132.8 | 138.2 |
| **7: 2** | **86** | 106.6 | 112.0 | 117.3 | 122.7 | 128.0 | 133.4 | 138.7 |

## Height-for-age BOYS

**5 to 19 years (z-scores)**

| | | Z-scores (height in cm) | | | | | | |
|---|---|---|---|---|---|---|---|---|
| Year: Month | Month | -3 SD | -2 SD | -1 SD | Median | 1 SD | 2 SD | 3 SD |
| **7: 3** | **87** | 107.0 | 112.4 | 117.8 | 123.1 | 128.5 | 133.9 | 139.3 |
| **7: 4** | **88** | 107.4 | 112.8 | 118.2 | 123.6 | 129.0 | 134.4 | 139.8 |
| **7: 5** | **89** | 107.8 | 113.2 | 118.6 | 124.1 | 129.5 | 134.9 | 140.4 |
| **7: 6** | **90** | 108.1 | 113.6 | 119.1 | 124.5 | 130.0 | 135.5 | 140.9 |
| **7: 7** | **91** | 108.5 | 114.0 | 119.5 | 125.0 | 130.5 | 136.0 | 141.5 |
| **7: 8** | **92** | 108.9 | 114.4 | 119.9 | 125.5 | 131.0 | 136.5 | 142.0 |
| **7: 9** | **93** | 109.2 | 114.8 | 120.4 | 125.9 | 131.5 | 137.0 | 142.6 |
| **7:10** | **94** | 109.6 | 115.2 | 120.8 | 126.4 | 132.0 | 137.5 | 143.1 |
| **7:11** | **95** | 110.0 | 115.6 | 121.2 | 126.8 | 132.4 | 138.1 | 143.7 |
| **8: 0** | **96** | 110.3 | 116.0 | 121.6 | 127.3 | 132.9 | 138.6 | 144.2 |
| **8: 1** | **97** | 110.7 | 116.4 | 122.0 | 127.7 | 133.4 | 139.1 | 144.7 |
| **8: 2** | **98** | 111.0 | 116.7 | 122.5 | 128.2 | 133.9 | 139.6 | 145.3 |
| **8: 3** | **99** | 111.4 | 117.1 | 122.9 | 128.6 | 134.3 | 140.1 | 145.8 |
| **8: 4** | **100** | 111.7 | 117.5 | 123.3 | 129.0 | 134.8 | 140.6 | 146.4 |
| **8: 5** | **101** | 112.1 | 117.9 | 123.7 | 129.5 | 135.3 | 141.1 | 146.9 |
| **8: 6** | **102** | 112.4 | 118.3 | 124.1 | 129.9 | 135.8 | 141.6 | 147.4 |
| **8: 7** | **103** | 112.8 | 118.7 | 124.5 | 130.4 | 136.2 | 142.1 | 148.0 |
| **8: 8** | **104** | 113.1 | 119.0 | 124.9 | 130.8 | 136.7 | 142.6 | 148.5 |
| **8: 9** | **105** | 113.5 | 119.4 | 125.3 | 131.3 | 137.2 | 143.1 | 149.0 |
| **8:10** | **106** | 113.8 | 119.8 | 125.7 | 131.7 | 137.6 | 143.6 | 149.5 |
| **8:11** | **107** | 114.2 | 120.2 | 126.1 | 132.1 | 138.1 | 144.1 | 150.1 |
| **9: 0** | **108** | 114.5 | 120.5 | 126.6 | 132.6 | 138.6 | 144.6 | 150.6 |
| **9: 1** | **109** | 114.9 | 120.9 | 127.0 | 133.0 | 139.0 | 145.1 | 151.1 |
| **9: 2** | **110** | 115.2 | 121.3 | 127.4 | 133.4 | 139.5 | 145.6 | 151.7 |
| **9: 3** | **111** | 115.6 | 121.7 | 127.8 | 133.9 | 140.0 | 146.1 | 152.2 |

## Height-for-age BOYS

**5 to 19 years (z-scores)**

| | | Z-scores (height in cm) | | | | | | |
|---|---|---|---|---|---|---|---|---|
| Year: Month | Month | -3 SD | -2 SD | -1 SD | Median | 1 SD | 2 SD | 3 SD |
| 9: 4 | 112 | 115.9 | 122.0 | 128.2 | 134.3 | 140.4 | 146.6 | 152.7 |
| 9: 5 | 113 | 116.3 | 122.4 | 128.6 | 134.7 | 140.9 | 147.1 | 153.2 |
| 9: 6 | 114 | 116.6 | 122.8 | 129.0 | 135.2 | 141.4 | 147.6 | 153.8 |
| 9: 7 | 115 | 116.9 | 123.2 | 129.4 | 135.6 | 141.8 | 148.1 | 154.3 |
| 9: 8 | 116 | 117.3 | 123.5 | 129.8 | 136.1 | 142.3 | 148.6 | 154.8 |
| 9: 9 | 117 | 117.6 | 123.9 | 130.2 | 136.5 | 142.8 | 149.1 | 155.3 |
| 9:10 | 118 | 118.0 | 124.3 | 130.6 | 136.9 | 143.2 | 149.5 | 155.9 |
| 9:11 | 119 | 118.3 | 124.7 | 131.0 | 137.3 | 143.7 | 150.0 | 156.4 |
| 10: 0 | 120 | 118.7 | 125.0 | 131.4 | 137.8 | 144.2 | 150.5 | 156.9 |
| 10: 1 | 121 | 119.0 | 125.4 | 131.8 | 138.2 | 144.6 | 151.0 | 157.4 |
| 10: 2 | 122 | 119.3 | 125.8 | 132.2 | 138.6 | 145.1 | 151.5 | 157.9 |
| 10: 3 | 123 | 119.7 | 126.2 | 132.6 | 139.1 | 145.5 | 152.0 | 158.5 |
| 10: 4 | 124 | 120.0 | 126.5 | 133.0 | 139.5 | 146.0 | 152.5 | 159.0 |
| 10: 5 | 125 | 120.4 | 126.9 | 133.4 | 140.0 | 146.5 | 153.0 | 159.5 |
| 10: 6 | 126 | 120.7 | 127.3 | 133.8 | 140.4 | 146.9 | 153.5 | 160.1 |
| 10: 7 | 127 | 121.1 | 127.7 | 134.3 | 140.8 | 147.4 | 154.0 | 160.6 |
| 10: 8 | 128 | 121.4 | 128.1 | 134.7 | 141.3 | 147.9 | 154.5 | 161.1 |
| 10: 9 | 129 | 121.8 | 128.5 | 135.1 | 141.7 | 148.4 | 155.0 | 161.7 |
| 10:10 | 130 | 122.2 | 128.8 | 135.5 | 142.2 | 148.9 | 155.5 | 162.2 |
| 10:11 | 131 | 122.5 | 129.2 | 135.9 | 142.7 | 149.4 | 156.1 | 162.8 |
| 11: 0 | 132 | 122.9 | 129.7 | 136.4 | 143.1 | 149.8 | 156.6 | 163.3 |
| 11: 1 | 133 | 123.3 | 130.1 | 136.8 | 143.6 | 150.3 | 157.1 | 163.9 |
| 11: 2 | 134 | 123.7 | 130.5 | 137.3 | 144.1 | 150.8 | 157.6 | 164.4 |
| 11: 3 | 135 | 124.1 | 130.9 | 137.7 | 144.5 | 151.3 | 158.2 | 165.0 |

## Height-for-age BOYS

**5 to 19 years (z-scores)**

| | | Z-scores (height in cm) | | | | | | |
|---|---|---|---|---|---|---|---|---|
| Year: Month | Month | -3 SD | -2 SD | -1 SD | Median | 1 SD | 2 SD | 3 SD |
| 11: 4 | 136 | 124.5 | 131.3 | 138.2 | 145.0 | 151.9 | 158.7 | 165.6 |
| 11: 5 | 137 | 124.9 | 131.7 | 138.6 | 145.5 | 152.4 | 159.3 | 166.1 |
| 11: 6 | 138 | 125.3 | 132.2 | 139.1 | 146.0 | 152.9 | 159.8 | 166.7 |
| 11: 7 | 139 | 125.7 | 132.6 | 139.6 | 146.5 | 153.4 | 160.4 | 167.3 |
| 11: 8 | 140 | 126.1 | 133.1 | 140.0 | 147.0 | 154.0 | 160.9 | 167.9 |
| 11: 9 | 141 | 126.5 | 133.5 | 140.5 | 147.5 | 154.5 | 161.5 | 168.5 |
| 11:10 | 142 | 126.9 | 134.0 | 141.0 | 148.0 | 155.0 | 162.1 | 169.1 |
| 11:11 | 143 | 127.4 | 134.4 | 141.5 | 148.5 | 155.6 | 162.7 | 169.7 |
| 12: 0 | 144 | 127.8 | 134.9 | 142.0 | 149.1 | 156.2 | 163.3 | 170.3 |
| 12: 1 | 145 | 128.3 | 135.4 | 142.5 | 149.6 | 156.7 | 163.9 | 171.0 |
| 12: 2 | 146 | 128.7 | 135.9 | 143.0 | 150.2 | 157.3 | 164.5 | 171.6 |
| 12: 3 | 147 | 129.2 | 136.4 | 143.6 | 150.7 | 157.9 | 165.1 | 172.2 |
| 12: 4 | 148 | 129.7 | 136.9 | 144.1 | 151.3 | 158.5 | 165.7 | 172.9 |
| 12: 5 | 149 | 130.2 | 137.4 | 144.6 | 151.9 | 159.1 | 166.3 | 173.6 |
| 12: 6 | 150 | 130.7 | 137.9 | 145.2 | 152.4 | 159.7 | 167.0 | 174.2 |
| 12: 7 | 151 | 131.2 | 138.5 | 145.7 | 153.0 | 160.3 | 167.6 | 174.9 |
| 12: 8 | 152 | 131.7 | 139.0 | 146.3 | 153.6 | 160.9 | 168.3 | 175.6 |
| 12: 9 | 153 | 132.2 | 139.5 | 146.9 | 154.2 | 161.6 | 168.9 | 176.3 |
| 12:10 | 154 | 132.7 | 140.1 | 147.5 | 154.8 | 162.2 | 169.6 | 176.9 |
| 12:11 | 155 | 133.2 | 140.6 | 148.0 | 155.4 | 162.8 | 170.2 | 177.6 |
| 13: 0 | 156 | 133.8 | 141.2 | 148.6 | 156.0 | 163.5 | 170.9 | 178.3 |
| 13: 1 | 157 | 134.3 | 141.7 | 149.2 | 156.7 | 164.1 | 171.6 | 179.0 |
| 13: 2 | 158 | 134.8 | 142.3 | 149.8 | 157.3 | 164.7 | 172.2 | 179.7 |
| 13: 3 | 159 | 135.4 | 142.9 | 150.4 | 157.9 | 165.4 | 172.9 | 180.4 |

## Height-for-age BOYS

**5 to 19 years (z-scores)**

| | | Z-scores (height in cm) | | | | | | |
|---|---|---|---|---|---|---|---|---|
| Year: Month | Month | -3 SD | -2 SD | -1 SD | Median | 1 SD | 2 SD | 3 SD |
| 13: 4 | 160 | 135.9 | 143.4 | 151.0 | 158.5 | 166.0 | 173.5 | 181.1 |
| 13: 5 | 161 | 136.4 | 144.0 | 151.5 | 159.1 | 166.6 | 174.2 | 181.8 |
| 13: 6 | 162 | 137.0 | 144.5 | 152.1 | 159.7 | 167.3 | 174.8 | 182.4 |
| 13: 7 | 163 | 137.5 | 145.1 | 152.7 | 160.3 | 167.9 | 175.5 | 183.1 |
| 13: 8 | 164 | 138.0 | 145.7 | 153.3 | 160.9 | 168.5 | 176.1 | 183.7 |
| 13: 9 | 165 | 138.6 | 146.2 | 153.8 | 161.5 | 169.1 | 176.7 | 184.4 |
| 13:10 | 166 | 139.1 | 146.7 | 154.4 | 162.1 | 169.7 | 177.4 | 185.0 |
| 13:11 | 167 | 139.6 | 147.3 | 154.9 | 162.6 | 170.3 | 178.0 | 185.6 |
| 14: 0 | 168 | 140.1 | 147.8 | 155.5 | 163.2 | 170.9 | 178.6 | 186.3 |
| 14: 1 | 169 | 140.6 | 148.3 | 156.0 | 163.7 | 171.4 | 179.1 | 186.9 |
| 14: 2 | 170 | 141.1 | 148.8 | 156.5 | 164.3 | 172.0 | 179.7 | 187.4 |
| 14: 3 | 171 | 141.6 | 149.3 | 157.1 | 164.8 | 172.5 | 180.3 | 188.0 |
| 14: 4 | 172 | 142.1 | 149.8 | 157.6 | 165.3 | 173.1 | 180.8 | 188.6 |
| 14: 5 | 173 | 142.5 | 150.3 | 158.1 | 165.8 | 173.6 | 181.3 | 189.1 |
| 14: 6 | 174 | 143.0 | 150.8 | 158.5 | 166.3 | 174.1 | 181.8 | 189.6 |
| 14: 7 | 175 | 143.4 | 151.2 | 159.0 | 166.8 | 174.6 | 182.3 | 190.1 |
| 14: 8 | 176 | 143.9 | 151.7 | 159.5 | 167.2 | 175.0 | 182.8 | 190.6 |
| 14: 9 | 177 | 144.3 | 152.1 | 159.9 | 167.7 | 175.5 | 183.3 | 191.1 |
| 14:10 | 178 | 144.7 | 152.5 | 160.3 | 168.1 | 175.9 | 183.7 | 191.5 |
| 14:11 | 179 | 145.1 | 152.9 | 160.7 | 168.5 | 176.3 | 184.1 | 191.9 |
| 15: 0 | 180 | 145.5 | 153.4 | 161.2 | 169.0 | 176.8 | 184.6 | 192.4 |
| 15: 1 | 181 | 145.9 | 153.7 | 161.5 | 169.4 | 177.2 | 185.0 | 192.8 |
| 15: 2 | 182 | 146.3 | 154.1 | 161.9 | 169.7 | 177.5 | 185.4 | 193.2 |
| 15: 3 | 183 | 146.7 | 154.5 | 162.3 | 170.1 | 177.9 | 185.7 | 193.5 |

## Height-for-age BOYS

**5 to 19 years (z-scores)**

| | | Z-scores (height in cm) | | | | | | |
|---|---|---|---|---|---|---|---|---|
| Year: Month | Month | -3 SD | -2 SD | -1 SD | Median | 1 SD | 2 SD | 3 SD |
| 15: 4 | 184 | 147.1 | 154.9 | 162.7 | 170.5 | 178.3 | 186.1 | 193.9 |
| 15: 5 | 185 | 147.4 | 155.2 | 163.0 | 170.8 | 178.6 | 186.4 | 194.2 |
| 15: 6 | 186 | 147.7 | 155.5 | 163.3 | 171.1 | 178.9 | 186.8 | 194.6 |
| 15: 7 | 187 | 148.1 | 155.9 | 163.7 | 171.5 | 179.3 | 187.1 | 194.9 |
| 15: 8 | 188 | 148.4 | 156.2 | 164.0 | 171.8 | 179.6 | 187.4 | 195.2 |
| 15: 9 | 189 | 148.7 | 156.5 | 164.3 | 172.1 | 179.9 | 187.7 | 195.4 |
| 15:10 | 190 | 149.0 | 156.8 | 164.6 | 172.4 | 180.1 | 187.9 | 195.7 |
| 15:11 | 191 | 149.3 | 157.1 | 164.9 | 172.6 | 180.4 | 188.2 | 196.0 |
| 16: 0 | 192 | 149.6 | 157.4 | 165.1 | 172.9 | 180.7 | 188.4 | 196.2 |
| 16: 1 | 193 | 149.9 | 157.6 | 165.4 | 173.1 | 180.9 | 188.7 | 196.4 |
| 16: 2 | 194 | 150.1 | 157.9 | 165.6 | 173.4 | 181.1 | 188.9 | 196.7 |
| 16: 3 | 195 | 150.4 | 158.1 | 165.9 | 173.6 | 181.4 | 189.1 | 196.9 |
| 16: 4 | 196 | 150.6 | 158.4 | 166.1 | 173.8 | 181.6 | 189.3 | 197.0 |
| 16: 5 | 197 | 150.9 | 158.6 | 166.3 | 174.0 | 181.8 | 189.5 | 197.2 |
| 16: 6 | 198 | 151.1 | 158.8 | 166.5 | 174.2 | 181.9 | 189.7 | 197.4 |
| 16: 7 | 199 | 151.3 | 159.0 | 166.7 | 174.4 | 182.1 | 189.8 | 197.5 |
| 16: 8 | 200 | 151.5 | 159.2 | 166.9 | 174.6 | 182.3 | 190.0 | 197.7 |
| 16: 9 | 201 | 151.7 | 159.4 | 167.1 | 174.7 | 182.4 | 190.1 | 197.8 |
| 16:10 | 202 | 151.9 | 159.6 | 167.2 | 174.9 | 182.6 | 190.2 | 197.9 |
| 16:11 | 203 | 152.1 | 159.7 | 167.4 | 175.0 | 182.7 | 190.3 | 198.0 |
| 17: 0 | 204 | 152.2 | 159.9 | 167.5 | 175.2 | 182.8 | 190.4 | 198.1 |
| 17: 1 | 205 | 152.4 | 160.0 | 167.7 | 175.3 | 182.9 | 190.5 | 198.2 |
| 17: 2 | 206 | 152.5 | 160.2 | 167.8 | 175.4 | 183.0 | 190.6 | 198.2 |
| 17: 3 | 207 | 152.7 | 160.3 | 167.9 | 175.5 | 183.1 | 190.7 | 198.3 |

## Height-for-age BOYS

**5 to 19 years (z-scores)**

| | | Z-scores (height in cm) | | | | | | |
|---|---|---|---|---|---|---|---|---|
| Year: Month | Month | -3 SD | -2 SD | -1 SD | Median | 1 SD | 2 SD | 3 SD |
| 17: 4 | 208 | 152.8 | 160.4 | 168.0 | 175.6 | 183.2 | 190.8 | 198.4 |
| 17: 5 | 209 | 153.0 | 160.5 | 168.1 | 175.7 | 183.3 | 190.8 | 198.4 |
| 17: 6 | 210 | 153.1 | 160.6 | 168.2 | 175.8 | 183.3 | 190.9 | 198.4 |
| 17: 7 | 211 | 153.2 | 160.8 | 168.3 | 175.8 | 183.4 | 190.9 | 198.5 |
| 17: 8 | 212 | 153.3 | 160.9 | 168.4 | 175.9 | 183.4 | 191.0 | 198.5 |
| 17: 9 | 213 | 153.4 | 160.9 | 168.5 | 176.0 | 183.5 | 191.0 | 198.5 |
| 17:10 | 214 | 153.5 | 161.0 | 168.5 | 176.0 | 183.5 | 191.0 | 198.5 |
| 17:11 | 215 | 153.6 | 161.1 | 168.6 | 176.1 | 183.6 | 191.1 | 198.6 |
| 18: 0 | 216 | 153.7 | 161.2 | 168.7 | 176.1 | 183.6 | 191.1 | 198.6 |
| 18: 1 | 217 | 153.8 | 161.3 | 168.7 | 176.2 | 183.6 | 191.1 | 198.6 |
| 18: 2 | 218 | 153.9 | 161.4 | 168.8 | 176.2 | 183.7 | 191.1 | 198.6 |
| 18: 3 | 219 | 154.0 | 161.4 | 168.9 | 176.3 | 183.7 | 191.1 | 198.6 |
| 18: 4 | 220 | 154.1 | 161.5 | 168.9 | 176.3 | 183.7 | 191.1 | 198.6 |
| 18: 5 | 221 | 154.2 | 161.6 | 169.0 | 176.4 | 183.8 | 191.1 | 198.5 |
| 18: 6 | 222 | 154.2 | 161.6 | 169.0 | 176.4 | 183.8 | 191.1 | 198.5 |
| 18: 7 | 223 | 154.3 | 161.7 | 169.0 | 176.4 | 183.8 | 191.2 | 198.5 |
| 18: 8 | 224 | 154.4 | 161.7 | 169.1 | 176.4 | 183.8 | 191.2 | 198.5 |
| 18: 9 | 225 | 154.5 | 161.8 | 169.1 | 176.5 | 183.8 | 191.2 | 198.5 |
| 18:10 | 226 | 154.5 | 161.8 | 169.2 | 176.5 | 183.8 | 191.1 | 198.5 |
| 18:11 | 227 | 154.6 | 161.9 | 169.2 | 176.5 | 183.8 | 191.1 | 198.5 |
| 19: 0 | 228 | 154.6 | 161.9 | 169.2 | 176.5 | 183.8 | 191.1 | 198.4 |

## Height-for-age GIRLS

**5 to 19 years (z-scores)**

| | | Z-scores (height in cm) | | | | | | |
|---|---|---|---|---|---|---|---|---|
| Year: Month | Month | -3 SD | -2 SD | -1 SD | Median | 1 SD | 2 SD | 3 SD |
| 5: 1 | 61 | 95.3 | 100.1 | 104.8 | 109.6 | 114.4 | 119.1 | 123.9 |
| 5: 2 | 62 | 95.7 | 100.5 | 105.3 | 110.1 | 114.9 | 119.7 | 124.5 |
| 5: 3 | 63 | 96.1 | 101.0 | 105.8 | 110.6 | 115.5 | 120.3 | 125.2 |
| 5: 4 | 64 | 96.5 | 101.4 | 106.3 | 111.2 | 116.0 | 120.9 | 125.8 |
| 5: 5 | 65 | 97.0 | 101.9 | 106.8 | 111.7 | 116.6 | 121.5 | 126.4 |
| 5: 6 | 66 | 97.4 | 102.3 | 107.2 | 112.2 | 117.1 | 122.0 | 127.0 |
| 5: 7 | 67 | 97.8 | 102.7 | 107.7 | 112.7 | 117.6 | 122.6 | 127.6 |
| 5: 8 | 68 | 98.2 | 103.2 | 108.2 | 113.2 | 118.2 | 123.2 | 128.2 |
| 5: 9 | 69 | 98.6 | 103.6 | 108.6 | 113.7 | 118.7 | 123.7 | 128.8 |
| 5:10 | 70 | 99.0 | 104.0 | 109.1 | 114.2 | 119.2 | 124.3 | 129.3 |
| 5:11 | 71 | 99.4 | 104.5 | 109.6 | 114.6 | 119.7 | 124.8 | 129.9 |
| 6: 0 | 72 | 99.8 | 104.9 | 110.0 | 115.1 | 120.2 | 125.4 | 130.5 |
| 6: 1 | 73 | 100.2 | 105.3 | 110.5 | 115.6 | 120.8 | 125.9 | 131.1 |
| 6: 2 | 74 | 100.5 | 105.7 | 110.9 | 116.1 | 121.3 | 126.4 | 131.6 |
| 6: 3 | 75 | 100.9 | 106.1 | 111.3 | 116.6 | 121.8 | 127.0 | 132.2 |
| 6: 4 | 76 | 101.3 | 106.6 | 111.8 | 117.0 | 122.3 | 127.5 | 132.7 |
| 6: 5 | 77 | 101.7 | 107.0 | 112.2 | 117.5 | 122.8 | 128.0 | 133.3 |
| 6: 6 | 78 | 102.1 | 107.4 | 112.7 | 118.0 | 123.3 | 128.6 | 133.9 |
| 6: 7 | 79 | 102.5 | 107.8 | 113.1 | 118.4 | 123.8 | 129.1 | 134.4 |
| 6: 8 | 80 | 102.9 | 108.2 | 113.6 | 118.9 | 124.3 | 129.6 | 135.0 |
| 6: 9 | 81 | 103.2 | 108.6 | 114.0 | 119.4 | 124.8 | 130.2 | 135.5 |
| 6:10 | 82 | 103.6 | 109.0 | 114.5 | 119.9 | 125.3 | 130.7 | 136.1 |
| 6:11 | 83 | 104.0 | 109.5 | 114.9 | 120.3 | 125.8 | 131.2 | 136.7 |
| 7: 0 | 84 | 104.4 | 109.9 | 115.3 | 120.8 | 126.3 | 131.7 | 137.2 |
| 7: 1 | 85 | 104.8 | 110.3 | 115.8 | 121.3 | 126.8 | 132.3 | 137.8 |
| 7: 2 | 86 | 105.2 | 110.7 | 116.2 | 121.8 | 127.3 | 132.8 | 138.3 |

## Height-for-age GIRLS

**5 to 19 years (z-scores)**

| Year: Month | Month | Z-scores (height in cm) | | | | | | |
|---|---|---|---|---|---|---|---|---|
| | | -3 SD | -2 SD | -1 SD | Median | 1 SD | 2 SD | 3 SD |
| **7: 3** | **87** | 105.6 | 111.1 | 116.7 | 122.2 | 127.8 | 133.3 | 138.9 |
| **7: 4** | **88** | 106.0 | 111.6 | 117.1 | 122.7 | 128.3 | 133.9 | 139.4 |
| **7: 5** | **89** | 106.4 | 112.0 | 117.6 | 123.2 | 128.8 | 134.4 | 140.0 |
| **7: 6** | **90** | 106.8 | 112.4 | 118.0 | 123.7 | 129.3 | 134.9 | 140.6 |
| **7: 7** | **91** | 107.2 | 112.8 | 118.5 | 124.1 | 129.8 | 135.5 | 141.1 |
| **7: 8** | **92** | 107.6 | 113.2 | 118.9 | 124.6 | 130.3 | 136.0 | 141.7 |
| **7: 9** | **93** | 108.0 | 113.7 | 119.4 | 125.1 | 130.8 | 136.5 | 142.3 |
| **7:10** | **94** | 108.4 | 114.1 | 119.8 | 125.6 | 131.3 | 137.1 | 142.8 |
| **7:11** | **95** | 108.8 | 114.5 | 120.3 | 126.1 | 131.8 | 137.6 | 143.4 |
| **8: 0** | **96** | 109.2 | 115.0 | 120.8 | 126.6 | 132.4 | 138.2 | 143.9 |
| **8: 1** | **97** | 109.6 | 115.4 | 121.2 | 127.0 | 132.9 | 138.7 | 144.5 |
| **8: 2** | **98** | 110.0 | 115.8 | 121.7 | 127.5 | 133.4 | 139.2 | 145.1 |
| **8: 3** | **99** | 110.4 | 116.3 | 122.1 | 128.0 | 133.9 | 139.8 | 145.7 |
| **8: 4** | **100** | 110.8 | 116.7 | 122.6 | 128.5 | 134.4 | 140.3 | 146.2 |
| **8: 5** | **101** | 111.2 | 117.1 | 123.1 | 129.0 | 134.9 | 140.9 | 146.8 |
| **8: 6** | **102** | 111.6 | 117.6 | 123.5 | 129.5 | 135.5 | 141.4 | 147.4 |
| **8: 7** | **103** | 112.0 | 118.0 | 124.0 | 130.0 | 136.0 | 142.0 | 147.9 |
| **8: 8** | **104** | 112.5 | 118.5 | 124.5 | 130.5 | 136.5 | 142.5 | 148.5 |
| **8: 9** | **105** | 112.9 | 118.9 | 125.0 | 131.0 | 137.0 | 143.1 | 149.1 |
| **8:10** | **106** | 113.3 | 119.4 | 125.4 | 131.5 | 137.5 | 143.6 | 149.7 |
| **8:11** | **107** | 113.7 | 119.8 | 125.9 | 132.0 | 138.1 | 144.2 | 150.2 |
| **9: 0** | **108** | 114.2 | 120.3 | 126.4 | 132.5 | 138.6 | 144.7 | 150.8 |
| **9: 1** | **109** | 114.6 | 120.7 | 126.9 | 133.0 | 139.1 | 145.3 | 151.4 |
| **9: 2** | **110** | 115.0 | 121.2 | 127.3 | 133.5 | 139.7 | 145.8 | 152.0 |
| **9: 3** | **111** | 115.5 | 121.6 | 127.8 | 134.0 | 140.2 | 146.4 | 152.6 |

## Height-for-age GIRLS

**5 to 19 years (z-scores)**

| Year: Month | Month | Z-scores (height in cm) | | | | | | |
|---|---|---|---|---|---|---|---|---|
| | | -3 SD | -2 SD | -1 SD | Median | 1 SD | 2 SD | 3 SD |
| **9: 4** | **112** | 115.9 | 122.1 | 128.3 | 134.5 | 140.7 | 146.9 | 153.1 |
| **9: 5** | **113** | 116.3 | 122.6 | 128.8 | 135.0 | 141.3 | 147.5 | 153.7 |
| **9: 6** | **114** | 116.8 | 123.0 | 129.3 | 135.5 | 141.8 | 148.1 | 154.3 |
| **9: 7** | **115** | 117.2 | 123.5 | 129.8 | 136.1 | 142.3 | 148.6 | 154.9 |
| **9: 8** | **116** | 117.7 | 124.0 | 130.3 | 136.6 | 142.9 | 149.2 | 155.5 |
| **9: 9** | **117** | 118.1 | 124.4 | 130.8 | 137.1 | 143.4 | 149.7 | 156.1 |
| **9:10** | **118** | 118.5 | 124.9 | 131.2 | 137.6 | 144.0 | 150.3 | 156.7 |
| **9:11** | **119** | 119.0 | 125.4 | 131.7 | 138.1 | 144.5 | 150.9 | 157.2 |
| **10: 0** | **120** | 119.4 | 125.8 | 132.2 | 138.6 | 145.0 | 151.4 | 157.8 |
| **10: 1** | **121** | 119.9 | 126.3 | 132.7 | 139.2 | 145.6 | 152.0 | 158.4 |
| **10: 2** | **122** | 120.4 | 126.8 | 133.2 | 139.7 | 146.1 | 152.6 | 159.0 |
| **10: 3** | **123** | 120.8 | 127.3 | 133.7 | 140.2 | 146.7 | 153.1 | 159.6 |
| **10: 4** | **124** | 121.3 | 127.8 | 134.2 | 140.7 | 147.2 | 153.7 | 160.2 |
| **10: 5** | **125** | 121.7 | 128.2 | 134.8 | 141.3 | 147.8 | 154.3 | 160.8 |
| **10: 6** | **126** | 122.2 | 128.7 | 135.3 | 141.8 | 148.3 | 154.8 | 161.4 |
| **10: 7** | **127** | 122.7 | 129.2 | 135.8 | 142.3 | 148.9 | 155.4 | 162.0 |
| **10: 8** | **128** | 123.2 | 129.7 | 136.3 | 142.9 | 149.4 | 156.0 | 162.6 |
| **10: 9** | **129** | 123.6 | 130.2 | 136.8 | 143.4 | 150.0 | 156.6 | 163.1 |
| **10:10** | **130** | 124.1 | 130.7 | 137.3 | 143.9 | 150.5 | 157.1 | 163.7 |
| **10:11** | **131** | 124.6 | 131.2 | 137.8 | 144.5 | 151.1 | 157.7 | 164.3 |
| **11: 0** | **132** | 125.1 | 131.7 | 138.3 | 145.0 | 151.6 | 158.3 | 164.9 |
| **11: 1** | **133** | 125.5 | 132.2 | 138.9 | 145.5 | 152.2 | 158.9 | 165.5 |
| **11: 2** | **134** | 126.0 | 132.7 | 139.4 | 146.1 | 152.7 | 159.4 | 166.1 |
| **11: 3** | **135** | 126.5 | 133.2 | 139.9 | 146.6 | 153.3 | 160.0 | 166.7 |

## Height-for-age GIRLS

**5 to 19 years (z-scores)**

| Year: Month | Month | Z-scores (height in cm) | | | | | | |
|---|---|---|---|---|---|---|---|---|
| | | -3 SD | -2 SD | -1 SD | Median | 1 SD | 2 SD | 3 SD |
| 11: 4 | 136 | 127.0 | 133.7 | 140.4 | 147.1 | 153.8 | 160.6 | 167.3 |
| 11: 5 | 137 | 127.4 | 134.2 | 140.9 | 147.7 | 154.4 | 161.1 | 167.9 |
| 11: 6 | 138 | 127.9 | 134.7 | 141.4 | 148.2 | 154.9 | 161.7 | 168.4 |
| 11: 7 | 139 | 128.4 | 135.2 | 141.9 | 148.7 | 155.5 | 162.2 | 169.0 |
| 11: 8 | 140 | 128.9 | 135.7 | 142.4 | 149.2 | 156.0 | 162.8 | 169.6 |
| 11: 9 | 141 | 129.3 | 136.1 | 142.9 | 149.7 | 156.5 | 163.3 | 170.1 |
| 11:10 | 142 | 129.8 | 136.6 | 143.4 | 150.2 | 157.1 | 163.9 | 170.7 |
| 11:11 | 143 | 130.3 | 137.1 | 143.9 | 150.7 | 157.6 | 164.4 | 171.2 |
| 12: 0 | 144 | 130.7 | 137.6 | 144.4 | 151.2 | 158.1 | 164.9 | 171.8 |
| 12: 1 | 145 | 131.2 | 138.0 | 144.9 | 151.7 | 158.6 | 165.4 | 172.3 |
| 12: 2 | 146 | 131.6 | 138.5 | 145.3 | 152.2 | 159.1 | 165.9 | 172.8 |
| 12: 3 | 147 | 132.0 | 138.9 | 145.8 | 152.7 | 159.5 | 166.4 | 173.3 |
| 12: 4 | 148 | 132.5 | 139.3 | 146.2 | 153.1 | 160.0 | 166.9 | 173.8 |
| 12: 5 | 149 | 132.9 | 139.8 | 146.7 | 153.6 | 160.5 | 167.4 | 174.3 |
| 12: 6 | 150 | 133.3 | 140.2 | 147.1 | 154.0 | 160.9 | 167.8 | 174.7 |
| 12: 7 | 151 | 133.7 | 140.6 | 147.5 | 154.4 | 161.3 | 168.3 | 175.2 |
| 12: 8 | 152 | 134.1 | 141.0 | 147.9 | 154.8 | 161.8 | 168.7 | 175.6 |
| 12: 9 | 153 | 134.5 | 141.4 | 148.3 | 155.2 | 162.2 | 169.1 | 176.0 |
| 12:10 | 154 | 134.8 | 141.8 | 148.7 | 155.6 | 162.6 | 169.5 | 176.4 |
| 12:11 | 155 | 135.2 | 142.1 | 149.1 | 156.0 | 162.9 | 169.9 | 176.8 |
| 13: 0 | 156 | 135.6 | 142.5 | 149.4 | 156.4 | 163.3 | 170.3 | 177.2 |
| 13: 1 | 157 | 135.9 | 142.8 | 149.8 | 156.7 | 163.7 | 170.6 | 177.6 |
| 13: 2 | 158 | 136.2 | 143.2 | 150.1 | 157.1 | 164.0 | 171.0 | 177.9 |
| 13: 3 | 159 | 136.5 | 143.5 | 150.4 | 157.4 | 164.3 | 171.3 | 178.2 |

## Height-for-age GIRLS

**5 to 19 years (z-scores)**

| Year: Month | Month | Z-scores (height in cm) | | | | | | |
|---|---|---|---|---|---|---|---|---|
| | | -3 SD | -2 SD | -1 SD | Median | 1 SD | 2 SD | 3 SD |
| 13: 4 | 160 | 136.9 | 143.8 | 150.8 | 157.7 | 164.7 | 171.6 | 178.6 |
| 13: 5 | 161 | 137.2 | 144.1 | 151.1 | 158.0 | 165.0 | 171.9 | 178.9 |
| 13: 6 | 162 | 137.4 | 144.4 | 151.3 | 158.3 | 165.3 | 172.2 | 179.2 |
| 13: 7 | 163 | 137.7 | 144.7 | 151.6 | 158.6 | 165.5 | 172.5 | 179.4 |
| 13: 8 | 164 | 138.0 | 144.9 | 151.9 | 158.8 | 165.8 | 172.7 | 179.7 |
| 13: 9 | 165 | 138.2 | 145.2 | 152.1 | 159.1 | 166.0 | 173.0 | 179.9 |
| 13:10 | 166 | 138.5 | 145.4 | 152.4 | 159.3 | 166.3 | 173.2 | 180.2 |
| 13:11 | 167 | 138.7 | 145.7 | 152.6 | 159.6 | 166.5 | 173.5 | 180.4 |
| 14: 0 | 168 | 139.0 | 145.9 | 152.8 | 159.8 | 166.7 | 173.7 | 180.6 |
| 14: 1 | 169 | 139.2 | 146.1 | 153.1 | 160.0 | 166.9 | 173.9 | 180.8 |
| 14: 2 | 170 | 139.4 | 146.3 | 153.3 | 160.2 | 167.1 | 174.1 | 181.0 |
| 14: 3 | 171 | 139.6 | 146.5 | 153.5 | 160.4 | 167.3 | 174.2 | 181.2 |
| 14: 4 | 172 | 139.8 | 146.7 | 153.6 | 160.6 | 167.5 | 174.4 | 181.3 |
| 14: 5 | 173 | 140.0 | 146.9 | 153.8 | 160.7 | 167.7 | 174.6 | 181.5 |
| 14: 6 | 174 | 140.1 | 147.1 | 154.0 | 160.9 | 167.8 | 174.7 | 181.6 |
| 14: 7 | 175 | 140.3 | 147.2 | 154.1 | 161.0 | 168.0 | 174.9 | 181.8 |
| 14: 8 | 176 | 140.5 | 147.4 | 154.3 | 161.2 | 168.1 | 175.0 | 181.9 |
| 14: 9 | 177 | 140.6 | 147.5 | 154.4 | 161.3 | 168.2 | 175.1 | 182.0 |
| 14:10 | 178 | 140.8 | 147.7 | 154.5 | 161.4 | 168.3 | 175.2 | 182.1 |
| 14:11 | 179 | 140.9 | 147.8 | 154.7 | 161.6 | 168.4 | 175.3 | 182.2 |
| 15: 0 | 180 | 141.0 | 147.9 | 154.8 | 161.7 | 168.5 | 175.4 | 182.3 |
| 15: 1 | 181 | 141.2 | 148.0 | 154.9 | 161.8 | 168.6 | 175.5 | 182.4 |
| 15: 2 | 182 | 141.3 | 148.1 | 155.0 | 161.9 | 168.7 | 175.6 | 182.5 |
| 15: 3 | 183 | 141.4 | 148.2 | 155.1 | 162.0 | 168.8 | 175.7 | 182.5 |

## Height-for-age GIRLS

**5 to 19 years (z-scores)**

| Year: Month | Month | Z-scores (height in cm) | | | | | | |
|---|---|---|---|---|---|---|---|---|
| | | -3 SD | -2 SD | -1 SD | Median | 1 SD | 2 SD | 3 SD |
| **15: 4** | **184** | 141.5 | 148.3 | 155.2 | 162.0 | 168.9 | 175.7 | 182.6 |
| **15: 5** | **185** | 141.6 | 148.4 | 155.3 | 162.1 | 169.0 | 175.8 | 182.6 |
| **15: 6** | **186** | 141.7 | 148.5 | 155.4 | 162.2 | 169.0 | 175.9 | 182.7 |
| **15: 7** | **187** | 141.8 | 148.6 | 155.4 | 162.3 | 169.1 | 175.9 | 182.7 |
| **15: 8** | **188** | 141.9 | 148.7 | 155.5 | 162.3 | 169.1 | 176.0 | 182.8 |
| **15: 9** | **189** | 141.9 | 148.7 | 155.6 | 162.4 | 169.2 | 176.0 | 182.8 |
| **15:10** | **190** | 142.0 | 148.8 | 155.6 | 162.4 | 169.2 | 176.0 | 182.8 |
| **15:11** | **191** | 142.1 | 148.9 | 155.7 | 162.5 | 169.3 | 176.1 | 182.9 |
| **16: 0** | **192** | 142.2 | 148.9 | 155.7 | 162.5 | 169.3 | 176.1 | 182.9 |
| **16: 1** | **193** | 142.2 | 149.0 | 155.8 | 162.6 | 169.3 | 176.1 | 182.9 |
| **16: 2** | **194** | 142.3 | 149.1 | 155.8 | 162.6 | 169.4 | 176.1 | 182.9 |
| **16: 3** | **195** | 142.3 | 149.1 | 155.9 | 162.6 | 169.4 | 176.2 | 182.9 |
| **16: 4** | **196** | 142.4 | 149.2 | 155.9 | 162.7 | 169.4 | 176.2 | 182.9 |
| **16: 5** | **197** | 142.4 | 149.2 | 155.9 | 162.7 | 169.4 | 176.2 | 182.9 |
| **16: 6** | **198** | 142.5 | 149.2 | 156.0 | 162.7 | 169.5 | 176.2 | 182.9 |
| **16: 7** | **199** | 142.5 | 149.3 | 156.0 | 162.7 | 169.5 | 176.2 | 182.9 |
| **16: 8** | **200** | 142.6 | 149.3 | 156.0 | 162.8 | 169.5 | 176.2 | 182.9 |
| **16: 9** | **201** | 142.6 | 149.4 | 156.1 | 162.8 | 169.5 | 176.2 | 182.9 |
| **16:10** | **202** | 142.7 | 149.4 | 156.1 | 162.8 | 169.5 | 176.2 | 182.9 |
| **16:11** | **203** | 142.7 | 149.4 | 156.1 | 162.8 | 169.5 | 176.2 | 182.9 |
| **17: 0** | **204** | 142.8 | 149.5 | 156.2 | 162.9 | 169.5 | 176.2 | 182.9 |
| **17: 1** | **205** | 142.8 | 149.5 | 156.2 | 162.9 | 169.6 | 176.2 | 182.9 |
| **17: 2** | **206** | 142.9 | 149.5 | 156.2 | 162.9 | 169.6 | 176.2 | 182.9 |
| **17: 3** | **207** | 142.9 | 149.6 | 156.2 | 162.9 | 169.6 | 176.3 | 182.9 |

## Height-for-age GIRLS

**5 to 19 years (z-scores)**

| Year: Month | Month | Z-scores (height in cm) | | | | | | |
|---|---|---|---|---|---|---|---|---|
| | | -3 SD | -2 SD | -1 SD | Median | 1 SD | 2 SD | 3 SD |
| **17: 4** | **208** | 142.9 | 149.6 | 156.3 | 162.9 | 169.6 | 176.3 | 182.9 |
| **17: 5** | **209** | 143.0 | 149.6 | 156.3 | 162.9 | 169.6 | 176.3 | 182.9 |
| **17: 6** | **210** | 143.0 | 149.7 | 156.3 | 163.0 | 169.6 | 176.3 | 182.9 |
| **17: 7** | **211** | 143.1 | 149.7 | 156.3 | 163.0 | 169.6 | 176.3 | 182.9 |
| **17: 8** | **212** | 143.1 | 149.7 | 156.4 | 163.0 | 169.6 | 176.3 | 182.9 |
| **17: 9** | **213** | 143.1 | 149.8 | 156.4 | 163.0 | 169.6 | 176.3 | 182.9 |
| **17:10** | **214** | 143.2 | 149.8 | 156.4 | 163.0 | 169.7 | 176.3 | 182.9 |
| **17:11** | **215** | 143.2 | 149.8 | 156.4 | 163.0 | 169.7 | 176.3 | 182.9 |
| **18: 0** | **216** | 143.2 | 149.8 | 156.5 | 163.1 | 169.7 | 176.3 | 182.9 |
| **18: 1** | **217** | 143.3 | 149.9 | 156.5 | 163.1 | 169.7 | 176.3 | 182.9 |
| **18: 2** | **218** | 143.3 | 149.9 | 156.5 | 163.1 | 169.7 | 176.3 | 182.9 |
| **18: 3** | **219** | 143.3 | 149.9 | 156.5 | 163.1 | 169.7 | 176.3 | 182.9 |
| **18: 4** | **220** | 143.4 | 149.9 | 156.5 | 163.1 | 169.7 | 176.3 | 182.9 |
| **18: 5** | **221** | 143.4 | 150.0 | 156.5 | 163.1 | 169.7 | 176.3 | 182.9 |
| **18: 6** | **222** | 143.4 | 150.0 | 156.6 | 163.1 | 169.7 | 176.3 | 182.9 |
| **18: 7** | **223** | 143.4 | 150.0 | 156.6 | 163.1 | 169.7 | 176.3 | 182.8 |
| **18: 8** | **224** | 143.5 | 150.0 | 156.6 | 163.1 | 169.7 | 176.3 | 182.8 |
| **18: 9** | **225** | 143.5 | 150.0 | 156.6 | 163.1 | 169.7 | 176.3 | 182.8 |
| **18:10** | **226** | 143.5 | 150.0 | 156.6 | 163.2 | 169.7 | 176.3 | 182.8 |
| **18:11** | **227** | 143.5 | 150.1 | 156.6 | 163.2 | 169.7 | 176.2 | 182.8 |
| **19: 0** | **228** | 143.5 | 150.1 | 156.6 | 163.2 | 169.7 | 176.2 | 182.8 |

## Weight-for-age BOYS

**5 to 10 years (z-scores)**

| | | Z-scores (weight in kg) | | | | | | |
|---|---|---|---|---|---|---|---|---|
| Year: Month | Month | -3 SD | -2 SD | -1 SD | Median | 1 SD | 2 SD | 3 SD |
| 5: 1 | 61 | 12.7 | 14.4 | 16.3 | 18.5 | 21.1 | 24.2 | 27.8 |
| 5: 2 | 62 | 12.8 | 14.5 | 16.4 | 18.7 | 21.3 | 24.4 | 28.1 |
| 5: 3 | 63 | 13.0 | 14.6 | 16.6 | 18.9 | 21.5 | 24.7 | 28.4 |
| 5: 4 | 64 | 13.1 | 14.8 | 16.7 | 19.0 | 21.7 | 24.9 | 28.8 |
| 5: 5 | 65 | 13.2 | 14.9 | 16.9 | 19.2 | 22.0 | 25.2 | 29.1 |
| 5: 6 | 66 | 13.3 | 15.0 | 17.0 | 19.4 | 22.2 | 25.5 | 29.4 |
| 5: 7 | 67 | 13.4 | 15.2 | 17.2 | 19.6 | 22.4 | 25.7 | 29.8 |
| 5: 8 | 68 | 13.6 | 15.3 | 17.4 | 19.8 | 22.6 | 26.0 | 30.1 |
| 5: 9 | 69 | 13.7 | 15.4 | 17.5 | 19.9 | 22.8 | 26.3 | 30.4 |
| 5:10 | 70 | 13.8 | 15.6 | 17.7 | 20.1 | 23.1 | 26.6 | 30.8 |
| 5:11 | 71 | 13.9 | 15.7 | 17.8 | 20.3 | 23.3 | 26.8 | 31.2 |
| 6: 0 | 72 | 14.1 | 15.9 | 18.0 | 20.5 | 23.5 | 27.1 | 31.5 |
| 6: 1 | 73 | 14.2 | 16.0 | 18.2 | 20.7 | 23.7 | 27.4 | 31.9 |
| 6: 2 | 74 | 14.3 | 16.2 | 18.3 | 20.9 | 24.0 | 27.7 | 32.2 |
| 6: 3 | 75 | 14.5 | 16.3 | 18.5 | 21.1 | 24.2 | 28.0 | 32.6 |
| 6: 4 | 76 | 14.6 | 16.5 | 18.7 | 21.3 | 24.4 | 28.3 | 33.0 |
| 6: 5 | 77 | 14.7 | 16.6 | 18.8 | 21.5 | 24.7 | 28.6 | 33.3 |
| 6: 6 | 78 | 14.9 | 16.8 | 19.0 | 21.7 | 24.9 | 28.9 | 33.7 |
| 6: 7 | 79 | 15.0 | 16.9 | 19.2 | 21.9 | 25.2 | 29.2 | 34.1 |
| 6: 8 | 80 | 15.1 | 17.1 | 19.3 | 22.1 | 25.4 | 29.5 | 34.5 |
| 6: 9 | 81 | 15.3 | 17.2 | 19.5 | 22.3 | 25.6 | 29.8 | 34.9 |
| 6:10 | 82 | 15.4 | 17.4 | 19.7 | 22.5 | 25.9 | 30.1 | 35.3 |
| 6:11 | 83 | 15.5 | 17.5 | 19.9 | 22.7 | 26.1 | 30.4 | 35.7 |
| 7: 0 | 84 | 15.7 | 17.7 | 20.0 | 22.9 | 26.4 | 30.7 | 36.1 |
| 7: 1 | 85 | 15.8 | 17.8 | 20.2 | 23.1 | 26.6 | 31.0 | 36.5 |
| 7: 2 | 86 | 15.9 | 18.0 | 20.4 | 23.3 | 26.9 | 31.3 | 36.9 |

## Weight-for-age BOYS

**5 to 10 years (z-scores)**

| | | Z-scores (weight in kg) | | | | | | |
|---|---|---|---|---|---|---|---|---|
| Year: Month | Month | -3 SD | -2 SD | -1 SD | Median | 1 SD | 2 SD | 3 SD |
| 7: 3 | 87 | 16.1 | 18.1 | 20.6 | 23.5 | 27.1 | 31.7 | 37.4 |
| 7: 4 | 88 | 16.2 | 18.3 | 20.7 | 23.7 | 27.4 | 32.0 | 37.8 |
| 7: 5 | 89 | 16.3 | 18.4 | 20.9 | 23.9 | 27.7 | 32.3 | 38.2 |
| 7: 6 | 90 | 16.5 | 18.6 | 21.1 | 24.1 | 27.9 | 32.6 | 38.7 |
| 7: 7 | 91 | 16.6 | 18.7 | 21.3 | 24.3 | 28.2 | 33.0 | 39.1 |
| 7: 8 | 92 | 16.7 | 18.9 | 21.4 | 24.6 | 28.4 | 33.3 | 39.6 |
| 7: 9 | 93 | 16.9 | 19.0 | 21.6 | 24.8 | 28.7 | 33.7 | 40.1 |
| 7:10 | 94 | 17.0 | 19.2 | 21.8 | 25.0 | 29.0 | 34.0 | 40.5 |
| 7:11 | 95 | 17.1 | 19.3 | 22.0 | 25.2 | 29.2 | 34.4 | 41.0 |
| 8: 0 | 96 | 17.3 | 19.5 | 22.1 | 25.4 | 29.5 | 34.7 | 41.5 |
| 8: 1 | 97 | 17.4 | 19.6 | 22.3 | 25.6 | 29.8 | 35.1 | 42.0 |
| 8: 2 | 98 | 17.5 | 19.8 | 22.5 | 25.9 | 30.1 | 35.5 | 42.5 |
| 8: 3 | 99 | 17.7 | 19.9 | 22.7 | 26.1 | 30.3 | 35.8 | 43.1 |
| 8: 4 | 100 | 17.8 | 20.1 | 22.9 | 26.3 | 30.6 | 36.2 | 43.6 |
| 8: 5 | 101 | 17.9 | 20.2 | 23.0 | 26.5 | 30.9 | 36.6 | 44.1 |
| 8: 6 | 102 | 18.1 | 20.4 | 23.2 | 26.7 | 31.2 | 37.0 | 44.7 |
| 8: 7 | 103 | 18.2 | 20.5 | 23.4 | 27.0 | 31.5 | 37.4 | 45.2 |
| 8: 8 | 104 | 18.3 | 20.7 | 23.6 | 27.2 | 31.8 | 37.8 | 45.8 |
| 8: 9 | 105 | 18.4 | 20.8 | 23.8 | 27.4 | 32.1 | 38.2 | 46.4 |
| 8:10 | 106 | 18.6 | 21.0 | 23.9 | 27.6 | 32.4 | 38.6 | 47.0 |
| 8:11 | 107 | 18.7 | 21.1 | 24.1 | 27.9 | 32.7 | 39.0 | 47.6 |
| 9: 0 | 108 | 18.8 | 21.3 | 24.3 | 28.1 | 33.0 | 39.4 | 48.2 |
| 9: 1 | 109 | 18.9 | 21.4 | 24.5 | 28.3 | 33.3 | 39.9 | 48.8 |
| 9: 2 | 110 | 19.1 | 21.6 | 24.7 | 28.6 | 33.6 | 40.3 | 49.5 |
| 9: 3 | 111 | 19.2 | 21.7 | 24.9 | 28.8 | 33.9 | 40.7 | 50.1 |

## Weight-for-age BOYS

**5 to 10 years (z-scores)**

| | | Z-scores (weight in kg) | | | | | | |
|---|---|---|---|---|---|---|---|---|
| Year: Month | Month | -3 SD | -2 SD | -1 SD | Median | 1 SD | 2 SD | 3 SD |
| 9: 4 | 112 | 19.3 | 21.9 | 25.1 | 29.1 | 34.3 | 41.2 | 50.8 |
| 9: 5 | 113 | 19.5 | 22.1 | 25.3 | 29.3 | 34.6 | 41.7 | 51.5 |
| 9: 6 | 114 | 19.6 | 22.2 | 25.5 | 29.6 | 34.9 | 42.1 | 52.1 |
| 9: 7 | 115 | 19.7 | 22.4 | 25.7 | 29.8 | 35.3 | 42.6 | 52.8 |
| 9: 8 | 116 | 19.9 | 22.5 | 25.9 | 30.1 | 35.6 | 43.1 | 53.5 |
| 9: 9 | 117 | 20.0 | 22.7 | 26.1 | 30.4 | 36.0 | 43.5 | 54.2 |
| 9:10 | 118 | 20.1 | 22.9 | 26.3 | 30.6 | 36.3 | 44.0 | 55.0 |
| 9:11 | 119 | 20.3 | 23.0 | 26.5 | 30.9 | 36.7 | 44.5 | 55.7 |
| 10: 0 | 120 | 20.4 | 23.2 | 26.7 | 31.2 | 37.0 | 45.0 | 56.4 |

## Weight-for-age GIRLS

**5 to 10 years (z-scores)**

| | | Z-scores (weight in kg) | | | | | | |
|---|---|---|---|---|---|---|---|---|
| Year: Month | Month | -3 SD | -2 SD | -1 SD | Median | 1 SD | 2 SD | 3 SD |
| 5: 1 | 61 | 12.4 | 14.0 | 15.9 | 18.3 | 21.2 | 24.8 | 29.5 |
| 5: 2 | 62 | 12.5 | 14.1 | 16.0 | 18.4 | 21.4 | 25.1 | 29.8 |
| 5: 3 | 63 | 12.6 | 14.2 | 16.2 | 18.6 | 21.6 | 25.4 | 30.2 |
| 5: 4 | 64 | 12.7 | 14.3 | 16.3 | 18.8 | 21.8 | 25.6 | 30.5 |
| 5: 5 | 65 | 12.8 | 14.4 | 16.5 | 19.0 | 22.0 | 25.9 | 30.9 |
| 5: 6 | 66 | 12.9 | 14.6 | 16.6 | 19.1 | 22.2 | 26.2 | 31.3 |
| 5: 7 | 67 | 13.0 | 14.7 | 16.8 | 19.3 | 22.5 | 26.5 | 31.6 |
| 5: 8 | 68 | 13.1 | 14.8 | 16.9 | 19.5 | 22.7 | 26.7 | 32.0 |
| 5: 9 | 69 | 13.2 | 14.9 | 17.0 | 19.6 | 22.9 | 27.0 | 32.3 |
| 5:10 | 70 | 13.3 | 15.0 | 17.2 | 19.8 | 23.1 | 27.3 | 32.7 |
| 5:11 | 71 | 13.4 | 15.2 | 17.3 | 20.0 | 23.3 | 27.6 | 33.1 |
| 6: 0 | 72 | 13.5 | 15.3 | 17.5 | 20.2 | 23.5 | 27.8 | 33.4 |
| 6: 1 | 73 | 13.6 | 15.4 | 17.6 | 20.3 | 23.8 | 28.1 | 33.8 |
| 6: 2 | 74 | 13.7 | 15.5 | 17.8 | 20.5 | 24.0 | 28.4 | 34.2 |
| 6: 3 | 75 | 13.8 | 15.6 | 17.9 | 20.7 | 24.2 | 28.7 | 34.6 |
| 6: 4 | 76 | 13.9 | 15.8 | 18.0 | 20.9 | 24.4 | 29.0 | 35.0 |
| 6: 5 | 77 | 14.0 | 15.9 | 18.2 | 21.0 | 24.6 | 29.3 | 35.4 |
| 6: 6 | 78 | 14.1 | 16.0 | 18.3 | 21.2 | 24.9 | 29.6 | 35.8 |
| 6: 7 | 79 | 14.2 | 16.1 | 18.5 | 21.4 | 25.1 | 29.9 | 36.2 |
| 6: 8 | 80 | 14.3 | 16.3 | 18.6 | 21.6 | 25.3 | 30.2 | 36.6 |
| 6: 9 | 81 | 14.4 | 16.4 | 18.8 | 21.8 | 25.6 | 30.5 | 37.0 |
| 6:10 | 82 | 14.5 | 16.5 | 18.9 | 22.0 | 25.8 | 30.8 | 37.4 |
| 6:11 | 83 | 14.6 | 16.6 | 19.1 | 22.2 | 26.1 | 31.1 | 37.8 |
| 7: 0 | 84 | 14.8 | 16.8 | 19.3 | 22.4 | 26.3 | 31.4 | 38.3 |
| 7: 1 | 85 | 14.9 | 16.9 | 19.4 | 22.6 | 26.6 | 31.8 | 38.7 |
| 7: 2 | 86 | 15.0 | 17.1 | 19.6 | 22.8 | 26.8 | 32.1 | 39.2 |

## Weight-for-age GIRLS

**5 to 10 years (z-scores)**

| Year: Month | Month | Z-scores (weight in kg) | | | | | | |
|---|---|---|---|---|---|---|---|---|
| | | -3 SD | -2 SD | -1 SD | Median | 1 SD | 2 SD | 3 SD |
| 7: 3 | 87 | 15.1 | 17.2 | 19.8 | 23.0 | 27.1 | 32.5 | 39.6 |
| 7: 4 | 88 | 15.2 | 17.3 | 19.9 | 23.2 | 27.4 | 32.8 | 40.1 |
| 7: 5 | 89 | 15.4 | 17.5 | 20.1 | 23.4 | 27.6 | 33.1 | 40.6 |
| 7: 6 | 90 | 15.5 | 17.6 | 20.3 | 23.6 | 27.9 | 33.5 | 41.1 |
| 7: 7 | 91 | 15.6 | 17.8 | 20.5 | 23.9 | 28.2 | 33.9 | 41.5 |
| 7: 8 | 92 | 15.7 | 17.9 | 20.7 | 24.1 | 28.5 | 34.2 | 42.0 |
| 7: 9 | 93 | 15.9 | 18.1 | 20.9 | 24.3 | 28.8 | 34.6 | 42.6 |
| 7:10 | 94 | 16.0 | 18.3 | 21.0 | 24.5 | 29.1 | 35.0 | 43.1 |
| 7:11 | 95 | 16.2 | 18.4 | 21.2 | 24.8 | 29.4 | 35.4 | 43.6 |
| 8: 0 | 96 | 16.3 | 18.6 | 21.4 | 25.0 | 29.7 | 35.8 | 44.1 |
| 8: 1 | 97 | 16.4 | 18.8 | 21.6 | 25.3 | 30.0 | 36.2 | 44.7 |
| 8: 2 | 98 | 16.6 | 18.9 | 21.8 | 25.5 | 30.3 | 36.6 | 45.2 |
| 8: 3 | 99 | 16.7 | 19.1 | 22.0 | 25.8 | 30.6 | 37.0 | 45.8 |
| 8: 4 | 100 | 16.9 | 19.3 | 22.3 | 26.0 | 30.9 | 37.4 | 46.3 |
| 8: 5 | 101 | 17.0 | 19.5 | 22.5 | 26.3 | 31.2 | 37.8 | 46.9 |
| 8: 6 | 102 | 17.2 | 19.6 | 22.7 | 26.6 | 31.6 | 38.3 | 47.5 |
| 8: 7 | 103 | 17.3 | 19.8 | 22.9 | 26.8 | 31.9 | 38.7 | 48.1 |
| 8: 8 | 104 | 17.5 | 20.0 | 23.1 | 27.1 | 32.2 | 39.1 | 48.7 |
| 8: 9 | 105 | 17.7 | 20.2 | 23.3 | 27.4 | 32.6 | 39.6 | 49.3 |
| 8:10 | 106 | 17.8 | 20.4 | 23.6 | 27.6 | 32.9 | 40.0 | 49.9 |
| 8:11 | 107 | 18.0 | 20.6 | 23.8 | 27.9 | 33.3 | 40.5 | 50.5 |
| 9: 0 | 108 | 18.1 | 20.8 | 24.0 | 28.2 | 33.6 | 41.0 | 51.1 |
| 9: 1 | 109 | 18.3 | 21.0 | 24.3 | 28.5 | 34.0 | 41.4 | 51.8 |
| 9: 2 | 110 | 18.5 | 21.2 | 24.5 | 28.8 | 34.4 | 41.9 | 52.4 |
| 9: 3 | 111 | 18.7 | 21.4 | 24.7 | 29.1 | 34.7 | 42.4 | 53.1 |

## Weight-for-age GIRLS

**5 to 10 years (z-scores)**

| Year: Month | Month | Z-scores (weight in kg) | | | | | | |
|---|---|---|---|---|---|---|---|---|
| | | -3 SD | -2 SD | -1 SD | Median | 1 SD | 2 SD | 3 SD |
| 9: 4 | 112 | 18.8 | 21.6 | 25.0 | 29.4 | 35.1 | 42.9 | 53.7 |
| 9: 5 | 113 | 19.0 | 21.8 | 25.2 | 29.7 | 35.5 | 43.3 | 54.4 |
| 9: 6 | 114 | 19.2 | 22.0 | 25.5 | 30.0 | 35.9 | 43.8 | 55.0 |
| 9: 7 | 115 | 19.4 | 22.2 | 25.7 | 30.3 | 36.2 | 44.3 | 55.7 |
| 9: 8 | 116 | 19.5 | 22.4 | 26.0 | 30.6 | 36.6 | 44.8 | 56.4 |
| 9: 9 | 117 | 19.7 | 22.6 | 26.2 | 30.9 | 37.0 | 45.3 | 57.1 |
| 9:10 | 118 | 19.9 | 22.8 | 26.5 | 31.2 | 37.4 | 45.8 | 57.8 |
| 9:11 | 119 | 20.1 | 23.0 | 26.8 | 31.5 | 37.8 | 46.4 | 58.5 |
| 10: 0 | 120 | 20.3 | 23.3 | 27.0 | 31.9 | 38.2 | 46.9 | 59.2 |

# Index

## A

**B**

## C



## D



## E

## F

## J



## K



## L

## M



## N

## O



## P



## Q



## R

## T

## U

## V



## W



## Z